PEDIATRIC COLLECTIONS

Breastfeeding: Support, Challenges, and Benefits

About AAP Pediatric Collections

Pediatric Collections is a series of selected pediatric articles that highlight different facets of information across various AAP publications, including AAP Journals, AAP News, Blog Articles, and eBooks. Each series of collections focuses on specific topics in the field of pediatrics so that you can keep up with best practices, and make an informed response to public health matters, trending news, and current events. Each collection includes previously published content focusing on specific topics and articles selected by AAP editors.

Visit http://collections.aap.org to view a list of upcoming collections.

TABLE OF CONTENTS

go.aap.org/connect

TABLE OF CONTENTS

TABLE OF CONTENTS

Benefits

Introduction

Why a collection of recently published articles on breastfeeding? Breastfeeding is a health care intervention of profound significance. Optimal breastfeeding practices, defined as exclusive breastfeeding through 6 months of age followed by continued breastfeeding with introduction of solid foods, save lives. Worldwide, in children 0–23 months, careful meta-analysis demonstrates a significantly decreased mortality rate with dose response in both all-cause and infection-related mortality among infants and children who received recommended breastfeeding, compared to those who received partial or no breastfeeding.[1] Mothers benefit from optimal breastfeeding practices too, and recent analysis of data from high-, middle-, and low-income countries shows that universal optimal breastfeeding could prevent 20,000 deaths due to breast cancer (breastfeeding has been clearly shown to decrease risk of breast cancer in a dose-related manner).[2] Breastfeeding may be the least expensive yet most cost-effective health intervention known. Both in the United States and abroad, the calculated cost of not breastfeeding is extraordinary, estimated to represent economic losses of about $302 billion annually worldwide or 0.49% of world gross national income.[3] In the United States alone, the medical cost of suboptimal breastfeeding is estimated at $3 billion, and to bring this all the way home for you, consider that for every 597 women who optimally breastfeed their infant, one death of a child or mother is prevented.[4] I'd call this data absolutely staggering.

So, I would argue that this group of breastfeeding-related articles, blogs, news articles, and commentaries is just a beginning, hopefully, in raising awareness about a basic health practice that makes huge differences globally. The editors have carefully curated a broad array of pragmatic articles and research that samples the current literature and focuses on 3 areas: support, challenges, and benefits.

Until Healthy People 2020 goals[5] for breastfeeding initiation and exclusive continuation have been met and exceeded, and conversely goal rates of formula supplementation have been met and lowered, it's relatively easy to agree that additional support for breastfeeding is needed. Dr. Joan Meek, Chairperson of the AAP Section on Breastfeeding, kicks off with a comprehensive, practical, and evidence-based outline explaining how to move your office practice toward "breastfeeding friendly"—a nice riff on the Baby-Friendly Hospital Initiative. Several commentaries respond to concerning findings in an original article by Drs. Lori Feldman-Winter, Richard Schanler, and colleagues: even as pediatricians' recommendations and practices regarding breastfeeding have improved from 1995 to 2014, their attitudes about the likelihood that mothers will actually achieve breastfeeding success have declined. Section Executive Member Dr. Maya Bunik reaches out a helping hand with "The Pediatrician's Role in Encouraging Exclusive Breastfeeding," offering "can-do" pragmatic advice for all of us. The bane of exclusive breastfeeding is formula supplementation, and Dr. Trang Nguyen and colleagues examine the prevalence of formula supplementation among breastfed infants in maternity hospitals in New York state. Using birth certificate–based information, they ask the important question: what factors impact this key hospital practice? Finally, acknowledging increasing awareness of the vital role that fathers/partners play in supporting breastfeeding, a randomized controlled trial by Dr. Jennifer Abbass-Dick and colleagues evaluate the effectiveness of a coparenting intervention on exclusive breastfeeding among primiparous couples: significant improvements in paternal breastfeeding self-efficacy were just one of the study benefits. Support from all directions is imperative if we hope to move the breastfeeding needle forward. What I love about these articles is that a broad range of approaches and angles are brought together here.

The second section of articles focuses on epidemiological and societal challenges to achieving full breastfeeding. Longstanding variations in rates of breastfeeding between groups of individuals with differing social, economic, educational, and racial backgrounds represent not only health disparities or inequalities (read, differences), but rather need to be recognized as health inequities, meaning that those differences are unfair, unethical, and avoidable. Companion articles from Germany by Dr. Chad Logan et al, and from the United States by Dr. Chelsea O. McKinney et al, each focus on this critical phenomenon of breastfeeding inequities. Both identified demographic factors that explained differences in breastfeeding intent, initiation, and duration between groups, and McKinney et al additionally find that early in-hospital formula supplementation played a unique role in perpetuating inequities in breastfeeding duration. Both are must-read articles, and a commentary is included. Finally, a well done oral health study from Brazil yielded provocative results regarding severe caries among children breastfed for more than 2 years—will this result be meaningful for your practice?

Finally, the third section of articles describes new benefits (and non-benefits) of breastfeeding. Dr. Lisa-Christine Girard and colleagues examined the impact of breastfeeding on cognitive and behavioral outcomes at ages 3–5 years, and to the surprise of many, could not find an enduring benefit of breastfeeding after careful statistical correction for underlying breastfed versus not breastfed differences in the studied children. We can learn a lot from negative studies, and a commentary and blog highlight this. Two other articles and accompanying comments identify meaningful new benefits of breastfeeding: Dr. Fern Hauck et al used individual participant data meta-analysis to examine the specific role of breastfeeding duration in SIDS, and Dr. Takashi Yorifuji et al found a remarkable protective effect of breastfeeding against Kawasaki syndrome in Japan, the country in which the disease is most common. A unique article from Dr. Stacey A. Carling and colleagues studied the role of breastfeeding in obesity prevention by scrutinizing early weight for length increases among infants at high-risk for obesity due to multiple maternal factors: those infants at highest risk benefitted significantly from just 4+ months of breastfeeding, a highly instructive result.

In summary, enjoy the depth and breadth of these articles related to breastfeeding. Each one will give you a boost in your understanding of one of the most meaningful and important health practices we know.

—**Lydia Furman, MD, FAAP,**
Associate Editor, *Pediatrics*

REFERENCES

1. Sankar MJ, Sinha B, Chowdhury R, et al. Optimal breastfeeding practices and infant and child mortality: a systematic review and meta-analysis. *Acta Paediatr.* 2015;104(467):3-13
2. Victora CG, Bahl R, Barros AJ, et al; Lancet Breastfeeding Series Group. Breastfeeding in the 21st century: epidemiology, mechanisms, and lifelong effect. *Lancet.* 2016;387(10017):475-90
3. Rollins NC, Bhandari N, Hajeebhoy N, et al; Lancet Breastfeeding Series Group. Why invest, and what it will take to improve breastfeeding practices? *Lancet.* 2016;387(10017):491-504
4. Bartick MC, Schwarz LB, Green BD, et al. Suboptimal breastfeeding in the United States: maternal and pediatric health outcomes and costs. *Matern Child Nutr.* 2017;13(1)
5. HealthyPeople.gov. 2020 Topics and Objectives. US Department of Health and Human Services. https://www. healthypeople.gov/2020/topics-objectives/ topic/maternal-infant-and-child-health/ objectives. Accessed 7-3-2018

How to Establish a Breastfeeding-Friendly Pediatric Office

Joan Younger Meek, M.D., M.S., FAAP

Breastfeeding initiation rates in the U.S. are the highest in decades at 81%, yet less than a quarter of infants are breastfed exclusively at 6 months. In addition, there are significant disparities based on race, ethnicity, education and socioeconomic status, according to the Centers for Disease Control and Prevention (CDC).

Pediatricians are positioned to play a pivotal role in supporting breastfeeding families in the office practice. Recommendations on creating a breastfeeding-supportive environment are highlighted in the clinical report *The Breastfeeding-Friendly Pediatric Office Practice* from the AAP Section on Breastfeeding (https://doi.org/10.1542/peds.2017-0647).

The Academy has long supported breastfeeding as the optimal infant nutrition. It recommends exclusive breastfeeding for about six months and continued breastfeeding for at least one year. Among its many benefits, breastfeeding helps prevent acute infectious disease and development of chronic disease, reduces risk of sudden infant death syndrome, and promotes optimal outcomes for both mothers and children. The Academy advocates that breastfeeding should be considered a public health imperative and not merely a lifestyle choice.

WHY IS OFFICE SUPPORT IMPORTANT?

Pediatric care professionals see healthy infants frequently in the office during the first year of life, giving them many opportunities to provide anticipatory guidance that supports and encourages breastfeeding.

Pediatricians must be trained to assess breastfeeding adequacy in the mother-baby pair, troubleshoot problems and refer mothers to community resources, as needed. Pediatricians also must be knowledgeable about how over-the-counter and prescription drugs may affect the breastfeeding infant (see resources).

It is important that breastfeeding be evaluated formally with observation during the first office visit, when any issues can be identified early. Mothers who note difficulty with latch, pain or milk supply need timely intervention, as do infants with inadequate weight gain.

Pediatricians should advise mothers on breastfeeding after returning to work and refer to community-based support personnel such as lactation consultants, nutrition staff from the Special Supplemental Nutrition Program for *Women, Infants and Children*, peer counselors and support groups.

AAP Clinical Report

Dr. Meek is co-author of the clinical report and chair of the AAP Section on Breastfeeding Executive Committee.

A culture of breastfeeding support in the pediatric office begins with a welcoming environment that encourages mothers to breastfeed in the waiting room or separate area, if privacy is desired.

All staff must understand the practice's support of breastfeeding mothers and babies, and clinical staff should be trained in breastfeeding support and telephone triage guidelines. At least one person trained in lactation support, such as a nurse or other staff member, should routinely provide breastfeeding support under the guidance of the pediatrician. If possible, consider employing a board-certified lactation consultant in the office.

Pediatricians should make sure that formula is not being advertised through posters, publications and other materials in the office, and should not distribute free formula or coupons for formula.

FEDERAL INITIATIVES SUPPORT BREASTFEEDING

In 2011, then-Surgeon General Regina M. Benjamin, M.D., M.B.A., issued the first Call to Action to support breastfeeding, urging greater support for breastfeeding women; education and training for all health care providers; and systems to ensure continuity of care between the hospital and community settings.

The CDC supports breastfeeding by providing tools for providers and families, collecting statistics and promoting population health measures.

The CDC monitors hospital maternity care practices and provides funding to improve these practices through assistance to facilities in implementing the WHO/UNICEF Ten Steps to Successful Breastfeeding. The number of births in hospitals that have implemented the Ten Steps and become designated as Baby-Friendly Hospitals increased from 2.9% in 2007 to 20.1% as of January 2017, according to Baby-Friendly USA.

Due to the impact of federal programs, as well as state and local initiatives, many newborns leave the hospital breastfeeding after their brief postpartum stays.

Most mothers want to breastfeed, but many do not meet their personal breast-feeding goals. The breastfeeding-friendly pediatric office practice is well-suited to provide the support that women need to meet their goals and to improve the health outcomes of their pediatric patients. It even can be a way to grow and market the practice to new mothers.

RECOMMENDATIONS

- Have a written breastfeeding-friendly office policy.
- Train staff in breastfeeding support skills.
- Discuss breastfeeding during prenatal visits and at each well-child visit.
- Encourage exclusive breastfeeding for about six months and provide anticipatory guidance that supports the continuation of breastfeeding as long as desired.
- Incorporate breastfeeding observation into routine care.
- Educate mothers on breast milk expression and return to work.
- Provide noncommercial breast-feeding educational resources for parents.
- Encourage breastfeeding in the waiting room, but provide private space on request.
- Eliminate distribution of free formula.
- Train staff to follow telephone triage protocols to address breastfeeding concerns.
- Collaborate with the local hospital or birthing center and obstetric commu-nity regarding breastfeeding-friendly care.
- Link with breastfeeding community resources.
- Monitor breastfeeding rates in the practice.

American Academy
of Pediatrics

DEDICATED TO THE HEALTH OF ALL CHILDREN™

The Breastfeeding-Friendly Pediatric Office Practice

Joan Younger Meek, MD, MS, RD, FAAP, IBCLC, Amy J. Hatcher, MD, FAAP, SECTION ON BREASTFEEDING

abstract

The landscape of breastfeeding has changed over the past several decades as more women initiate breastfeeding in the postpartum period and more hospitals are designated as Baby-Friendly Hospitals by following the evidence-based Ten Steps to Successful Breastfeeding. The number of births in such facilities has increased more than sixfold over the past decade. With more women breastfeeding and stays in the maternity facilities lasting only a few days, the vast majority of continued breastfeeding support occurs in the community. Pediatric care providers evaluate breastfeeding infants and their mothers in the office setting frequently during the first year of life. The office setting should be conducive to providing ongoing breastfeeding support. Likewise, the office practice should avoid creating barriers for breastfeeding mothers and families or unduly promoting infant formula. This clinical report aims to review practices shown to support breastfeeding that can be implemented in the outpatient setting, with the ultimate goal of increasing the duration of exclusive breastfeeding and the continuation of any breastfeeding.

Department of Clinical Sciences, Florida State University College of Medicine, Tallahassee, Florida

Drs Meek and Hatcher conceptualized the review, developed the search criteria, contributed to drafting the initial manuscript and to manuscript revisions, and responded to questions and comments from reviewers and the Board of Directors; and both authors approved the final manuscript as submitted.

DOI: 10.1542/peds.2017-0647

Address correspondence to Joan Younger Meek, MD, MS, RD, FAAP, IBCLC. E-mail: joan.meek@med.fsu.edu

PEDIATRICS (ISSN Numbers: Print, 0031-4005; Online, 1098-4275).

To cite: Meek JY, Hatcher AJ, AAP SECTION ON BREAST-FEEDING. The Breastfeeding-Friendly Pediatric Office Practice. Pediatrics. 2017;139(5):e20170647

BACKGROUND/CURRENT RECOMMENDATIONS

Breastfeeding has long been documented as the ideal method for feeding and promoting the optimal development of infants and children, with rare exceptions (see Recommendation 3 below). The American Academy of Pediatrics (AAP) describes breastfeeding as the normative method of infant feeding. There are countless medical, emotional, and economic benefits of breastfeeding as described in the 2012 AAP statement "Breastfeeding and the Use of Human Milk."[1] Benefits of breastfeeding include decreased risk of lower respiratory infections, gastroenteritis, otitis media, and necrotizing enterocolitis, the latter being especially important in preterm infants. Because breastfeeding is the norm for infant feeding, comparatively there are risks associated with the lack of breastfeeding, which include an increase in sudden infant death syndrome, obesity, asthma, certain childhood cancers, diabetes, and postneonatal death.[1–3] Breastfeeding promotes attachment and optimal cognitive development. In women, lack of breastfeeding is associated with an increase in the risk of breast and ovarian cancer, type 2 diabetes, heart disease, and postpartum depression.[4–7]

The AAP recommends exclusive breastfeeding for approximately 6 months, followed by continued breastfeeding for 1 year or longer, as mutually desired by mother and child.[1] The *Surgeon General's Call to Action To Support Breastfeeding*[8] in 2011 emphasized the importance of breastfeeding as a public health imperative. Breastfeeding is strongly promoted, supported, and encouraged by the AAP, the Academy of Breastfeeding Medicine,[9] the American College of Obstetricians and Gynecologists,[10,11] and the American Academy of Family Physicians.[12] Each of these organizations calls on its members to be actively engaged in promoting and supporting breastfeeding among their patients.

EPIDEMIOLOGY

The rate of initiation of any breastfeeding in the US population is 81.1% according to data from the National Immunization Survey (2016, birth cohort from 2013).[13] Although the rate of breastfeeding initiation approaches the Healthy People 2020 target[14] of 81.9%, only 22.3% of US infants are breastfed exclusively at age 6 months. There are significant disparities in terms of breastfeeding rates in the country; among black infants, only 66.3% are breastfed at all, and only 14.6% are exclusively breastfed through the first 6 months of life. Among Native American and Alaska Native infants, breastfeeding initiation is 68.3% and exclusive breastfeeding rates at 6 months are 17.9%. Mothers are more likely to breastfeed if they are married, have a college education, live in metropolitan areas, do not experience poverty, and do not

TABLE 1 The Ten Steps to Successful Breastfeeding

1. Have a written breastfeeding-friendly policy that is routinely communicated to all health care staff.
2. Train all health care staff in the skills necessary to implement this policy.
3. Inform all pregnant women about the benefits and management of breastfeeding.
4. Help mothers initiate breastfeeding within 1 hour of birth.
5. Show mothers how to breastfeed and how to maintain lactation, even if they are separated from their infants.
6. Give infants no food or drink other than breast milk, unless medically indicated.
7. Practice rooming in: allow mothers and infants to remain together 24 hours a day.
8. Encourage breastfeeding on demand.
9. Give no pacifiers or artificial nipples to breastfeeding infants.[a]
10. Foster the establishment of breastfeeding support groups and refer mothers to them on discharge from the hospital or birth center.

[a] The AAP does not support a categorical ban on pacifiers because of their role in SIDS risk reduction and their analgesic benefit during painful procedures when breastfeeding cannot provide the analgesia. Pacifier use in the hospital in the neonatal period should be limited to specific medical indications, such as pain reduction, calming in a drug-exposed infant, etc. For breastfed infants, pacifier introduction should be delayed until breastfeeding is firmly established. Infants who are not being directly breastfed can begin pacifier use as soon as desired.

receive benefits from the Special Supplemental Nutrition Program for Women, Infants, and Children (WIC). WIC provides targeted breastfeeding support and peer-counseling services for mothers who qualify for their services. Infants most likely to experience toxic stress are least likely to be breastfed. According to the 2005–2007 Infant Feeding Practices Study II, 85% of US mothers intended to breastfeed exclusively for ≥3 months; however, only 32.4% achieved their intended exclusive breastfeeding duration.[15]

CURRENT INITIATIVES TO INCREASE BREASTFEEDING RATES

There have been numerous initiatives to increase breastfeeding exclusivity and duration both in hospitals and in the outpatient setting. US hospitals accredited by The Joint Commission with maternity units that have at least 1100 births per year are required to report data on the Perinatal Care Core Measure Set, which includes a measure on Exclusive Breast Milk Feeding.[16] There have been major initiatives to increase the number of maternity facilities designated as Baby-Friendly. The first of these was Best Fed Beginnings,[17] a collaboration of the National Initiative for Children's Healthcare Quality, the Centers for Disease Control and Prevention

(CDC), and Baby-Friendly USA, in a national effort to improve maternity care practices and achieve designation as Baby-Friendly. Through Best Fed Beginnings, hospitals implemented the evidence-based and AAP-endorsed Ten Steps to Successful Breastfeeding (Table 1), as established in the Baby-Friendly Hospital Initiative, developed by the World Health Organization (WHO)/ United Nations Children's Fund.[18–20] Additional maternity care facilities are pursuing the Baby-Friendly designation by participating in EMPower Breastfeeding: Enhancing Maternity Practices,[21] in cooperation with the CDC's Division of Nutrition, Physical Activity, and Obesity, and in partnership with the Carolina Global Breastfeeding Institute and Population Health Improvement Partners. EMPower similarly provides support to hospitals in quality-improvement methodology and breastfeeding support to improve maternity care practices and achieve Baby-Friendly USA designation. The number of births in designated facilities increased from 2.9% in 2007 to 20.01% in January 2017,[22] surpassing the Healthy People 2020 goal of 8.1%.[14]

For the national breastfeeding targets to be met, outpatient support from pediatricians and other pediatric care providers is imperative. As more infants are being discharged from hospitals designated as Baby-Friendly and having successfully initiated breastfeeding, it is essential that the pediatricians with whom they will follow up are knowledgeable about breastfeeding and that their office practices are prepared to support these breastfeeding dyads. The *Surgeon General's Call to Action To Support Breastfeeding* lists specific action steps that apply directly to the pediatric outpatient practice (Table 2).

Many pediatricians have little experience in clinical breastfeeding management. Analysis of an AAP Periodic Survey of Fellows regarding breastfeeding in 2004, compared with a similar survey in 1995, showed that pediatricians were less likely to believe that the benefits of breastfeeding outweighed the difficulties or inconvenience, and fewer believed that almost all mothers were able to succeed.[23] Unfortunately, more pediatricians in 2004 reported reasons to recommend against breastfeeding compared with the cohort who responded in 1995. A 2014 AAP Periodic Survey confirmed that some of these attitudes persist (unpublished data from American Academy of Pediatrics Periodic Survey of Fellows No. 89).

Szucs et al[24] found that there were gaps in providers' breastfeeding knowledge, counseling skills, and professional education and training. The authors showed that providers' cultures and attitudes affected breastfeeding promotion and support and that the providers used their own breastfeeding experiences to replace evidence-based knowledge and AAP policy statement recommendations. Both the Academy of Breastfeeding Medicine (ABM)[25] and the US Breastfeeding Committee[26] have published recommendations regarding the education and training of health care professionals, including pediatric care providers,

TABLE 2 Relevant Steps in the US Surgeon General's Call to Action to Support Breastfeeding

1. Give mothers the support they need to breastfeed their infants.
6. Ensure that the marketing of infant formula is conducted in a way that minimizes its negative impacts on exclusive breastfeeding.
8. Develop systems to guarantee continuity of skilled support for lactation between hospitals and health care settings in the community.
9. Provide education and training in breastfeeding for all health professionals who care for women and children.
10. Include basic support for breastfeeding as a standard of care for midwives, obstetricians, family physicians, nurse practitioners, and pediatricians.
11. Ensure access to services provided by IBCLCs.

Shown are action steps that apply directly to the pediatric outpatient practice, numbered according to the original steps in the Call to Action.[8]

in breastfeeding support and management.

The ABM's clinical protocol "The Breastfeeding-Friendly Physician's Office: Optimizing Care for Infant and Children"[27] details specific steps that a practice can take to become more breastfeeding friendly. These guidelines can inform the guidance for pediatric offices. Corriveau et al[28] sought to determine whether implementing a program based on this clinical protocol affected breastfeeding rates within the pediatric primary care setting. Even with a diverse patient population, rates of both initiation of and exclusive breastfeeding increased after the implementation of the ABM breastfeeding-friendly protocol. Feldman-Winter[29] outlined methods to increase breastfeeding initiation and duration in "Evidence-Based Interventions To Support Breastfeeding." In a comprehensive evidence review for the US Preventive Services Task Force, Chung et al[30] provided evidence that breastfeeding interventions, including both pre- and postnatal interventions, were more influential than either alone and that interventions including a component of lay support, such as peer counselors, are more effective than usual care in increasing short- and long-term breastfeeding rates. The US Preventive Services Task Force recommends interventions during pregnancy and after birth to support breastfeeding and concludes that coordinated interventions can

increase breastfeeding initiation, duration, and exclusivity (Evidence Grade B).[31]

THE BREASTFEEDING-FRIENDLY PEDIATRIC OFFICE PRACTICE

Because of the importance of breastfeeding to maternal and infant health outcomes, all pediatric care providers should aim to improve breastfeeding rates in their practices, with the goal of achieving the AAP breastfeeding recommendations for exclusive breastfeeding until approximately 6 months, followed by continued breastfeeding for 1 year or longer, as mutually desired by the mother and infant.[1] Pediatric care providers should help mothers identify and reach their own breastfeeding goals.

The following evidence-based recommendations for the pediatric outpatient practice should be considered as part of the practice-improvement process to increase breastfeeding rates to meet or exceed the AAP recommendations and the Healthy People 2020 goals. These recommendations provide guidance for clinical care and are not intended to imply a standard of care, nor does this report provide a strict weighing of the evidence:

1. Establish a written breastfeeding-friendly office policy that includes the provisions as outlined in this document and in Table 3.[27,32,33] Provide a lactation room with

supplies for employees who breastfeed or express breast milk at work. This room could also be used by breastfeeding mothers (refer to recommendation 12). Collaborate with the entire team, including colleagues and office staff. All employees should be aware of the policy, and copies of the policy should be provided to all staff, including anyone who answers the telephone or retrieves messages, such as front office staff.

2. Train staff in the skills necessary to support breastfeeding, especially nurses and medical assistants.[33] Identify ≥1 breastfeeding resource personnel on staff. If possible, consider employing an International Board Certified Lactation Consultant (IBCLC), or a nurse or other staff member trained in lactation support. Trained staff members may be able to perform much of the routinely provided breastfeeding support under the guidance of the pediatrician or other health care provider. The staff should be aware of community resources, including IBCLCs and other lactation support personnel, especially if one is not available in the practice (see recommendation 15).

3. Become knowledgeable regarding the rare but true contraindications to breastfeeding, which include infants with the classic form of galactosemia, maternal HIV or antiretroviral therapy, untreated active tuberculosis, human T-cell lymphotropic virus type I or II, use of illicit drugs, or mothers undergoing chemotherapy or radiation treatment.[34] Most maternal medications are compatible with breastfeeding. Specific drug information can be verified through the National Institutes of Health Toxicology

TABLE 3 Summary of Breastfeeding Supportive Office Practices

1. Have a written breastfeeding-friendly office policy
2. Train staff in breastfeeding support skills
3. Discuss breastfeeding during prenatal visits and at each well-child visit
4. Encourage exclusive breastfeeding for ~6 months
5. Provide appropriate anticipatory guidance that supports the continuation of breastfeeding as long as desired
6. Incorporate breastfeeding observation into routine care
7. Educate mothers on breast-milk expression and return to work
8. Provide noncommercial breastfeeding educational resources for parents
9. Encourage breastfeeding in the waiting room, but provide private space on request
10. Eliminate the distribution of free formula
11. Train staff to follow telephone triage protocols to address breastfeeding concerns
12. Collaborate with the local hospital or birthing center and obstetric community regarding breastfeeding-friendly care
13. Link with breastfeeding community resources
14. Monitor breastfeeding rates in your practice

Data Network, LactMed, which is accessible online or through a mobile device application.[35]

4. Introduce the subject of breastfeeding as early as possible, ideally with prenatal visits and early postpartum visits.[27] Use open-ended questions to inquire about feeding plans for the child, such as "What are your thoughts about feeding your baby?" or "Tell me about your previous infant feeding experiences." Encourage attendance by both parents and/or partners at all visits, and consider discussions with grandparents or other important decision-makers in the family.[36]

5. Encourage breastfeeding mothers to feed newborn infants only human milk and to avoid offering supplements, including formula, glucose water, or other liquids, unless medically indicated.[1] This education ideally should begin prenatally, in anticipation of the newborn infant's stay in the maternity hospital, and should continue through the early postnatal visits.

6. Work with committees within the local hospital or birthing center to implement breastfeeding-friendly care.[1,17,18]

Provide the hospital or birthing center with your office policies regarding breastfeeding. If the facility is not aware of the WHO/United Nations Children's Fund Ten Steps to Successful Breastfeeding, the pediatrician can provide education and help to develop breastfeeding-friendly order sets for the hospital. Encourage the facility to pursue the Baby-Friendly USA designation so that mothers and infants are exposed to maternal and newborn care that supports and encourages breastfeeding, beginning with skin-to-skin care in the immediate postpartum period and early initiation of breastfeeding.[20] Show support for breastfeeding during hospital rounds by reinforcing the benefits of breastfeeding, encouraging exclusive breastfeeding, educating about the importance of frequent breastfeeding, and assessing the adequacy of breastfeeding. During rounds, either evaluate a feeding directly or review the chart for documentation of adequacy of feeding. Encourage mothers to attend breastfeeding classes. Advocate for lactation consultation for mothers who are experiencing any breastfeeding problems or who have concerns.

7. Schedule the first newborn visit by the third to fifth day of life, or approximately 24 to 48 hours from the time the newborn infant is discharged depending on the length of the hospital stay. At office visits, incorporate anticipatory guidance that supports exclusive breastfeeding until infants are approximately 6 months old, followed by continued breastfeeding for 1 year or longer, as mutually desired by the infant and mother.[1] Anticipatory guidance should include appropriate guidance about weight-gain expectations with the use of appropriate growth charts, such as the WHO growth standards for ages 0 to 2 years recommended by the CDC.[37]

8. Educate mothers regarding the provisions of the Patient Protection and Affordable Care Act (Pub L No. 111-148 [2010]), which cover access to breastfeeding support services, breaks to breastfeed or pump at work, as applicable,[38] and the ability to obtain breast pumps through insurance.[39]

9. Provide mothers with anticipatory guidance about returning to work. Workplace support in the pediatric practice and in other work environments can be optimized through the implementation of guidance from the Health Resources and Services Administration Maternal and Child Health Bureau's Business Case for Breastfeeding.[32] Provide information and education to mothers about both the expression and the storage of human milk, which may include providing parents with handouts detailing the recommendations regarding expression and storage.[40]

10. Have the front office staff advise the family, when the first follow-up appointment is scheduled, that the pediatrician or other trained office staff may wish to observe a feeding during the first visit, so that the family will be aware. Encourage the family to let the staff know when the infant is ready to feed while waiting for the appointment. For the first and subsequent appointments, feedings should be observed when the mother identifies any breastfeeding problem, or if weight gain is not appropriate.

11. Provide appropriate educational resources for parents.[41,42] These resources could cover, at a minimum, the benefits of breastfeeding for mother and child, AAP recommendations for duration of breastfeeding, education regarding feeding cues, how to tell whether the infant is getting enough milk, latch and holding techniques, and a list of peer support groups and local breastfeeding resources. The literature should be culturally sensitive and appropriate for the literacy of the patient population. Consider linking to appropriate resources on the practice Web site. Avoid distributing literature provided by manufacturers of infant formula.

12. Allow and encourage breastfeeding in the waiting room.[33] Display noncommercial posters and pamphlets that encourage mothers to breastfeed in waiting areas and examination rooms. Include graphics that show diversity and include fathers, who are valuable partners in the success of the breastfeeding dyad. Do not interrupt or discourage breastfeeding, either in the waiting room or in the examination room. Provide a comfortable, private area for mothers to breastfeed if they prefer privacy. This room may include a rocking chair, pillows, music, water fountain, or whatever helps to create a warm and relaxing environment. An examination room may suffice as a private room for breastfeeding.

13. Eliminate the practice of distribution of free formula and other infant items from formula companies to parents.[43,44] In accordance with the WHO International Code of Marketing of Breast-milk Substitutes,[45] the storage of formula supplies, which may be purchased by the practice as applicable for formula-fed infants, should be out of the view of patients. The breastfeeding-friendly pediatric office practice should not accept gifts (formula and other feeding supplies, pens, writing pads, calendars, mugs, etc) from companies manufacturing infant formula, feeding bottles, or pacifiers. Consumer publications that advertise infant formula or have tear-off cards or inserts to receive free or discounted formula should be discouraged.

14. Train staff to follow telephone triage protocols to address breastfeeding concerns and problems. Train staff on providing appropriate breastfeeding telephone advice, including when to refer to an IBCLC or to a physician with special expertise in breastfeeding management.[46] Telehealth consults may be an option in some locations.

15. Acquire or maintain a list of community resources and be knowledgeable about referral procedures. Refer expectant and new parents to peer, community support, and resource groups.[33] Get to know peer and community support groups in your area. WIC breastfeeding support services, La Leche League International, and peer counselors are

some options. Not all groups may provide evidence-based information, so it is useful if the pediatric care provider or members of the clinic staff have attended and maintain good communication with the leaders of these support groups. Consider inviting successfully breastfeeding mothers to join any advisory groups associated with the practice.

16. Frenulum clipping of the tongue/upper lip has become a popular practice, which may improve infant latch and the effectiveness of breastfeeding and milk transfer. Work closely with local lactation consultants or breastfeeding specialists to determine if frenotomy is appropriate. If so, refer to otolaryngologists and/or dentists with experience in clipping the frenulum in a timely fashion, if the physicians in the practice do not perform the procedure.

17. Collaborate with the obstetric community to develop optimal breastfeeding support programs, because it is clearly documented that a mother's decision to breastfeed starts in the prenatal period and, in many cases, before pregnancy.[10,36]

18. Provide support and education to local child care centers on the importance of breastfeeding and the handling, storage, and feeding of expressed human milk.[47]

19. Monitor breastfeeding initiation and duration rates in the pediatric practice. Be able to access state and national trends as tracked by the CDC through the National Immunization Survey[11] and hospital practices through the Maternity Practices in Infant Nutrition and Care biannual survey data.[48]

BARRIERS TO IMPLEMENTING BREASTFEEDING-FRIENDLY OFFICE PRACTICES

There are challenges to implementing the steps as outlined above for the breastfeeding-friendly pediatric office practice. Breastfeeding care delivered by physicians in the outpatient practice may be limited by lack of knowledge, skills, time, and cultural sensitivity.[23] Breastfeeding management and counseling can be both time consuming and labor intensive. In many health care systems, especially in the United States, practice revenue currently is dependent on volume of visits and patients seen instead of the outcomes of those patients. The AAP Section on Breastfeeding has developed a guide on coding and billing[49] as a tool to optimize reimbursement for time spent in breastfeeding support in the office. Coding guidance also is available through the American College of Obstetricians and Gynecologists for maternal conditions.[50] If additional office visits are required beyond those covered for well-child visits, then diagnosis codes should be used for conditions such as jaundice, newborn feeding problem, infection associated with lactation, etc. Extended visits that require repeated evaluation of breastfeeding and extensive counseling should be billed according to time-based codes.

Even if payment were not an issue, time constraints may be. Complicated breastfeeding problems may require immediate attention and can monopolize staff time and space. Some of these more complex issues may exceed the knowledge level or skill set of the general pediatric care provider. Identifying health care providers and lactation support personnel in the community as sources for referral is important for timely intervention. Lactation support personnel may be limited in certain geographic distributions, especially

rural areas, as well as in certain communities. There are different skill levels among lactation support personnel. These may include, among others, volunteer or paid peer counselors, lactation educators, certified lactation counselors, IBCLCs, and breastfeeding medicine specialists. The extent of training required by the lactation specialist may vary depending on the needs of the mother and/or infant and the particular clinical or community setting. There exists a need for greater availability of culturally appropriate and ethnically diverse lactation support personnel in a variety of community and health care settings. Home visitation, where available, is a family-friendly way to provide lactation support. Pediatric care providers need to be knowledgeable about common complications that can affect both mother and infant and either treat these conditions in the mother or become aware of obstetrician/gynecologists, family physicians, or breastfeeding medicine specialists in the community who are comfortable and knowledgeable in treating the maternal conditions.

Clearly, there will be obstacles to implementing the steps outlined in this report; however, these obstacles are not insurmountable. With ongoing advocacy for the support of breastfeeding, there should be fewer barriers over time.

FURTHER RESEARCH

It would be valuable to study the cost-effectiveness and impact of the routine presence of trained lactation support personnel, such as IBCLCs, versus no specific lactation support in the outpatient pediatric practice on breastfeeding exclusivity and duration. In addition, further research is needed on the effectiveness and intensity of other interventions to support breastfeeding, such as in-person consultation, group sessions, online resources, or use of telehealth, as well as community support interventions. Another area for research is the best method for improving pediatric care provider education in breastfeeding management and support during undergraduate and graduate medical education, as well as continuing medical education for practicing physicians. Education of other members of the health care team who may interact with breastfeeding mothers or children is also important. Finally, similar to the research published in *Pediatrics* entitled "Evaluation of an Office Protocol To Increase Exclusivity of Breastfeeding,"[28] in which the authors evaluated the ABM's clinical protocol for the Breastfeeding-Friendly Physician's Office,[27] an evaluation of the impact of implementation in pediatric office practices of the steps outlined in this clinical report on rates of exclusive breastfeeding and duration of breastfeeding would be beneficial.

CONCLUSIONS

The benefits of breastfeeding and the potential risks of not breastfeeding are numerous, and increasing breastfeeding initiation, duration, and exclusivity has been the focus of multiple recent initiatives in the health care setting, workplace, and community, as recommended by the *Surgeon General's Call to Action To Support Breastfeeding*. With national goals as outlined in Healthy People 2020, an increase in overall breastfeeding initiation, and more Baby-Friendly–designated hospitals, the need for increased support from all members of the health care team is clear. The pediatric care provider is well suited to play a primary role in this effort. The steps outlined in this document provide clear and concise ways for the pediatric office practice to support breastfeeding mothers, infants, and families; increase breastfeeding exclusivity and duration in their patients; and improve health outcomes for the population.

AUTHORS

Joan Younger Meek, MD, MS, RD, FAAP, IBCLC
Amy J. Hatcher, MD, FAAP

SECTION ON BREASTFEEDING EXECUTIVE COMMITTEE, 2015–2016

Joan Younger Meek, MD, MS, RD, FAAP, IBCLC, Chairperson

Margreete Johnston, MD, MPH, FAAP
Mary O'Connor, MD, MPH, FAAP
Lisa Stellwagen, MD, FAAP
Jennifer Thomas, MD, MPH, FAAP
Julie Ware, MD, FAAP
Richard Schanler, MD, FAAP, Immediate Past Chairperson

SUBCOMMITTEE CHAIRPERSONS

Lawrence Noble, MD, FAAP — Policy Chairperson
Krystal Revai, MD, MPH, FAAP — Chief Chapter Breastfeeding Coordinator
Natasha Sriraman, MD, MPH, FAAP — Education Program Chairperson

STAFF

Ngozi Onyema-Melton, MPH, CHES

ABBREVIATIONS

AAP: American Academy of Pediatrics
ABM: Academy of Breastfeeding Medicine
CDC: Centers for Disease Control and Prevention
IBCLC: International Board Certified Lactation Consultant
WHO: World Health Organization
WIC: Special Supplemental Nutrition Program for Women, Infants, and Children

---

FUNDING: No external funding.

POTENTIAL CONFLICT OF INTEREST: The authors have indicated they have no potential conflicts of interest to disclose.

REFERENCES

1. Eidelman AI, Schanler RJ, Johnston M, et al; Section on Breastfeeding. Breastfeeding and the use of human milk. *Pediatrics*. 2012; 129(3). :Available at: www.pediatrics. org/cgi/content/full/ 129/3/e827

2. Chen A, Rogan WJ. Breastfeeding and the risk of postneonatal death in the United States. *Pediatrics*. 2004;113(5). Available at: www.pediatrics.org/cgi/ content/full/113/5/e435

3. Grummer-Strawn LM, Rollins N. Summarising the health effects of breastfeeding. *Acta Paediatr*. 2015;104(467):1–2

4. Collaborative Group on Hormonal Factors in Breast Cancer. Breast cancer and breastfeeding: collaborative reanalysis of individual data from 47 epidemiological studies in 30 countries, including 50302 women with breast cancer and 96973 women without the disease. *Lancet*. 2002;360(9328):187–195

5. Stuebe AM, Rich-Edwards JW, Willett WC, Manson JE, Michels KB. Duration of lactation and incidence of type 2 diabetes. *JAMA*. 2005;294(20):2601–2610

6. Schwarz EB, Ray RM, Stuebe AM, et al. Duration of lactation and risk factors for maternal cardiovascular disease. *Obstet Gynecol*. 2009;113(5):974–982

7. Victora CG, Bahl R, Barros AJ, et al; Lancet Breastfeeding Series Group. Breastfeeding in the 21st century: epidemiology, mechanisms, and lifelong effect. *Lancet*. 2016;387(10017):475–490

8. US Department of Health and Human Services. The Surgeon General's Call to Action To Support Breastfeeding. Washington, DC: US Department of Health and Human Services, Office of the Surgeon General; 2011. Available at: www.surgeongeneral.gov/library/

calls/breastfeeding/. Accessed August 10, 2016

9. Academy of Breastfeeding Medicine Board of Directors. Position on breastfeeding. *Breastfeed Med.* 2008;3(4):267–270

10. American College of Obstetricians and Gynecologists. Optimizing support for breastfeeding as part of obstetric practice. Committee Opinion No. 658. *Obstet Gynecol.* 2016;127(2):e86–e92

11. American College of Obstetricians and Gynecologists. Breastfeeding in underserved women: increasing initiation and continuation of breastfeeding. Committee Opinion No. 570. *Obstet Gynecol.* 2013;122(2 pt 1):423–428

12. American Academy of Family Physicians. Breastfeeding, family physicians supporting [position paper]. Available at: www.aafp.org/about/policies/all/breastfeeding-support.html. Accessed August 10, 2016

13. Centers for Disease Control and Prevention. National immunization survey. Available at: www.cdc.gov/breastfeeding/data/nis_data/rates-any-exclusive-bf-socio-dem-2013.htm. Accessed August 10, 2016

14. US Department of Health and Human Services. Healthy People 2020: maternal, infant, and child health. Available at: https://www.healthypeople.gov/2020/topics-objectives/topic/maternal-infant-and-child-health. Accessed August 10, 2016

15. Perrine CG, Scanlon KS, Li R, Odom E, Grummer-Strawn LM. Baby-friendly hospital practices and meeting exclusive breastfeeding intention. *Pediatrics.* 2012;130(1):54–60

16. The Joint Commission. Perinatal care core measures. Available at: www.jointcommission.org/perinatal_care/. Accessed August 10, 2016

17. National Institute for Children's Health Quality. Projects: Best Fed Beginnings. Available at: http://breastfeeding.nichq.org/solutions/best-fed-beginnings. Accessed August 10, 2016

18. World Health Organization. Evidence for the Ten Steps to Successful Breastfeeding. Available at: www.who.int/maternal_child_adolescent/documents/9241591544/en/. Accessed August 10, 2016

19. World Health Organization. Baby-Friendly Hospital Initiative: revised, updated and expanded for integrated care. Available at: www.who.int/nutrition/publications/infantfeeding/bfhi_trainingcourse/en/. Accessed August 10, 2016

20. World Health Organization. Baby-Friendly Hospital Initiative. Available at: www.who.int/nutrition/topics/bfhi/en/. Accessed August 10, 2016

21. EMPower Breastfeeding [home page]. Available at: http://empowerbreastfeeding.org/. Accessed August 10, 2016

22. Baby-Friendly USA [home page]. Available at: https://www.babyfriendlyusa.org/. Accessed August 10, 2016

23. Feldman-Winter LB, Schanler RJ, O'Connor KG, Lawrence RA. Pediatricians and the promotion and support of breastfeeding. *Arch Pediatr Adolesc Med.* 2008;162(12):1142–1149

24. Szucs KA, Miracle DJ, Rosenman MB. Breastfeeding knowledge, attitudes, and practices among providers in a medical home. *Breastfeed Med.* 2009;4(1):31–42

25. Academy of Breastfeeding Medicine. Educational objectives and skills for the physician with respect to breastfeeding. *Breastfeed Med.* 2011;6(2):99–105

26. US Breastfeeding Committee. *Core Competencies in Breastfeeding Care and Services for All Health Professionals, Revised Edition.* Washington, DC: US Breastfeeding Committee; 2010

27. Grawey AE, Marinelli KA, Holmes AV; Academy of Breastfeeding Medicine. ABM clinical protocol #14. Breastfeeding-friendly physician's office: optimizing care for infants and children, revised 2013. *Breastfeed Med.* 2013;8(2):237–242

28. Corriveau SK, Drake EE, Kellams AL, Rovnyak VG. Evaluation of an office protocol to increase exclusivity of breastfeeding. *Pediatrics.* 2013;131(5):942–950

29. Feldman-Winter L. Evidence-based interventions to support breastfeeding. *Pediatr Clin North Am.* 2013;60(1):169–187

30. Chung M, Raman G, Trikalinos T, Lau J, Ip S. Interventions in primary care to promote breastfeeding: an evidence review for the U.S. Preventive Services Task Force. *Ann Intern Med.* 2008;149(8):565–582

31. US Preventive Services Task Force. Final recommendation statement: breastfeeding: counseling. Available at:www.uspreventiveservicestaskforce.org/Page/Document/RecommendationStatementFinal/breastfeeding-counseling. Accessed August 10, 2016

32. US Department of Health and Human Services; Health Resources and Service Administration, Maternal and Child Health Bureau. The business case for breastfeeding. Available at: www.womenshealth.gov/breastfeeding/government-in-action/business-case-for-breastfeeding/business-case-for-breastfeeding-for-business-managers.pdf. Accessed August 10, 2016

33. American Academy of Pediatrics Section on Breastfeeding. 10 Steps to support parent's choice to breastfeed their baby. Available at: http://www2.aap.org/breastfeeding/files/pdf/TenStepsPoster.pdf. Accessed August 10, 2016

34. Centers for Disease Control and Prevention. Breastfeeding: diseases and conditions. When should a mother avoid breastfeeding? Available at: www.cdc.gov/breastfeeding/disease/index.htm. Accessed August 10, 2016

35. National Institutes of Health; US National Library of Medicine. LactMed: a TOXNET database. Available at: http://toxnet.nlm.nih.gov/newtoxnet/lactmed.htm. Accessed August 10, 2016

36. American College of Obstetricians and Gynecologists. Physician conversation guide on support for breastfeeding. Available at: www.acog.org/About-ACOG/ACOG-Departments/Toolkits-for-Health-Care-Providers/Breastfeeding-Toolkit/Physician-Conversation-Guide-on-Support-for-Breastfeeding. Accessed August 10, 2016

37. Centers for Disease Control and Prevention. The WHO growth charts. Available at: www.cdc.

gov/growthcharts/who_charts.
htm#The%20WHO%20Growth%20
Charts. Accessed August 10, 2016

38. US Department of Labor, Wage and
Hour Division. Break time for nursing
mothers. Available at: www.dol.gov/
whd/nursingmothers/. Accessed
August 10, 2016

39. HealthCare.gov. Breastfeeding benefits.
Available at: https://www.healthcare.
gov/coverage/breast-feeding-benefits/.
Accessed August 10, 2016

40. Academy of Breastfeeding Medicine
Protocol Committee. ABM clinical
protocol #8: human milk storage
information for home use for full-
term infants. *Breastfeed Med.*
2010;5(3):127–130

41. US Health and Human Services Office
on Women's Health. Breastfeeding.
Available at: www.womenshealth.gov/
breastfeeding/. Accessed August 10,
2016

42. Healthychildren.org; American
Academy of Pediatrics. Breastfeeding.
Available at: https://www.
healthychildren.org/English/

ages-stages/baby/breastfeeding/.
Accessed August 10, 2016

43. Rosenberg KD, Eastham CA, Kasehagen
LJ, Sandoval AP. Marketing infant
formula through hospitals: the impact
of commercial hospital discharge
packs on breastfeeding. *Am J Public
Health.* 2008;98(2):290–295

44. Howard C, Howard F, Lawrence R,
Andresen E, DeBlieck E, Weitzman
M. Office prenatal formula
advertising and its effect on breastfeeding patterns. *Obstet Gynecol.*
2000;95(2):296–303

45. World Health Organization.
International code of marketing of
breast-milk substitutes. Available
at: www.unicef.org/nutrition/files/
nutrition_code_english.pdf. Accessed
August 10, 2016

46. Bunik M. *Breastfeeding Telephone
Triage and Advice.* 2nd ed. Elk Grove
Village, IL: American Academy of
Pediatrics; 2016

47. UNC Gillings School of Global
Public Health; Carolina Global
Breastfeeding Institute. Tools for

action-breastfeeding and child care.
Available at: http://breastfeeding.sph.
unc.edu/what-we-do/programs-and-
initiatives/breastfeeding-and-child-
care-toolkit/. Accessed August 10,
2016

48. Centers for Disease Control and
Prevention. Maternity Practices
in Infant Nutrition and Care
(mPINC) survey. Available at: www.
cdc.gov/breastfeeding/data/mpinc/
index.htm. Accessed August 10,
2016

49. American Academy of Pediatrics.
Supporting breastfeeding and
lactation: the primary care
pediatrician's guide to getting paid.
Available at: http://www2.aap.org/
breastfeeding/files/pdf/coding.pdf.
Accessed August 10, 2016

50. American College of Obstetricians and
Gynecologists. Breastfeeding coding.
Available at: www.acog.org/About-
ACOG/ACOG-Departments/Toolkits-for-
Health-Care-Providers/Breastfeeding-
Toolkit/Breastfeeding-Coding. Accessed
August 10, 2016

Get Comfortable With Giving Breastfeeding Support

Dr Heather Campbell, MD, Early Career Physician, *Pediatrics in Review*

During my pediatric residency, I noticed something odd.

I don't have asthma, but I had no problem discussing the importance of using a daily controller medication or demonstrating the use of a spacer with my patients.

I'm not a smoker, but I always felt comfortable reviewing the risks of secondhand smoke exposure with parents and exploring ways to cut down on cigarette use.

I was not a parent, and yet I incorporated anticipatory guidance about child behavioral milestones in nearly all of my patient encounters.

But when it came time for me to counsel breastfeeding mothers, I, as a person who had never breastfed a child, often felt completely out of my league.

Many mothers who struggle with breastfeeding also struggle with a surfeit of information and opinions about breastfeeding. By the time they arrive in a pediatrician's office with concerns, many mothers have been overwhelmed by advice from family, friends, books, strangers, and the Internet.

For a pediatrician, sorting through this information and providing reassurance and actionable advice for breastfeeding mothers can be challenging.

In August 2017 *Pediatrics in Review*, the article by Maya Bunik, MD, MSPH, and its accompanying PowerPoint Teaching Slides provide a comprehensive guide to addressing the many barriers to exclusive breastfeeding.

Given the many recognized benefits of breastfeeding--from early immunoprotection to enhanced maturity of the infant gut--it is essential that all pediatricians learn how to support mothers through their breastfeeding difficulties.

This article will be a handy resource for any pediatrician to incorporate breastfeeding support during their clinic visits.

The Pediatrician's Role in Encouraging Exclusive Breastfeeding

Maya Bunik, MD, MSPH*

*Department of Pediatrics, University of Colorado School of Medicine, Children's Hospital Colorado, Aurora, CO

Practice Gap

Although most pregnant women in the United States plan to breastfeed, there is a clear gap between the proportion of women who prenatally intend to breastfeed and those who actually meet their goals postpartum. (1,2) Pediatricians are often challenged by providing support and management for nursing issues.

Objectives   After completing this article, readers should be able to:

1. Describe differences between human milk and formula and the practice of breastfeeding and formula feeding.

2. Identify the factors that interfere with breastfeeding.

3. Discuss management of maternal nipple pain, low milk supply, late preterm infants, infants with allergic colitis, and problems with maternal milk oversupply.

4. Learn the best ways to support the mother-baby dyad through the birth, hospital, and postpartum periods.

5. Recognize the effects of maternal ingestion of drugs and other substances.

AUTHOR DISCLOSURE Dr Bunik has disclosed no financial relationships relevant to this article. This commentary does not contain a discussion of an unapproved/investigative use of a commercial product/device.

ABBREVIATIONS

BFHI   Baby-Friendly Hospital Initiative
CDC   Centers for Disease Control and Prevention
THC   tetrahydrocannabinol

INTRODUCTION

According to the US Centers for Disease Control and Prevention (CDC), many mothers initiate breastfeeding at birth, but only 22% of infants are exclusively breastfed for 6 months, and only 29% experience any breastfeeding in the first 12 months. (3) This falls short of the Healthy People 2020 goals of 25.5% exclusively breastfeeding for 6 months and 34.1% breastfeeding in the first 12 months (Fig 1). (4) Disparities exist, including differences related to race and ethnicity. For example, Hispanics have higher breastfeeding initiation and duration rates than the black population but lower exclusivity rates than the white population. (5) Moreover, lower breastfeeding rates are also associated with socioeconomic disparities, such as lower education level, poverty, young age, high body mass index, not abstaining from alcohol use, smoking within 6 weeks of delivery, and living in rural areas. These disparities in breastfeeding affect subsequent child health.

The US Preventive Services Task Force recently gave primary care breastfeeding support a "B" recommendation, meaning there is strong evidence that office-based health care promotion should be a priority. (6) Therefore, pediatricians, as advocates and partners for the health of children, should support and promote breastfeeding in mother-infant dyads. Most current intervention efforts are not adequately communicating to families the importance of breastfeeding exclusivity and duration as the norm for all mother-infant dyads. (7,8) Professional education in breastfeeding and helping mothers get access to professional support are provider responsibilities highlighted in the CDC's "Guide to Strategies to Support Breastfeeding Mothers and Babies." (9) In addition, providers should make sure that support for breastfeeding starts in the hospital at birth and then continues with office-based support and peer support at discharge. If a mother is returning to work, she will need support from her employer, as well as her childcare provider.

In this review article, the main objective is to present ways for pediatricians to address the current continued barriers for exclusive breastfeeding, to describe early management challenges, and to provide key tools to foster the rewarding relationship that results when pediatricians and/or staff in their practice play a main role in breastfeeding success.

UNDERSTANDING THE DIFFERENCES BETWEEN HUMAN MILK AND FORMULA

Content Comparison

Human milk is superior to formula because of the immunologic properties that are passed on to the infant and are the basis for disease prevention. Human milk has bioactive factors such as living cells, enzymes, and antibodies that offer immune protection and support the physiological microbes of the gastrointestinal tract. Tow stated in her breastfeeding review that the "most significant inheritance a child will ever receive is the maternal microbiome." (10) Immunoglobulins in human milk are predominantly secretory immunoglobulin A, with smaller amounts of immunoglobulin M and immunoglobulin G. Cells in the breasts interact with maternal plasma from the bronchial tree and intestine to produce immunoglobulin A antibodies that offer specific protection against pathogens in the mother's environment.

High concentration and structural diversity of human milk oligosaccharides, as a group of more than 200 identified complex and diverse glycans, are resistant to gastrointestinal digestion and reach the colon as the first prebiotics. Many human milk oligosaccharides are known to directly interact with the surface of pathogenic bacteria, such as *Haemophilus influenzae* and *Streptococcus pneumoniae*, and inhibit binding and toxins to the host receptors. (11)

In this way, human milk oligosaccharides act as decoys to protect infants from infectious diseases. They are also responsible for a diverse spectrum of functions that include the compositional development of gut microbiota, prevention of intestinal infections, and development of the brain. (12) Lactoferrin, lysozyme, complement, α-lactalbumin, and casein are other important bioactive proteins that act in concert with the complex immune framework. (13)

The composition of human milk varies somewhat from feeding to feeding but usually ranges from 19 to 21 calories per ounce. Volumes can vary throughout the day and also from mother to mother.

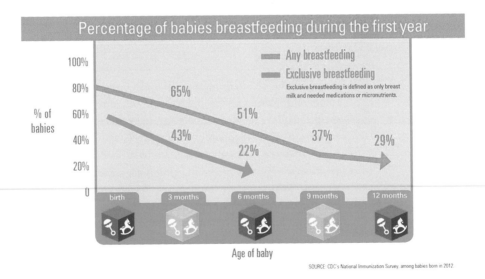

Figure 1. CDC graph of the percentage of babies breastfeeding during the first year.

Formula companies are constantly improving on nutritional content to make formula closer to human milk—for example, by adding docosahexaenoic acid and probiotics. Unfortunately, various labeling and advertising on their products can lead families to believe that certain formulas can eliminate infants' gastrointestinal symptoms, such as gas and reflux. In terms of other nutritional components, formulas contain slightly higher levels of protein than human milk (1.5 g vs 1.1 g per 110 mL, respectively).

Infant Early Weight Loss Nomograms

In a large Kaiser study, investigators found that 5% of exclusively breastfed, vaginally delivered newborns and 10% of cesarean-delivered newborns lost 10% or more of their birth weight 48 hours after delivery. Formula-fed newborns had much lower weight loss rates of 2.9% and 3.5%, respectively. These nomograms (see Fig 2) should be used for early identification of newborns on a trajectory of greater weight loss and follow-up for associated morbidities. (14,15)

Return to Birth Weight and Weight Gain

Some exclusively breastfed newborns may require slightly longer than 2 weeks to return to their birth weight. (16) Close monitoring with frequent weight checks is preferable in this situation because the addition of supplementation may cause more morbidity than watchful waiting.

Infant Temperament and Maternal Bonding

Mothers often report that breastfeeding is an enjoyable bonding time with their infants. (17) Functional brain magnetic resonance imaging has been used to compare exclusively breastfeeding mothers with exclusively formula-feeding mothers as they listened to their infants' own cries versus a control infant's cry. Breastfeeding mothers showed greater brain activations on images while listening to their own baby cry. Studies have also supported the fact that breastfeeding mothers have a higher-rated sensitivity score and are more in tune with infant temperament than mothers who are formula feeding. (18,19)

Milk Volumes

Volume intake varies somewhat with breastfed infants because of the diurnal nature of maternal milk supply (with higher prolactin levels at night). In formula-fed infants, the bottle feedings are controlled by the parent or caregiver, who determines volume, frequency, hunger, and satiety cues. Conversely, infants who are actively feeding and are not sleepy at the breast are in control of the volume of the milk that they transfer from the mother.

Stool Production Patterns

Stool production patterns depend on adequate human milk intake and age of a baby. Expect one stool for each day of life until day 4, when a mother's milk is fully in, leading to a transition in stool color, from meconium black to green to yellow during this time. In the first few weeks, stools commonly occur with every feeding or every other feeding. The "breastfed stool variant" occurs in about one-third of breastfed infants starting at 4 to 6 weeks of age. (20) One soft, voluminous stool occurs usually every 3 to 4 days (but can take up to 12–14 days), and this is thought to be due to almost complete absorption of human milk. At times, the infant can appear uncomfortable, but more commonly, the infant is asymptomatic. It is not known why this occurs in only some breastfed infants.

Vitamin D Supplementation

Vitamin D is generated through the skin from exposure to the sun, and owing to concurrent recommendations for judicious use of sunscreen and sun avoidance, breastfeeding infants require 400 IU of vitamin D supplementation per day. However, adherence to these recommendations has been low. (21,22) Recent work suggests that maternal vitamin D at levels of 6400 IU per day are adequate for transfer of vitamin D to the infant. (23) Most infant formulas contain the added 400 IU of vitamin D with an intake range of 26 to 32 oz.

Developmental Phases

Developmental phases can sometimes interfere with breastfeeding and may differ from infants who are bottle-fed human milk or formula fed. At 4 to 5 months of age, when the infant's vision improves, most infants can become distracted during a feeding, and it can be challenging to keep the infant on the task of completing a full feeding. This may result in more hunger, more frequent feedings, more feeding in the nighttime, and, in rare cases, slower weight gain. Nursing in a quiet, dark room with minimal distractions can help. When infants begin teething, biting can also become a problem. Mechanically, the infant cannot bite and ingest milk at the same time. Infants who bite at the breast when the breast is offered are usually not ready to feed, and biting at the end of the nursing session may mean that they are full. Anticipating this biting behavior may be helpful, and disengaging the infant quickly and ending the feeding usually sends the message that this is an undesirable behavior. Again, perception that the infant is not satisfied by breast milk alone is cited consistently as one of the top reasons for stopping breastfeeding, regardless of weaning

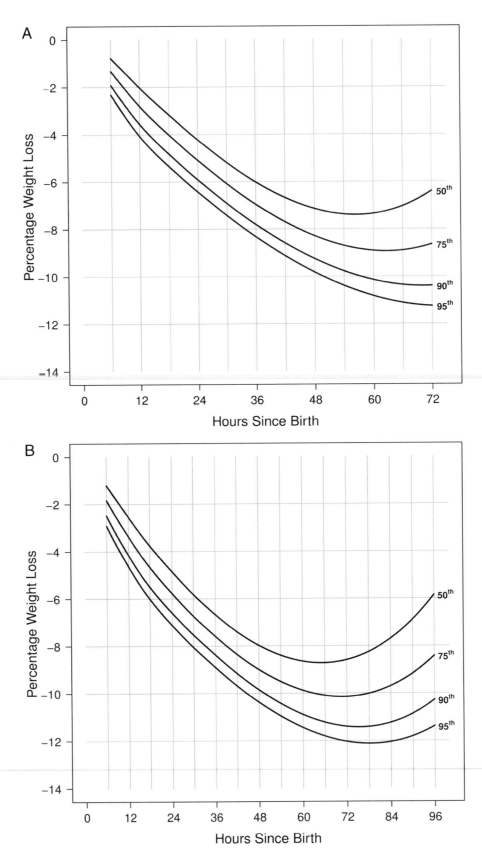

Figure 2. Nomograms for early neonate weight loss (14). A. Estimated percentile curves of percentage weight loss according to time after birth for vaginal deliveries. B. Estimated percentile curves of percentage weight loss according to time after birth for cesarean deliveries.

age. (24) As infants become older, they are usually more effective at breastfeeding and can transfer milk in less than 5 minutes. Mothers' breasts feel emptier, too, but the infant can usually extract the milk even if the suckling seems less effective. This concern about decrease in milk supply is a common misconception with older infants at the 9-month milestone. Providing reassurance at all of these phases can be comforting to the mother and prevent early cessation of breastfeeding.

Risk of not Breastfeeding for Infant and Mother

The dose-responsive benefits of breastfeeding for both the infant and mother are well known and well established and should be the basis for encouraging mothers to breastfeed exclusively. (25,26) The Surgeon General's Report in 2011 and others suggest reframing this argument as the "risk of not breastfeeding." (27,28) The risks of not breastfeeding for infants are shown in Table 1. Mothers who do not breast-feed do not return to prepregnancy weight as quickly and do not have the associated decreased incidence of type 2 diabetes, osteoporosis, hypertension, heart attack, stroke, postpartum depression, breast cancer, and ovarian cancer, as do mothers who breastfeed. (29–34)

ADDRESSING BARRIERS TO EXCLUSIVE BREASTFEEDING

Pain and Low Milk Supply

Pain, sore nipples, and perceived or real insufficient milk supply are the main reasons for early cessation of breast-feeding. (24,35) Sore nipples occur in about one-third of mothers. (36) To avoid pain and trauma, it is best to ensure proper latching by encouraging the newborn to open the mouth wide by tickling his or her lips with a finger or nipple. The mother should pull the baby in close to the mother's abdomen and support the back, so that the newborn's chin dives into the breast and the newborn's nose touches the breast at the nipple. Once latched, the baby's lips should be untucked and flared, like "fish lips." (Fig 3). Although neonates may spend up to 45 to 60 minutes nursing at a time, some of this time may not be nutritive, which is referred to as sleepy "flutter feeding." Prolonged time spent suckling can result in nipple soreness in the early days of breastfeeding, so limiting the time to 30 minutes total, while keeping the neonate on task by tickling or keeping his or her arm up in the air, helps. (20) The mother should break the newborn's strong mouth suction by putting her finger in the corner of the baby's mouth. If the mother has nipple red-ness or cracks, she should find some relief by applying

TABLE 1. Highlighted Risks of Not Breastfeeding for Infants

OUTCOME	EXCESS RISK, %
Full-term infants	
Acute ear infection (otitis media)	100
Eczema (atopic dermatitis)	47
Diarrhea and vomiting (gastrointestinal infection)	178
Hospitalization for lower respiratory tract diseases in the first year	257
Asthma, with family history	67
Asthma, no family history	35
Childhood obesity	32
Type 2 diabetes mellitus	64
Acute lymphocytic leukemia	23
Acute myelogenous leukemia	18
Sudden infant death syndrome	56
Preterm infants	
Necrotizing enterocolitis	138

Adapted from US Department of Health & Human Services. The Surgeon General's Call to Action to Support Breastfeeding. Accessed at http://www.surgeongeneral.gov/library/calls/breastfeeding/ on June 15, 2016 (27)

lanolin, as well as hydrogel or soothing pads. Most post-partum nipple discomfort usually improves by day 7 to day 10. A quick list of common causes of sore nipples is shown in Table 2. (20)

Many mothers perceive that human milk coming from the breasts is not enough to exclusively feed or satisfy an infant. Pediatricians should address this concern early on. At first, human milk comes in small yellow volumes as colostrum, and then in 3 to 4 days, the milk becomes more white and watery in appearance. Most women have a hard time believing that all the nutrition a baby needs can come from her breast, and formula is a readily available option when there is maternal doubt. (37,38) Causes for irrevers-ible low milk production include primary glandular insuf-ficiency (<5% of women), previous breast surgeries and associated scarring, and severe postpartum birth compli-cations, which usually involve hypertension or blood loss. Evaluation for poor latch, sleepy behavior at the breast, and inadequate milk removal will help identify the most likely reversible causes for milk supply concerns. Occasionally, oral contraceptives or pseudoephedrine decongestants can cause a decrease in milk supply. Frequent weight checks in the office, pre- and postfeeding weight checks on a sensitive scale (a scale made to weigh to the nearest gram), and an early-morning pumping session are ways to assess and reassure mothers about milk supply. It is critical to address all of these milk supply issues so as to not unnecessarily disrupt the path toward exclusive breastfeeding.

Breastfeeding Intention and Self-efficacy

Studies continue to show that mothers who have a strong intention to breastfeed prenatally are more likely to achieve their breastfeeding goals. They are more likely to overcome some variables that could affect their success, such as pain, fear of difficulty, birth method, partner support, and even medical complications. However, according to the latest infant feeding study, two-thirds of mothers who intend to exclusively breastfeed are not meeting their intended duration. (39) Increased Baby-Friendly Hospital Initiative (BFHI) practices, particularly giving neonates only breast milk in the hospital, may help more mothers achieve their exclusive breastfeeding intentions. (39) Prenatal maternal knowledge about infant health benefits and developing a level of comfort with breastfeeding in social settings was found to be directly related to the intention to exclusively breastfeed. (40,41) Numerous studies by Dennis and

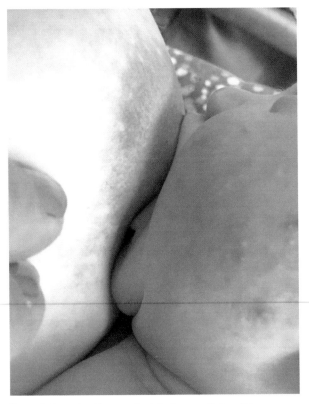

Figure 3. A good, wide, open latch is shown with flared lips.

colleagues in the past decade have shown that having early breastfeeding confidence in the first weeks is associated with longer breastfeeding duration. The validated short form, 14-item Breastfeeding Self-Efficacy Scale (42), includes statements such as, "I can always successfully cope with breastfeeding like I have other challenging tasks," and can be used to evaluate maternal level of confidence with breastfeeding.

IMPROVING ACCESS TO PROFESSIONAL SUPPORT

Birth Hospital Practices Matter

Hospital practices supportive of breastfeeding in the hours and days after birth make a difference in breastfeeding rates. Currently, 18% of US births occur in 11% of BFHI–designated facilities. (43) Yotebieng et al (44) showed that the number of specific BFHI practices had a cumulative effect on exclusivity of breastfeeding. To achieve breastfeeding exclusivity, hospitals should be encouraged to adopt some of these BFHI practices, if not all of them.

The following are the BFHI Ten Steps associated with increased breastfeeding exclusivity:

Written breastfeeding policy. The process of developing policy brings clarification to all staff levels. One example of this success is the decline in distribution of infant formula company discharge bags and sample packs over the past 9 years. (45)

Staff competency assessment. All staff should be trained in the skills and messaging necessary to support new mothers and breastfeeding.

Prenatal breastfeeding education. To affect maternal knowledge and intent as described previously, providing education prior to delivery can help mothers overcome the unexpected challenges of early latch and breastfeeding. One study indicated that 17% of mothers reported that their physician, nurse, or other health care worker missed the opportunity to talk about breastfeeding during any of their prenatal visits. (46)

Early initiation for latch, skin-to-skin kangaroo care, and nursing immediately after birth. Newborns who nurse in the first hours after birth appear to be more successful with latching and nursing later on, and putting the newborn on the mother skin to skin cues the mother and newborn to nurse. (47) Early work on skin-to-skin contact indicates that it may lead to exclusive breastfeeding. (48)

Teaching breastfeeding techniques. Whenever possible, the hospital staff should review what mothers learned prenatally. Observing the mother and practicing latch and

TABLE 2. Quick Reference for Pain with Breastfeeding (20)

INQUIRY	CAUSE OF PAIN	RECOMMENDATION
Lips tucked under—"grandpa lips"? Not opening the mouth wide enough and getting only the nipple in the mouth?	Poor latch	Untuck the lips Wait for a wide-open mouth; may need the baby to start feeding before becoming too awake and hungry to increase cooperation
Early days' discomfort from baby's vacuum suction? Any blanching?	Discomfort in the first weeks vs high suckling pressure	Lanolin Deep breathing Review of good latch
Blister-like lesions on breast?	Herpes	Avoid nursing on the affected side
Pink-tinged nipples? Itching? Shooting pain in the breast?	*Candida* infection	Simultaneous antifungal treatment of mother and baby (all-purpose nipple ointment[a] not adequate)
Does baby's tongue extend beyond the gums? Does baby's tongue move up and sideways when you rub the gums?	Tongue-tie, other mouth abnormalities	If any suspicion, get a formal evaluation (The author's experience is that tongue-tie is currently a popular overdiagnosis)
Shiny white dot on the tip of the nipple?	Bleb	Open up with a sterile needle; has a high rate of reoccurrence
Dry, flaky rash? History of allergies or eczema?	Eczema or irritant dermatitis	Apply over-the-counter hydrocortisone and, if there's no improvement, may need a more potent version via prescription May have allergy to lanolin, detergents/bleach, soaps
Sensitivity of nipples to cold or stimulation? Color change of nipple after nursing?	Vasospasm of nipple/Raynaud phenomenon	Needs evaluation, will likely need prescription for nifedipine
Plentiful milk supply? Baby pulls off with squirts of milk a few minutes into a nursing session?	Clamping down due to oversupply	Lean back with nursing, because it affords baby better control of fast flow
Soreness beyond the nipple? Area of redness of the breast? Fever?	Mastitis	Needs evaluation, will likely need antibiotics

[a]*All-purpose nipple ointment consists of compounded antibiotic, antifungal, and anti-inflammatory ointments.*

techniques to keep the newborn on task when breastfeeding empowers the mother to continue nursing after discharge from the hospital.

Limiting non–human milk feedings. Modeling the hospital use of mother's own milk whenever possible sends a strong message to families, such that they are less likely to use formula supplementation when they go home from the hospital. Although some birth hospitals are providing donor milk to term neonates, (49) there are no studies to support this practice, which is costly and not covered by insurance. In high-risk neonates, donor human milk is best provided from an established not-for-profit milk bank that is part of the Human Milk Banking Association of North America. (50) Donors are not paid and are carefully screened. Milk is collected according to guidelines and pasteurized. Although pasteurization provided by milk banks may affect some of the immune properties of human milk, much is still preserved. Milk sharing or purchasing on the Internet should be avoided, since there is potential for infections or contamination of milk with drugs. (51–54)

Rooming-in, including performing milk expression with the newborn nearby. Newborns and their mothers should be kept in close proximity for as much time as possible in the early breastfeeding days. (55) The newborn should also be close by when the mother uses a breast pump. (56) Neonate safety should be considered when there are medical issues with the maternal-infant dyad.

Teaching feeding cues. Getting the newborn to the breast early, usually every 1.5 to 2 hours, can help the latch process be less stressful for both mother and baby. Crying is a late hunger cue that can add to everyone's frustrations and desire to stop the crying with bottle feeding, thereby giving the newborn unnecessary supplementation.

Limiting pacifier use. The American Academy of Pediatrics suggests that there are exceptions to limiting pacifier use, such as when an infant has to undergo painful procedures and when an infant needs calming. It is best to introduce pacifiers after breastfeeding is established, so that feedings are not missed in the early weeks. (57)

Postdischarge support. After hospital discharge, mothers need to know who to call if they have questions, as well as have a plan for routine follow-up checks and breastfeeding problems. Postdischarge support is an important "outpatient extension" of BFHI.

Peer-to-Peer Support

Peer support by "mentor mothers" who have breastfed and are from the same community or ethnic group can be provided in several ways, including support groups (eg, La Leche League International or the birth hospital) and one-on-one support through telephone calls or visits in a home or clinical setting. Systematic reviews have demonstrated peer counselor programs to be effective in increasing breastfeeding exclusivity. (58,59) Women who provide peer support receive specific training for the best ways to offer emotional support, encouragement, education, and help with breastfeeding problems. (60,61)

Breastfeeding-Friendly Office Practice

The steps for creating a breastfeeding-friendly office practice are shown in Fig 4.

Evaluate early and often in the first weeks. Maternal milk supply is established in the first 3 to 4 weeks postpartum, thereby mandating close evaluation and follow-up to ensure continued breastfeeding. Screening questions (Fig 5) were developed for telephone triage and can be used to determine the level of concern for urgent evaluation. Breastfeeding difficulties usually cause substantial distress in a new family, so determining the level of urgency can help with scheduling an earlier assessment if needed. If there is uncertainty about milk supply or problems with latch, the mother should be seen in the pediatric office or by an outside lactation specialist.

Decide about supplementation. Supplementation with human milk is preferable to formula in times when there is concern about infant weight gain, because even a small amount of cow milk can disrupt the intestinal microbe environment. (62) Moreover, some infants can develop a preference early on in the feeding process, since the bottle method of feeding has a faster flow than the breast. "Slow-flow" nipples (which do not drip when the bottle is turned upside down) can help, but feeding from the breast is commonly slower than any bottle system.

Address combination feeding. In some cultures, the issues of combination feeding are widely accepted and associated with acculturation in the United States. "Las dos cosas" (literally, "those two things," or both breast milk and bottle formula) has been a well-described practice, particularly in Latinas, because mothers want their infants to have the "best of both worlds." (63) In addition, there is a common perception that breast milk is not enough for the infant after 3 months of age. (64,65) Meta-analyses have demonstrated that interventions to encourage exclusive breastfeeding among Latinas should ideally begin in the prenatal setting and involve frequent contact, especially with an International Board-Certified Lactation Consultant. (66)

Advocate for maternity leave and support the return-to-work transition. Studies show that women who intend to return to work within a year of their child's birth are less likely to initiate breastfeeding, and those who work full-time tend to breastfeed for shorter periods than those who work part-time or do not work out of the home. (67,68) Not surprisingly, women in salaried jobs and those with longer maternity leaves are more likely to breastfeed. (69) Unfortunately, planning for return to work seems to affect mothers' decision-making early in the postpartum period. (70) Many women worry about having enough milk stored and having to express milk at work. A double-sided pump is the best choice for a working mother because of its efficiency. Under the Affordable Care Act of 2014, insurance companies provide pumps as a covered benefit, but anecdotal experience suggests that these pumps may not always be of the best caliber. (71) Mothers should be encouraged to talk to their employers early during pregnancy and try to take at least 6 postpartum weeks off of work, if possible. Maternity leave of up to 6 weeks compared to 6 to 12 weeks after delivery was associated with higher odds of failure to establish breastfeeding. (72) Under the Affordable Care Act, working mothers should be provided with accommodations,

OFFERING BREASTFEEDING SUPPORT IN YOUR OFFICE IS AS EASY AS 1-2-3

#1 Train internal staff or provide early referral for breastfeeding management and support. This is also known as extending the Baby-Friendly Hospital Initiative to your office.

#2 Provide resources for mothers, such as hospital-based drop-in clinics or groups or other mother support groups. It is always a good idea to attend or have one of your staff attend these sites so that you are sure that the advice and any concerns raised are addressed appropriately and in line with general American Academy of Pediatrics recommendations.

#3 Avoid storing and giving out formula samples in your office. It may seem supportive, but it gives the wrong message about breastfeeding exclusivity. Providing information about pumps, pump rental stations, or hand expression is a better idea.

Figure 4. Offering breastfeeding support in your office is as easy as "1-2-3."

such as time and a private 4-foot by 6-foot space in which to pump. (73)

OTHER BREASTFEEDING CHALLENGES THAT PROVIDERS NEED TO ADDRESS

Oversupply

Most newborns, even when they are older, only ingest a maximum of 3.0 to 3.5 oz of milk at the breast, (74) so mothers who are producing more than that amount usually have a state of oversupply. Not only does oversupply cause uncomfortable fullness and leakage for the mother, but milk could be continuously "leftover" in the breast, leading to possible stasis, plugged ducts, and even mastitis. Mothers with milk oversupply should lean back as much as possible when nursing so that the infant has some ability to respond better to the fast flow, which occurs with let-down. In this position, the infant is less likely to pull off of the breast. The process of slowly and carefully down-regulating the milk supply, with less pumping and trending toward one-sided

1. **What is your baby's age and gestational age? Was your baby born early or on time? If early, how early? Do you have discharge sheets at home? Did the hospital tell you your newborn's gestational age?** (Late preterm is high risk.)
2. **Is your baby acting sick or abnormal in any way (eg, weak, decreased activity)?** Rule out sepsis, particularly in babies 4 weeks of age and younger.
3. **Is breastfeeding going well?** If not perceived as going well, mother and baby may need to be seen in the office today or tomorrow (within 24 hours).
4. **How many times have you breastfed in the past day?** Ten to 12 times per 24 hours is optimal; 8 times is minimal. Suboptimal nursing sessions require evaluation.
5. **How long is your baby awake and actively suckling and swallowing at the breast during a feeding?** Baby should be actively feeding at the breast without long pauses or flutter feeding for at least 10 minutes. Just as with microwave popcorn, pauses or extended time (ie, "cooking the popcorn" too long) are not effective (analogy courtesy of Sheela Geraghty, MD, MS, IBCLC, FAAP). The mother may need assistance with latch and keeping baby on task for nursing sessions.
6. **What color are your baby's stools?** By day 4, stools should be yellow and seedy, not black or green transitional stools.
7. **How many stools has your baby had in the past day?** The goal is 1 stool per day of life up to day 4 (ie, by day 4, the baby should have at least 4 stools daily). A suboptimal stool pattern requires evaluation.
8. **How many wet urine diapers has your baby had in the past day?** Seven to 8 wet urine diapers is normal (exception: 3 wet diapers per day can be normal for the first 5 days). A suboptimal urine pattern requires evaluation.
9. **Do your breasts feel full before feedings and softer afterward?** The optimal answer is yes. Before the milk is in, most mothers will not notice any change. If baby is close to 2 weeks of age, the mother's breasts may be adjusting to what the baby's needs are, and she may experience only mild symptoms of engorgement.
10. **How many times have you supplemented with formula in the past day?** Supplementation more than once in 24 hours can affect milk supply or may indicate breastfeeding difficulties.

Figure 5. Triage assessment questions are given for the early postpartum period—the first 2 weeks. When using these advice topics, it is best to begin each call with the following 10 screening questions and then ask, "What is your main breastfeeding question or concern?" Adapted from the Screening Form for Early Follow-Up of Breastfed Newborns on the Dr. Mom Web site at http://www.dr-mom.com. Reproduced with permission.

TABLE 3. Touch Points for Overcoming Obstacles to Breastfeeding Exclusivity (20)

TIME POINT	PARENTAL CONCERN	MAIN OBSTACLE	PROVIDER ADVICE
Prenatal	"I want to breastfeed, but since I am going to work, I need to be able to formula feed, too."	Lack of information about combining breastfeeding and working	Strongly encourage attendance at a prenatal breastfeeding class (deserves equal time to birthing class education)
		Lack of information about milk expression and access to breast pumps	Consider a longer maternity leave, if possible Prepare to simplify life during the transition to parenting
	"My husband/partner and other family members will want to help feed the baby. Won't they feel excluded if I only breastfeed?"	Family members wanting to feed the baby	Enlist father's/partner's help in supporting the nursing partner; fathers/partners can interact with their newborn by holding the baby skin to skin or taking the baby out while mom sleeps After breastfeeding is well established, others can feed the baby expressed milk by bottle
	"I want to do combination feeding, or las dos cosas."	Desire for "the best of both worlds" by combination feeding	"Puro pecho," or only mother's own milk, provides greater health benefits and helps maintain an abundant milk supply
		Lack of knowledge about the importance of frequent and exclusive breastfeeding during the early postpartum weeks for establishing mother's milk supply	If eligible, enrollment in the Special Supplemental Nutrition Program for Women, Infants, and Children (WIC) offers breastfeeding mothers a substantial food package, counseling, breast pumps, and peer counselors
Birth	"My friend says it is a good idea to ask the nurses to care for my baby at night so I can get some sleep."	Unrealistic expectations for the postbirth hospital stay	Promote immediate skin-to-skin contact after birth to facilitate the initiation of breastfeeding within the first hour
		Lack of prenatal education	Teach the mother to interpret her newborn's feeding cues and breastfeed as often as baby wants; advocate for no routine formula use in the system of care
		Frequent interruptions and excessive visitors deplete new mothers	Advise the mother to request help in the hospital with breastfeeding to promote task mastery
		Increased risk of formula supplements for nighttime births from 9 pm to 6 am	Encourage continuous rooming-in, where the mother can practice being with her baby in a controlled setting and learn to latch baby comfortably and effectively
	"The yellow milk does not look like much. A little formula won't hurt, will it?"	Belief that the small amount of colostrum is insufficient until the "milk comes in"	Explain the potency and adequacy of colostrum and the rapid increase in milk production from 36 to 96 h
3–5 d	"Now that we are home from the hospital, the baby seems to be feeding every hour. She or he doesn't seem satisfied with breast milk alone."	Lack of knowledge about normal frequency of feedings for breastfed newborns	Explain that 8–12 feedings in 24 h are typical and necessary to establish an abundant milk supply
		Newborns typically begin feeding more frequently the second night after birth, when the baby is at home	Provide a hand-pump or teach hand expression, so the mother can see that she has milk
		Concern about whether the newborn is getting enough milk, due to the mother's inability to see what the newborn takes at the breast	Explain normal newborn elimination patterns once the mother's milk comes in (3–5 voids and 3–4 stools per day by 3–5 d; onset of yellow, seedy milk stools by 4–5 d)
		Sleepy newborn	Perform newborn test weights (before and after feeding) to reassure the mother about baby's milk intake at a feeding Teach the mother the difference between newborn "flutter sucking" or "nibbling" that results in only a trickle of milk at the breast versus "drinking" milk, with active sucking and regular swallowing Tickling under the axilla or holding a hand up can help keep baby on task at the breast; or, compressing the breast when the baby stops slow, deep sucking can deliver a spray of milk to entice him or her to start drinking again Anticipate newborn appetite spurt at about 10–14 d of age

Continued

TABLE 3. (Continued)

TIME POINT	PARENTAL CONCERN	MAIN OBSTACLE	PROVIDER ADVICE
	"My nipples are sore and cracked. Can I take a break and give my baby a little formula?"	Sore nipples are usually attributable to incorrect latch-on technique and are a common reason that mothers discontinue breastfeeding early or start supplements	Observe a nursing session to evaluate latch; consider referring the mother to a lactation consultant for one-on-one assistance with latch
2 wk	"My breasts do not feel very full anymore. I'm afraid my milk went away."	As postpartum breast engorgement resolves and the breasts adjust to making and releasing milk, mothers may perceive that they have insufficient milk supply	Expect the newborn to be above birth weight by 10–14 d and reassure the mother about the newborn's rate of weight gain since the 3–5-d visit Although the mother's breasts are less swollen than during postpartum engorgement, they should feel fuller before feedings and softer afterward
	"How can I know my baby is getting enough?"	The 10–14-d appetite spurt can cause the mother to doubt the adequacy of her milk supply	Consider performing test weights (before and after feeding) to reassure the mother about her newborn's intake Anticipate another appetite spurt at about 3 wk of age
1 mo	"My baby is crying a lot, and I am tired and need sleep."	Normal infant crying peaks at about 6 wk (3–5 h in 24 h) Mother may attribute infant crying to hunger or an adverse reaction to her milk	Congratulate the mother on a full month of breastfeeding! If infant has gained weight appropriately, reassure the mother about the adequacy of her milk supply Offer coping strategies for infant crying, including holding the baby skin to skin; the 5 S's[a] (however, swaddle with the baby's hands up near the head to help assess feeding cues); use of an infant carrier; going for a stroller or car ride; observing a period of "purple crying"
	"Nothing seems to calm her/him except the bottle."	If the infant drinks milk from a bottle that is offered, the mother may assume that her infant is not satisfied by breastfeeding	Explain that infant sucking is reflexive, and drinking from an offered bottle doesn't always mean that the baby is hungry; baby "can't scream and suck at the same time," so the bottle may appear to calm baby, just as a pacifier might If mom desires to offer a bottle, use expressed milk as the supplement Forewarn the mother about cluster feedings (late afternoon/evening) and upcoming appetite spurts, occurring at about 6 wk and 3 mo
2 mo	"My mother said that, if I give my baby rice cereal in a bottle before bedtime, he or she may sleep longer at night."	Parental sleep deprivation The mother may have already returned to work, which often increases fatigue and leads to a decrease in milk supply	Explain the lack of evidence that rice cereal or other solid foods increase infant sleep Remind the mother that adding complementary foods is a project and increases the workload for parents Reinforce the benefits of exclusive breastfeeding for maternal-infant health and mother's milk supply
	"I am going back to work and am worried that I do not have enough frozen stores of milk. Are there any herbs I can take to keep my milk supply strong?"	Lack of knowledge about the principles of milk production and unrealistic beliefs about the effectiveness of galactogogues	Enlist help from others, including support for returning to work Explain that there is no "magic pill" or special tea to increase the mother's milk supply; the key to ongoing milk production is frequent, effective milk removal (every 3–4 h) Caution the mother to avoid going long intervals without draining her breasts
4 mo	"My baby seems to only eat for a few minutes, and when I try to put her/him back to the breast, she or he refuses."	Misinterpretation of infant's efficiency in nursing causes concern about infant milk intake	Explain that infants become more efficient at breastfeeding, and by 3 mo, they may drain the breast in 4–7 min Reinforce continuing to delay the introduction of solid foods

Continued

TABLE 3. (Continued)

TIME POINT	PARENTAL CONCERN	MAIN OBSTACLE	PROVIDER ADVICE
	"My baby seems more interested in everything around him or her than in nursing at the breast."	Normal infant distractibility causes the mother to believe her infant is self-weaning	Explain that distractibility is a normal developmental behavior at this age and that short, efficient feedings are common Nurse in a quiet, darkened room
6 mo	"My baby is drooling and rubbing on her or his gums all the time. I do not think that I can continue to breastfeed because my baby might bite me."	Common myth that a mother needs to wean when her baby gets teeth to avoid being bitten while breastfeeding	Congratulate the mother on 6 mo of exclusive breastfeeding! Explain that infants cannot bite and actively breastfeed at the same time. Biting tends to occur if the breast is offered when the infant is not interested or at the end of the feeding If the infant bites, say "No biting," touch the infant's lips, set the baby down, and briefly leave the room
	"My baby has refused to breastfeed for almost a whole day now. Is she or he ready to wean?"	Misinterpretation of sudden breastfeeding refusal ("nursing strike") to mean that a baby is self-weaning	Explain that some babies may suddenly refuse the breast between 4 and 7 mo of age for no apparent reason; common causes include upper respiratory infection, ear infection, teething, regular exposure to bottle-feeding, use of a new soap/perfume, maternal stress, or a decrease in milk supply Because many babies will nurse while asleep, try offering the breast when the baby is drowsy or asleep Regularly express milk if the baby won't nurse, and feed the pumped milk until the infant resumes breastfeeding

aThe 5 S's consist of swaddling, side lying, swaying, shushing, and sucking. From: Karp, Harvey. The Happiest Baby on the Block, 2nd Ed. New York: NY: [illegible]

feeding, is recommended but can be challenging because it seems counterintuitive to want to make less milk.

Tongue-Tie

It has become increasingly common for infants to have their tongue- or lip-tie diagnosed and clipped as part of a breastfeeding consultation. (75) Despite little evidence for these procedures, tongue and lip clipping have become widely accepted. (76)

Anterior lip-tie, which causes the tongue to have decreased lateral movement and decreased frontal movement up and over the gums, can cause pain and ineffective latch when breastfeeding. Anterior lip-tie can be associated with ineffective nursing and decreasing milk supply. (77) With posterior tongue-tie, the tongue is tacked down at the back of the mouth—a condition that is difficult to diagnose. This anatomic condition is not universally accepted by otolaryngologists and is not easily corrected with surgery, which involves releasing tissue at the base of the tongue. (78) Any infant who has undergone the procedure, by means of either incision or laser (now performed by many dentists and others), should be followed up closely. If breastfeeding does not improve after the procedure, more feeding evaluation and assistance may be needed.

Allergic Colitis

Allergic colitis is a cell-mediated hypersensitivity disorder that affects the large intestinal tract in less than 1% of exclusively breastfed infants. The most common symptom associated with food allergy in the infant is bloody stools. (79) Dietary proteins in the mother's milk are responsible, which are usually due to maternal ingestion of dairy products. Breastfed infants with allergic colitis are typically well appearing and rarely have reflux symptoms, such as vomiting, diarrhea, and abdominal distention. Elimination of cow milk from the maternal diet is the first step in treatment, and in most cases, symptoms in the infant should improve within 3 to 4 days. If continued mucus and blood are detected, then mothers need to eliminate soy products next, followed by the remaining causal agents: eggs, nuts, wheat, corn, strawberries, citrus, and chocolate. Compliance with these elimination diets is challenging initially and even more difficult to maintain, so mothers should be cautioned to eliminate only one item at a time to be sure that eliminating one particular food from the diet is necessary. Interestingly, most infants with allergic colitis tolerate cow milk after their first birthday. (80)

Fussiness

Just as breastfeeding is established at the end of the first month of life, many infants manifest common fussy behaviors that may be misinterpreted as gastroesophageal reflux or food allergies. Discussion about the normal crying curve that peaks at 6 weeks and about ways to soothe a crying infant should be part of anticipatory guidance for the breastfed infant. (81)(82) Mothers and family members (and medical providers) may erroneously blame breastfeeding in some way (diet, milk supply, medications) as a reason for the fussiness.

Reflux

Reflux symptoms, such as increased spitting up and fussiness, can cause unnecessary supplementation in the infant. Reflux can cause abdominal pain when the infant is not upright during nursing, which could mistakenly lead to elimination diets in the mother. About 50% of infants experience effortless spitting up of small amounts of breast milk (1–2 teaspoons). This spitting up should be distinguished from vomiting, which is forcefully throwing up more volume. It can be helpful to instruct the family that the stomach is like an "untied water balloon" and that any abrupt movement can cause "leakage." Providing the mother with reassurance that reflux will improve with age in most infants can help prevent the mother and infant from taking unnecessary paths toward medication use.

Maternal Medications

The need to prescribe almost any type of maternal medication can lead to erroneous early cessation of breastfeeding. The decision-making process around medication use while breastfeeding should be one of joint negotiation between mother and provider. (83) In general, the mother should avoid taking long-acting forms of medications and should watch her infant for any unusual signs and symptoms, such as sleepiness, irritability, or other known side effects of the prescribed medication. Acetaminophen and ibuprofen are well studied and safe. Some allergy medications can be sedating, so less sedating choices are better. Drugs contraindicated during breastfeeding include anti-cancer drugs, lithium, oral retinoids, iodine, amiodarone, and gold salts. (84) Online resources for guidance, such as LactMed, (85) InfantRisk Center (telephone 806/352-2519), (86) and the Postpartum Support International Warmline (telephone 800/944-4773) can help prevent giving incorrect advice about discontinuing a medication or discontinuing breastfeeding.

Herbs or Supplements

Lactation specialists have recommended herbs such as fenugreek and blessed thistle, usually as a last resort when other nonpharmacologic measures do not result in an increase in milk volume. (87) However, milk expression is the only successful, evidence-based method for increasing milk supply. During inquiry about maternal medication use, providers should question the mother about the use of herbal remedies or natural supplements. Appropriate counseling should be given to avoid the desire to take "magic bullets for milk supply."

Maternal Mental Health

Pregnancy-related depression and postpartum depression are associated with difficulty breastfeeding and shorter breastfeeding duration. Premature cessation of breastfeeding is also a risk factor for developing increased maternal anxiety. Women with high levels of anxiety and depression during pregnancy who stop breastfeeding early are at an additional multiplicative risk for postpartum anxiety and depression. (88) Best practice during a clinical visit is to screen the mother with a validated tool, such as the Edinburgh Postnatal Depression Scale, to ensure that maternal mental health is addressed adequately and objectively. (89)

Alcohol, Tobacco, and Marijuana Use

Alcohol is transferred readily into human milk at levels that match the mother's blood alcohol level. A safe rule, similar to the rule for safe drinking and driving a motor vehicle, is 1 drink consumed in 2 hours. Although alcohol test strips for breast milk are available for purchase, careful and limited consumption of alcohol is the best approach when breastfeeding. Tobacco smoking is not a contraindication to breastfeeding because the effects of smoking tobacco on the risk of sudden infant death syndrome and respiratory illness are almost negated if the infant has been breastfeeding. (90) However, nicotine can make an infant jittery, can interfere with let-down, and is associated with lower milk supply. Therefore, mothers who smoke should delay nursing as long as possible after smoking, and providers should provide motivational interviewing for smoking cessation assistance and/or suggest that a mother decrease the number of cigarettes she smokes or switch to cigarettes with lower nicotine content. Limited research is available on breastfeeding and marijuana use, including the amount of tetrahydrocannabinol (THC) in human milk, the length of time THC remains in the human milk after exposure, and the effects of THC on the infant. In a survey of more than 1,700 mothers in the Special Supplemental Nutrition Program for Women, Infants, and Children (WIC) in Colorado, 6% reported using THC during pregnancy for symptoms of nausea, depression, and anxiety. (91) Because of concern for the developing brain in infants, mothers should abstain from using marijuana while breastfeeding. (92,93)

Summary

- On the basis of strong evidence, the dose-responsive benefits of breastfeeding for both the infant and the mother are well established and should be the basis for recommending mothers to breastfeed exclusively. (25,26)

- On the basis of strong evidence, pain, sore nipples, and insufficient milk supply are the main reasons for early cessation of breastfeeding. (24,35)

- On the basis of strong evidence, hospital practices supportive of breastfeeding in the hours and days after birth make a difference in breastfeeding rates. However, currently, less than 20% of US births occur in Baby-Friendly Hospital Initiative–designated facilities.

- On the basis of consensus, in the first few weeks, stools commonly occur with every feeding or every other feeding. The "breastfed stool variant" occurs in about one-third of breastfed infants at about 4 to 6 weeks. One soft, voluminous stool occurs usually every 3 to 4 days, thought to be due to almost complete absorption of human milk.

- On the basis of consensus, developmental phases bring challenges for the breastfeeding dyad. Just when breastfeeding is getting established, infants go through a period of crying that may be misinterpreted as hunger and can lead to unnecessary supplementation. At about 4 months of age, most infants can become distracted during a feeding and are challenging to keep on the task of completing a full feeding. Nursing in a quiet, dark room with minimal distractions can help.

- On the basis of strong evidence and consensus, because milk supply is established in the first few weeks postpartum, access to trained internal staff or early referral for breastfeeding management and support is essential to ensure breastfeeding exclusivity. Hospital-based clinics or other maternal support groups provide additional support. (58,59)

- The breastfeeding touch points in Table 3 offer guidance for common issues that arise when supporting exclusive breastfeeding in the first 6 months postpartum and beyond.

To view teaching slides that accompany this article, visit http://pedsinreview.aappublications.org/content/38/8/353.supplemental.

The Pediatrician's Role in Encouraging Exclusive Breastfeeding

Maya Bunik, MD, MSPH

Pediatrics in Review   American Academy of Pediatrics

References for this article are at http://pedsinreview.aappublications.org/content/38/8/353.

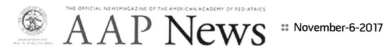

THE OFFICIAL NEWSMAGAZINE OF THE AMERICAN ACADEMY OF PEDIATRICS

AAP News :: November-6-2017

Study Looks at Trends in Breastfeeding Attitudes, Counseling Practices

from the AAP Department of Research

Research based on data from the AAP Periodic Survey of Fellows indicates that primary care pediatricians' recommendations regarding breastfeeding have become more reflective of AAP policy over the last two decades (Feldman-Winter L, et al. *Pediatrics*.2017;140:e20171229, http://bit.ly/2xQQWGs).

The authors found that 76% of pediatricians in 2014 recommended exclusive breastfeeding during the first month of life, up from 65% in 1995. Additionally, almost all pediatricians now recommend initiating breastfeeding within the first hour after delivery (92%) and keeping the newborn in the mother's room throughout the hospital stay (86%), whereas about half of pediatricians recommended these practices in 1995 (see figure). In 2014, more pediatricians reported that their main affiliated hospital had applied for a "baby-friendly" designation than in 1995 (57% vs. 12%, respectively).

The study also found that pediatricians' beliefs about breastfeeding success and the benefits of breastfeeding have declined slightly. In 2014, 57% of pediatricians believed that any mother can successfully breastfeed with persistence compared to 69% in 1995, and about half (53%) said breastfeeding benefits outweigh the difficulties and inconveniences faced by mothers compared to 68% in 1995.

Each Periodic Survey was mailed to approximately 1,600 non-retired U.S.-based AAP members. Response rates in 1995, 2004 and 2014 were 72%, 55% and 51%, respectively. Analyses were limited to pediatricians providing primary care to children 2 years old and younger. The 2014 survey was supported in part by Grant No. UC4MC21534 from the Maternal and Child Health Bureau (Title V, Social Security Act), Health Resources and Services Administration, Department of Health and Human Services. The conclusions are those of the authors and not necessarily those of the Maternal and Child Health Bureau.

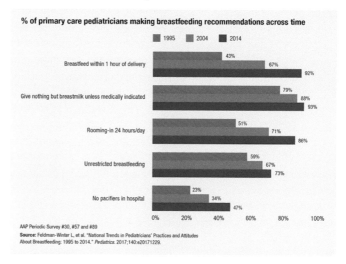

% of primary care pediatricians making breastfeeding recommendations across time

1995 ■ 2004 ■ 2014

Recommendation	1995	2004	2014
Breastfeed within 1 hour of delivery	43%	67%	92%
Give nothing but breastmilk unless medically indicated	79%	88%	93%
Rooming-in 24 hours/day	51%	71%	86%
Unrestricted breastfeeding	59%	67%	73%
No pacifiers in hospital	23%	34%	47%

AAP Periodic Survey #30, #57 and #89
Source: Feldman-Winter L, et al. "National Trends in Pediatricians' Practices and Attitudes About Breastfeeding: 1995 to 2014." *Pediatrics*. 2017;140:e20171229.

Research Update

When It Comes to Having a Positive Attitude About Breastfeeding Success, Pediatricians Have Some Work to Do

Dr Lewis First, MD, MA, Editor in Chief, *Pediatrics*

If any child health care professional is asked about what the ideal nutritional source is for ensuring the growth and development of a healthy infant, the response is certainly something like "of course, breastfeeding is best"! Yet just how optimistic are we that that saying that will result in exclusive breastfeeding for at least the first six months of an infant's life, and that mothers who breastfeed will be successful enough at it to persist with this important feeding practice? Feldman-Winter et al. (10.1542/peds.2017-1229) share with us some interesting data from a 2014 national survey of American Academy of Pediatrics (AAP) members looking at how pediatrician counseling practices and attitudes have changed from prior surveys dating back to 1995. While more of us are in hospitals with "Baby Friendly" designations and more of us are recommending exclusive breastfeeding, we have lost ground in thinking that mothers can actually be successful at exclusive breastfeeding or that the benefits of breastfeeding outweigh the difficulties. This is certainly disappointing data from the 620 respondents in this survey.

So who is less confident in their breastfeeding attitudes? Are these experienced or less experienced pediatricians in terms of years of practice? Can we do anything to change these attitudes so that the next survey does not continue to show even less positivity by pediatricians for endorsing, supporting, and believing that mothers can be successful with this feeding practice? To provide some perspective on these results and what we can do to improve our own competencies in breastfeeding support, we have asked pediatrician and board-certified lactation consultant Dr. Joan Meek to share her input through an accompanying commentary (10.1542/peds.2017-2509). Read this study and commentary and then reflect on just how you can improve your ability to troubleshoot breastfeeding problems in the mothers of your newest patients and in turn improve our overall support for this essential source of infant nutrition.

Pediatrician Competency in Breastfeeding Support Has Room for Improvement

Joan Younger Meek, MD, MS

The American Academy of Pediatrics (AAP) recommends breastfeeding as the preferred method of infant feeding. The protection, promotion, and support of breastfeeding are matters of public health policy and important roles for pediatricians.[1] In this issue of *Pediatrics*, Feldman-Winter et al[2] provide a summary and analysis of the data from 3 AAP Periodic Surveys of Fellows, conducted in 1995, 2004, and 2014, examining knowledge and attitudes of fellows of the AAP regarding breastfeeding. In examining the trends, the authors conclude that pediatricians' recommendations and practices have become more closely aligned with AAP policy between 1995 and 2014; however, their attitudes about the likelihood of breastfeeding success have worsened, so continued efforts to enhance pediatricians' training about breastfeeding are necessary.

Between 1995[3] and 2014[4] (most recent national data available), breastfeeding initiation rose from 60% to 82%, and 6-month breastfeeding rates for any (not exclusive) breastfeeding increased from 21% to 55%. These improvements in breastfeeding rates occurred across a backdrop of increased awareness regarding the importance of breastfeeding for women's and children's health outcomes while significant national initiatives promoted breastfeeding. In 2011, the US Department of Health and Human Services published "The Surgeon General's Call to Action to Support Breastfeeding,"[5] which established a national breastfeeding agenda with 20 action steps to encourage all segments of society to improve breastfeeding support. It called for all health professionals who care for women and children to receive education and training in breastfeeding and emphasized that basic support for breastfeeding should be considered a standard of care for pediatricians.

The Affordable Care Act included a provision covering breastfeeding counseling services and supplies and mandated breaks for milk expression for employed breastfeeding women.[6] The Department of Health and Human Services' "Business Case for Breastfeeding"[7] provides resources and innovative approaches to support breastfeeding women in the workplace. The US Department of Agriculture Food and Nutrition Service's Special Supplemental Nutrition Program for Women, Infants, and Children enhances breastfeeding support by providing anticipatory guidance, counseling, pumps, and education for pregnant and breastfeeding women.[8]

Hospital breastfeeding practices have changed as well. The Joint Commission adopted the perinatal care core measure on exclusive breastfeeding as a quality measure. The Centers for Disease Control and Prevention instituted the biannual Maternity Practices in Infant Nutrition and Care[8] surveys of maternity facilities in 2007. In that year, only 2.9% of births in the United States occurred in "Baby-Friendly"–designated facilities. By 2017, that number had

(FREE)

College of Medicine, Florida State University, Tallahassee, Florida

Opinions expressed in these commentaries are those of the author and not necessarily those of the American Academy of Pediatrics or its Committees.

DOI: https://doi.org/10.1542/peds.2017-2509

Accepted for publication Jul 25, 2017

Address correspondence to Joan Younger Meek, MD, MS, Florida State University College of Medicine, 1115 West Call St, Tallahassee, FL 32306. E-mail: joan.meek@med.fsu.edu

PEDIATRICS (ISSN Numbers: Print, 0031-4005; Online, 1098-4275).

FINANCIAL DISCLOSURE: The author has indicated she has no financial relationships relevant to this article to disclose.

FUNDING: No external funding.

POTENTIAL CONFLICT OF INTEREST: The author has indicated she has no potential conflicts of interest to disclose.

COMPANION PAPER: A companion to this article can be found online at www.pediatrics.org/cgi/doi/10.1542/peds.2017-1229.

To cite: Meek JY. Pediatrician Competency in Breastfeeding Support Has Room for Improvement. *Pediatrics*. 2017;140(4):e20172509

increased to 21.8%, accounting for 869 000 births.[9,10] The Centers for Disease Control and Prevention have funded 2 major national initiatives with the aims to improve maternity care practices and to increase the number of Baby-Friendly designated hospitals in the US. "Best Fed Beginnings,"[11] a nationwide quality improvement initiative, resulted in 80% of enrolled facilities achieving designation as Baby-Friendly.[12] "EMPower Breastfeeding: Enhancing Maternity Practices" has used a model of breastfeeding content experts and quality improvement coaches to guide enrolled facilities in improving maternity care practices and achieving designation as Baby-Friendly.[13] Baby-Friendly designated facilities must follow the "Ten Steps to Successful Breastfeeding."[14] Two of those steps include having a written breastfeeding policy routinely communicated to all health care staff and training all staff in the skills necessary to implement the policy. Pediatricians with privileges in newborn care must complete a minimum of 3 hours of education on breastfeeding management.

Residency training in breastfeeding is not universal. Freed et al[15] identified deficiencies in pediatric residency training in a national survey published in 1995. A survey of pediatric program directors in 2006 to 2007 concluded that pediatric residents received an average of only 3 hours of breastfeeding training per year.[16] The respondents reported that 67% of the pediatric residents have access to breastfeeding rooms, but only 10 programs had an official policy on breastfeeding accommodations for residents. Feldman-Winter et al[17] previously documented that the implementation of a breastfeeding curriculum improved breastfeeding knowledge, practice, and confidence.

Positive trends from the Periodic Survey of Fellows series were noted by Feldman-Winter et al.[2] More pediatricians are affiliated with Baby-Friendly–designated facilities. They were more likely to recommend both exclusive breastfeeding and an early first postnatal visit by the fifth day of life. Pediatricians reporting that breastfeeding should be initiated within the first hour after delivery increased significantly from 44% in 1995 to 92% in 2014.

Some concerning trends from the 2014 Periodic Survey of Fellows were that pediatricians were less likely to believe that the benefits of breastfeeding outweigh the difficulties or inconveniences encountered and that younger pediatricians felt less confident in their ability to manage breastfeeding despite being more predominantly women and having more personal breastfeeding experience. Fewer than half of the respondents in 2014 advised that families should delay the introduction of a pacifier until breastfeeding is well established, and 17% reported not making any recommendation about infant feeding in the first month of life.

The authors[2] indicated that pediatricians or residents affiliated with Baby-Friendly hospitals would be receiving the required provider breastfeeding education. As the trend toward staffing hospitals with pediatric hospitalists increases, it is important to remember that ambulatory pediatricians also need breastfeeding education because they are responsible for the ongoing follow-up care of breastfeeding families. The maintenance of certification and lifelong learning skills should include breastfeeding as a core competency for general pediatricians.

Although the 2014 Periodic Survey of Fellows shows progress in many areas, the importance of routine integration of breastfeeding into all aspects of medical education cannot be overstated.[18,19] Pediatric residents, especially, should receive targeted breastfeeding education (including clinical skills practice) not only during newborn nursery experiences but also in continuity clinic and inpatient pediatrics, where follow-up and newborn readmissions occur. Breastfeeding education should be as routine in the curriculum as other preventive health strategies, such as immunizations. Residents must develop the skills to assess breastfed infants and their lactating mothers and be confident in managing clinical breastfeeding problems. The residents' training programs should also provide a culture of support for residents who themselves are breastfeeding mothers because pediatric residents are the future providers, pediatric teaching faculty, and advocates for breastfeeding policy changes. Hopefully, by 2024, the Periodic Survey of Fellows will demonstrate that almost all practicing physicians have the breastfeeding knowledge, skills, attitudes, and confidence needed to provide competent breastfeeding support to their patients.

ABBREVIATION

AAP: American Academy of Pediatrics

REFERENCES

1. Section on Breastfeeding. Breastfeeding and the use of human milk. *Pediatrics*. 2012;129(3). Available at: www.pediatrics.org/cgi/content/full/129/3/e827

2. Feldman-Winter L, Szucs K, Milano A, Gottschlich E, Sisk B, Schanler RJ. National trends in pediatricians' practices and attitudes about breastfeeding: 1995 to 2014. *Pediatrics*. 2017;140(4):e20171229

3. Ryan AS. The resurgence of breastfeeding in the United States. *Pediatrics*. 1997;99(4):E12

4. Centers for Disease Control and Prevention. Percentage of U.S. Children Who Were Breastfeeding, by Birth

Year, National Immunization Survey. Available at: https://www.cdc.gov/breastfeeding/data/nis_data/index.htm. Accessed August 11, 2017

5. Office of the Surgeon General (US); Centers for Disease Control and Prevention (US); Office on Women's Health (US). *The Surgeon General's Call to Action to Support Breastfeeding.* Rockville, MD: Office of the Surgeon General; 2011. Available at: www.surgeongeneral.gov/library/calls/breastfeeding/. Accessed July 20, 2017

6. US Department of Labor. Section 7(r) of the Fair Labor Standards Act—Break Time for Nursing Mothers Provision. Available at https://www.dol.gov/whd/nursingmothers/Sec7rFLSA_btnm.htm. Accessed August 11, 2017

7. Office on Women's Health, US Department of Health and Human Services. Business case for breastfeeding. Available at: https://www.womenshealth.gov/breastfeeding/breastfeeding-home-work-and-public/breastfeeding-and-going-back-work/business-case. Accessed August 9, 2017

8. US Department of Agriculture Food and Nutrition Service. Women, Infants, and Children (WIC). Available at: https://www.fns.usda.gov/wic/women-infants-and-children-wic. Accessed August 8, 2017

9. Centers for Disease Control and Prevention. Maternity practices in infant nutrition and care (mPINC) survey. Available at: www.cdc.gov/breastfeeding/data/mpinc/index.htm. Accessed July 20, 2017

10. Baby-Friendly USA. Find facilities. Available at: https://www.babyfriendlyusa.org/find-facilities. Accessed July 20, 2017

11. National Institute for Children's Health Quality. Best Fed Beginnings. Available at: http://www.nichq.org/project/best-fed-beginnings. Accessed August 11, 2017

12. Feldman-Winter L, Ustianov J, Anastasio J, et al. Best Fed Beginnings: A Nationwide Quality Improvement Initiative to Increase Breastfeeding. *Pediatrics.* 2017;140(1):e20163121

13. EMPower Breastfeeding: Enhancing Maternity Practices. Available at: http://empowerbreastfeeding.org. Accessed August 11, 2017

14. Baby-Friendly USA. The ten steps to successful breastfeeding. Available at: https://www.babyfriendlyusa.org/about-us/baby-friendly-hospital-initiative/the-ten-steps. Accessed August 9, 2017

15. Freed GL, Clark SJ, Lohr JA, Sorenson JR. Pediatrician involvement in breastfeeding promotion: a national study of residents and practitioners. *Pediatrics.* 1995;96(3, pt 1):490–494

16. Osband YB, Altman RL, Patrick PA, Edwards KS. Breastfeeding education and support services offered to pediatric residents in the US. *Acad Pediatr.* 2011;11(1):75–79

17. Feldman-Winter L, Barone L, Milcarek B, et al. Residency curriculum improves breastfeeding care. *Pediatrics.* 2010;126(2):289–297

18. United States Breastfeeding Committee. *Core Competencies in Breastfeeding Care and Services for All Health Professionals.* Rev ed. Washington, DC: United States Breastfeeding Committee; 2010

19. Academy of Breastfeeding Medicine. Educational objectives and skills for the physician with respect to breastfeeding. *Breastfeed Med.* 2011;6(2):99–105

National Trends in Pediatricians' Practices and Attitudes About Breastfeeding: 1995 to 2014

Lori Feldman-Winter, MD, MPH, FAAP,[a] Kinga Szucs, MD, FAAP,[b] Aubri Milano, MD, FAAP,[a]
Elizabeth Gottschlich, MA,[c] Blake Sisk, PhD,[c] Richard J. Schanler, MD, FAAP[d]

abstract

BACKGROUND AND OBJECTIVES: The American Academy of Pediatrics (AAP) has affirmed breastfeeding as the preferred method of infant feeding; however, there has been little systematic examination of how pediatricians' recommendations, affiliated hospitals' policies, counseling practices, and attitudes toward breastfeeding have shifted over the past 2 decades. These trends were examined from 1995 to 2014.

METHODS: Data are from the Periodic Survey (PS) of Fellows, a nationally representative survey of AAP members. PS #30 (1995; response rate = 72%; N = 832), PS #57 (2004; response rate = 55%; N = 675), and PS #89 (2014; response rate = 51%; N = 620) collected demographics, patient and practice characteristics, and detailed responses on pediatricians' recommendations, affiliated hospitals' policies, counseling practices, and attitudes toward breastfeeding. By using bivariate statistics and logistic regression models, the analysis investigated changes over time with predicted values (PVs).

RESULTS: From 1995 to 2014, more pediatricians reported their affiliated hospitals applied for "baby-friendly" designation (PV = 12% in 1995, PV = 56% in 2014; P < .05), and more reported that they recommend exclusive breastfeeding (65% to 76% [P < .05]). However, fewer respondents indicated that mothers can be successful breastfeeding (PV = 70% in 1995, PV = 57% in 2014; P < .05) and that the benefits outweigh the difficulties (PV = 70% in 1995, PV = 50% in 2014; P < .05). Younger pediatricians were less confident than older pediatricians in managing breastfeeding problems (P < .01).

CONCLUSIONS: Pediatricians' recommendations and practices became more closely aligned with AAP policy from 1995 to 2014; however, their attitudes about the likelihood of breastfeeding success have worsened. These 2 divergent trends indicate that even as breastfeeding rates continue to rise, continued efforts to enhance pediatricians' training and attitudes about breastfeeding are necessary.

WHAT'S KNOWN ON THIS SUBJECT: Pediatricians' recommendations about breastfeeding have consistently improved over the past several decades and were closely aligned with guidelines issued by the American Academy of Pediatrics, yet attitudes about the potential for breastfeeding success and meeting goals for breastfeeding have declined.

WHAT THIS STUDY ADDS: Pediatricians have continued to improve their recommendations for breastfeeding in alignment with American Academy of Pediatrics policy and the "Ten Steps to Successful Breastfeeding"; however, there are modest declines in attitudes about breastfeeding, and younger pediatricians are less confident in managing breastfeeding problems.

To cite: Feldman-Winter L, Szucs K, Milano A, et al. National Trends in Pediatricians' Practices and Attitudes About Breastfeeding: 1995 to 2014. *Pediatrics.* 2017;140(4): e20171229

[a]Department of Pediatrics, Children' s Regional Hospital, Cooper University Health Care, Cooper Medical School, Rowan University, Camden, New Jersey; [b]Private Practice, Indianapolis, Indiana; [c]Department of Research, American Academy of Pediatrics, Elk Grove Village, Illinois; and [d]Cohen Children' s Medical Center, Northwell Health and Hofstra, Hofstra Northwell School of Medicine, Hofstra University, Hempstead, New York

Dr Feldman-Winter and Ms Gottschlich contributed to the conceptual study design, development and update of the Periodic Survey #89, data analysis and interpretation, and drafting of the initial manuscript; Dr Szucs made a substantial contribution to the concept and study design, including revision of the Periodic Survey #89 and drafting of the initial manuscript; Dr Milano contributed to the data analysis and interpretation and drafting of the initial manuscript; Drs Sisk and Schanler contributed to the conceptual study design, data analysis and interpretation, and drafting of the initial manuscript; and all authors approved the final version of the manuscript and are accountable for all aspects of the work.

ARTICLE

The American Academy of Pediatrics (AAP) has affirmed breastfeeding as the preferred method of infant feeding, providing ideal nutritional and optimal health outcomes.[1,2] In 2012, a new policy statement from the AAP reaffirmed the recommendation of exclusive breastfeeding for the first 6 months of life, citing universal agreement on this point, and acknowledged the critical role of the pediatrician in supporting and advocating breastfeeding at the hospital and community level.[2]

In 1995, a survey of pediatrician's attitudes and practices related to breastfeeding was conducted and the results were analyzed: 65% of the responding pediatricians recommended exclusive breastfeeding for the first month after birth, and only 38% recommended continued breastfeeding for the first year. Additionally, most responding pediatricians at the time of the survey were not familiar with the Baby-Friendly Hospital Initiative, and most were interested in additional education on breastfeeding management.[3] In the first decade after these data were collected and interpreted, there was an increase in research in which health benefits related to breastfeeding were delineated and methods of breastfeeding promotion and support were explored.[4] In 2004, a new survey was completed to trend the initial data in the face of this culture change; the authors of the survey concluded that there was a sense of improved preparedness among pediatricians to support breastfeeding and improved counseling strategies consistent with the "Ten Steps to Successful Breastfeeding," but it also concluded that the overall attitudes of these practitioners toward the benefits of breastfeeding and their commitment to advocating for it had deteriorated.[5]

In the decade since the 2004 survey, efforts toward increasing awareness, advocacy, and education among health professionals have continued and grown, both among professional societies and governmental entities.[6] In 2008, a formal curriculum for residency education in breastfeeding was developed through funding from the Maternal and Child Health Bureau in a project entitled "Breastfeeding Promotion in Physicians' Office Practices" for trainees in pediatrics, family medicine, internal medicine, and obstetrics and gynecology.[7] In 2009, the AAP gave its formal endorsement to the World Health Organization and United Nations Children's Fund's "Ten Steps to Successful Breastfeeding."[8] The "Ten Steps to Successful Breastfeeding" outlines the framework of systematic changes for delivery hospitals seeking "baby-friendly" designation. The role of primary care interventions in improving breastfeeding outcomes was studied,[9] and a focus on the primary care physicians' role in supporting this trend and driving it forward has evolved, with new research on methods and approaches to overcoming early barriers to breastfeeding.[4,10–12]

The Centers for Disease Control and Prevention Division of Nutrition, Physical Activity, and Obesity now collects and publishes yearly data on aspects of breastfeeding to monitor and encourage improvement in breastfeeding practices and support in the United States.[13] The percentage of US children who were ever breastfed increased from 71.4% for those born in 2002 to 81% for those born in 2013; the percentage who were exclusively breastfed for their first 6 months of life increased from 10.3% for those born in 2003 to 22.3% for those born in 2013.

The past decade has seen a rise in delivery hospitals implementing the "Ten Steps to Successful Breastfeeding" and becoming designated as baby-friendly hospitals.[14,15] Pediatrician education and training is an essential component of the Baby-Friendly Hospital Initiative and a requirement for designation. With more hospitals providing education and training about breastfeeding and more pediatricians working in environments with more women breastfeeding, enhanced knowledge and practices about breastfeeding would be expected. Given this assertion, we expected to find continued improvements in pediatricians' practices and a rebound toward positive attitudes with regards to advocating for and supporting breastfeeding. In this study, we followed preceding surveys of pediatricians to ascertain recommendations, affiliated hospitals' policies, counseling practices, and attitudes related to breastfeeding,[5] and we examined trends from 1995 to 2014.

METHODS

Data

This analysis used data from the Periodic Survey (PS) of Fellows, a nationally representative survey of randomly selected, nonretired US members of the AAP. PS #89 (2014) was administered to 1627 respondents, including residents and excluding those subboarded in a pediatric subspecialty. Seven mailed contacts were made to nonrespondents between July and December 2014 (in addition to 2 e-mails with a link to complete the survey electronically). The analysis also used data from 2 other similar PSs: PS #30 (1995) and PS #57 (2004). The 3 PSs collected demographic information on respondents, characteristics of their patients and practice, and detailed responses regarding breastfeeding recommendations, counseling, policies, and attitudes. The final survey response rates for 1995, 2004, and 2014 were 72%, 55%, and 51%, respectively. Restricting the analytic

TABLE 1 Pediatricians' Recommendations and Affiliated Hospitals' Policies Toward Breastfeeding: 1995, 2004, and 2014

	Descriptive Results[a]			Multivariable Results[b]					
	1995 (n = 821)	2004 (n = 670)	2014 (n = 6 13)	1995		2004		2014	
				PV	95% CI	PV	95% CI	PV	95% CI
Hospital policies									
Hospital has applied to be a "baby-friendly hospital"	11.9	22.6	56.9	12.2[c]	9.8–14.5	22.2[c]	18.9–25.5	55.6	51.4–59.9
Maintain written hospital policy that is available to all staff[d]	43.1	44.7	64.1	43.7[c]	40.0–47.5	45.1[c]	41.1–49.1	62.9	58.7–67.1
Establish support groups for parents within the community[e]	46.8	47.6	46.5	48.7	44.9–52.4	47.3	43.3–51.3	44.3	40.0–48.6
Recommendations									
Breastfeed within 1 h of delivery	43.4	67.0	92.3	44.3[c]	40.7–47.9	66.7[c]	63.0–70.5	91.9	89.7–94.2
Give nothing but breast milk unless medically indicated	78.9	88.2	92.6	80.2[c]	77.2–83.2	89.2	86.7–91.7	92.7	90.5–94.9
Rooming-in 24 h/d	51.0	70.8	86.3	49.4[c]	45.6–53.2	71.3[c]	67.7–74.9	87.3	84.6–90.0
Unrestricted breastfeeding	58.6	67.1	73.2	61.6[c]	58.0–65.2	66.5	62.7–70.3	71.3	67.4–75.2
No pacifiers in hospital	23.3	34.2	47.3	23.9[c]	20.9–27.1	33.4[c]	29.6–37.1	46.2	41.9–50.4
Inform all pregnant women about breastfeeding so they can make an informed decision (mean % of parents seen in prenatal visits)[b]	11.4	10.4	8.4	12.1[c]	10.7–13.5	10.8[c]	9.3–12.3	7.5	5.9–9.1

CI, confidence interval.

[a] Data presented in percentage of pediatricians reporting.

[b] Multivariable results are the PV of the dependent variable at each survey year holding all other variables at their means; model covariates include survey year, sex, age, personal breastfeeding experience, practicing general pediatrics >50% of the time, and total hours worked per week.

[c] Indicates the PV is significantly different ($P \leq .05$) from the PV in the 2014 survey year.

[d] 64.1% in 2014 reported that their hospital maintained a policy; 33.7% did not know if their hospital had a policy.

[e] Survey question was: "Practice refers or provides the following lactation service: breastfeeding support group."

sample to pediatricians who provide primary care to children from birth to 2 years of age yielded the following sample sizes for each survey: 1995 (N = 832), 2004 (N = 675), and 2014 (N = 620). The surveys were all approved by the AAP Institutional Review Board.

Dependent Variables

Three clusters of outcome variables were examined: policies, counseling, and attitudes. The policy outcomes indicate to what extent pediatricians' recommendations and affiliated hospital policies align with the "Ten Steps to Successful Breastfeeding" and whether the respondents' main hospital has applied to be a "baby-friendly hospital." The counseling variables were used to document respondents' breastfeeding counseling practices, including whether respondents advise

exclusive breastfeeding during the first month and schedule the first postnatal office visit within 5 days for breastfed infants. The attitudes cluster was used to measure agreement among respondents for a variety of statements regarding breastfeeding, such as "Almost any mother can be successful at breastfeeding if she keeps trying" and "Benefits of breastfeeding outweigh the difficulties or inconvenience mothers may encounter." We examined these 3 clusters of outcome variables across the 3 surveys, and with our analysis we investigated changes over time in pediatricians' affiliated hospitals' policies, counseling practices, and attitudes toward breastfeeding.

Independent Variables

The primary independent variable in this analysis was survey year (1995,

2004, and 2014). Other independent variables included as controls in multivariable models were sex, age, respondents' (both men and women) personal breastfeeding experience with their own children (including both exclusive and nonexclusive breastfeeding), practicing general pediatrics ≥50% of the time, and total hours worked per week; all the multivariable results presented in Tables 1, 2 and 3 include these independent variables as controls.

Nonresponse Bias

We assessed nonresponse bias for each of the 3 surveys based on key demographic variables available in the AAP administrative database. Each analytic sample was compared with its respective target sample by using a t test for age and 1-sample proportion tests for sex and US geographical region.

TABLE 2 Pediatricians' Counseling Practices Toward Breastfeeding: 1995, 2004, and 2014

	Descriptive Results[a]			Multivariable Results[b]					
	1995 (N = 794)	2004 (N = 657)	2014 (N = 615)	1995		2004		2014	
				PV	95% CI	PV	95% CI	PV	95% CI
Feeding during the first month[c]									
Formula feeding exclusively	2.0	2.9	2.3	1.9	0.1–2.9	2.7	1.4–3.9	2.3	1.0–3.5
Breastfeeding exclusively	65.0	74	75.7	66.4[d]	62.9–69.9	74.8	71.4–78.2	75.2	71.6–78.9
Breastfeeding with formula supplementation	12.8	7.5	4.9	12.3[d]	9.8–14.7	6.9	4.9–8.9	4.5	2.8–6.1
No recommendation	20.2	15.6	17.1	18.8	15.9–21.7	15.1	12.3–17.9	17.7	14.5–20.9
First postnatal office visit scheduled within 5 d after birth[e]									
Breastfed infants	—	51.8	90.1	—	—	53.3[d]	49.2–57.3	90.3	87.8–92.7
Formula-fed infants	—	31.5	80.1	—	—	31.9[d]	28.2–35.7	80.1	76.7–83.4

CI, confidence interval; —, not applicable.

[a] Data presented in percentage of pediatricians reporting.

[b] Multivariable results are the PV of the dependent variable at each survey year holding all other variables at their means; model covariates include survey year, sex, age, personal breastfeeding experience, practicing general pediatrics >50% of the time, and total hours worked per week.

[c] Initial breastfeeding should be exclusive without supplements.

[d] Indicates the PV is significantly different (P ≤ .05) from the PV in the 2014 survey year.

[e] If discharged <48 h after delivery, all breastfeeding mothers and their newborn infants should be seen when their infants are 2–4 d of age.

TABLE 3 Pediatricians' Attitudes Toward Breastfeeding: 1995, 2004, and 2014

	Descriptive Results[a]			Multivariable Results[b]					
	1995 (N = 821)	2004 (N = 670)	2014 (N = 613)	1995		2004		2014	
				PV	95% CI	PV	95% CI	PV	95% CI
Almost any mother can be successful at breastfeeding if she keeps trying (% agree)[c]	69.4	62.2	57.2	69.9[d]	66.7–73.3	62.1	58.3–65.9	56.6	52.4–60.8
Breastfeeding and formula feeding are equally acceptable methods for feeding infants (% agree)[c]	45.0	45.1	39.5	43.7	40.1–47.3	44.9	41.1–48.9	40.8	36.7–45.0
Benefits of breastfeeding outweigh the difficulties or inconvenience mothers may encounter (% agree)[c]	68.3	58.0	52.9	70.1[d]	66.8–73.4	58.2	54.4–62.1	50.3	46.0–54.5
In the long run, formula-fed infants are just as healthy as breastfed infants (% agree)[c]	34.5	26.0	23.6	33.0[d]	29.6–36.4	24.1	22.7–29.6	24.3	20.6–27.9
Advice from family and friends is the most important influence in the decision to breastfeed (% agree)[c]	72.4	55.1	57.7	71.6[d]	68.3–74.8	54.5	50.6–58.4	59.7	55.5–63.8
Pediatricians have little influence on whether mothers initiate breastfeeding (% agree)[c]	18.1	5.8	8.6	18.2[d]	15.4–21.1	5.6	3.8–7.4	7.4	5.3–9.6
Confidence in ability to competently manage common breastfeeding problems (% confident)[e]	76.5	79.4	82.9	83.0	80.3–85.8	82.8	79.8–85.9	81.1	77.6–84.7

CI, confidence interval.

[a] Data presented in percentage of pediatricians reporting.

[b] Multivariable results are the PV of the dependent variable at each survey year holding all other variables at their means; model covariates include survey year, sex, age, personal breastfeeding experience, practicing general pediatrics >50% of the time, and total hours worked per week.

[c] Responses are given on a scale of 1 (agree) to 3 (disagree); disagree and neutral responses are not shown.

[d] Indicates PV is significantly different (P ≤ .05) from the PV in the 2014 survey year.

[e] Pediatricians reporting that they were either confident or very confident (combined).

Analysis Plan

The first analysis step was to provide a descriptive overview of the sample. Then, logistic regression models were separately estimated for each individual outcome within the 3 clusters of dependent variables, controlling for the set of independent variables described above. The focus of the analysis is how pediatricians' responses to the outcomes shifted over time. Descriptive responses to each outcome in 1995, 2004, and 2014 are presented, along with the predicted value (PV) for each outcome for each survey year, generated from the multivariable model holding all other independent variables at their respective sample means.[16] This comprises the bulk of the analysis and establishes to what extent attitudes and behaviors related to breastfeeding have changed across surveys. To explore if the changing landscape of policies and education related to breastfeeding over time has created generational differences in pediatrician attitudes, an independent descriptive analysis was conducted for respondents to the 2014 survey by age (<45 vs 45 years or older), examining differences in 2 key outcomes: pediatricians' confidence in managing breastfeeding problems and ability to answer questions about breastfeeding. Data were analyzed by using IBM SPSS Statistics 24 (IBM SPSS Statistics, IBM Corporation) and Stata 12 (Stata Corp, College Station, TX).

RESULTS

Nonresponse Bias

In 2014, respondents were significantly older than the eligible target sample (mean ages of 45.5 and 43.0, respectively; $P < .001$) but there were no differences for sex and region. For 2004, there was a significantly larger proportion of women in the analytic sample than the target sample (59% and 53%, respectively; $P < .01$), but we found no age or region differences. In 1995, there were also more women in the analytic sample compared with the target sample (48% and 45%, respectively; $P < .05$), but again, no age or region differences were found.

Respondents' Practice and Personal Characteristics

Table 4 provides a descriptive overview of the analytic samples from the 3 surveys. In 2014, respondents were more likely than in 1995 or 2004 to be female, have a higher mean age, have any previous personal experience with breastfeeding, to spend a majority of their time in general pediatrics, and to have worked fewer hours per week on average.

Recommendations and Affiliated Hospitals' Policies

Table 1 displays results for pediatricians' recommendations and affiliated hospitals' policies toward breastfeeding in 1995, 2004, and 2014. Collectively, the results in Table 1 indicate a shift toward hospital policies and pediatrician recommendations that are more closely aligned with AAP recommendations. In 2014, pediatricians were significantly more likely than in 1995 or 2004 to report that their affiliated hospitals had applied to be a baby-friendly hospital (PV = 12% in 1995, PV = 22% in 2004, PV = 56% in 2014; $P < .05$) and that practices for the establishment of breastfeeding were more aligned with the "Ten Steps to Successful Breastfeeding." Nevertheless, fewer pediatricians had opportunities to discuss breastfeeding in the prenatal period in 2014 relative to 1995, as the predicted mean percentage of parents seen in prenatal visits declined from 12.1 to 7.5 ($P < .05$). Furthermore, there has been no change in the proportion of pediatricians referring mothers for breastfeeding support in the community.

Counseling Practices

Table 2 displays results for pediatricians' counseling practices regarding breastfeeding across the 3 surveys. Overall, results from Table 2 indicate that pediatricians' counseling practices in 2014 are more aligned with AAP policy than in the past; in 2014, a PV of 75% of pediatricians reported that they advise exclusive breastfeeding during the first month, up from 66% in 1995 ($P < .05$). Conversely, pediatricians in 2014 were less likely to report recommending breastfeeding with formula supplementation than in 1995 (PV = 12% in 1995, PV = 4.5% in 2014; $P < .05$). Moreover, the PV of respondents reporting that they schedule the first newborn follow-up visit within 5 days of life increased by 37 percentage points for breastfed infants and 48 percentage points for formula-fed infants ($P < .05$).

Attitudes

Table 3 displays results for pediatricians' attitudes toward breastfeeding. Across survey years, fewer respondents reported that

TABLE 4 Practice and Personal Characteristics of Respondents: 1995, 2004, and 2014

	1995 (N = 832)	2004 (N = 675)	2014 (N = 620)
Female (%)	47.7*	59.7*	67.7
Age (mean)	41.6*	41.7*	45.4
Any personal experience with breastfeeding (%)	41.7*	58.9*	68.2
Time in general pediatrics (mean %)	84.2*	88.4*	91.4
Practicing general pediatrics ≥50% of the time (%)	87.7*	92.1	93.6
Total hours worked per week (mean)	52.5*	47.7*	43.4

* Indicates a statistically significant difference ($P ≤ .05$) from the 2014 survey year.

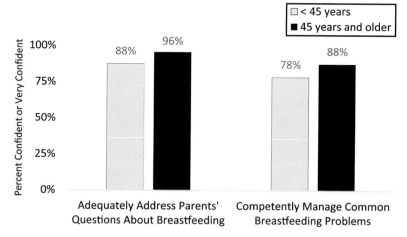

FIGURE 1

Pediatricians' confidence in their ability to care for breastfeeding concerns by age. * indicates a statistically significant difference between age groups ($P < .01$, χ^2 test). Data are from 2014 only.

almost any mother can be successful at breastfeeding if she keeps trying (PV = 70% in 1995, PV = 56% in 2014; $P < .05$). Similarly, fewer reported that the benefits of breastfeeding outweigh the difficulties mothers may encounter (PV = 70% in 1995, PV = 50% in 2014; $P < .05$). In 1995, a PV of 33% of pediatricians reported that formula-fed infants are just as healthy as breastfed infants in the long run, but by 2014 that decreased to 24% ($P < .05$).

Table 3 indicates that there has been no statistically significant change in the overall percent of pediatricians feeling confident in their ability to manage breastfeeding problems over the past 2 decades. Figure 1 displays pediatricians' reported confidence in their ability to care for breastfeeding concerns stratified by age group (2014 only). Results in Fig 1 indicate that, relative to older pediatricians, younger pediatricians are less confident in their ability to manage common breastfeeding problems ($P < .01$) and adequately address parents' questions about breastfeeding ($P < .01$).

DISCUSSION

Over the past 20 years, the share of pediatricians who report their affiliated hospitals seek baby-friendly designation has increased from

12% to 57%, with a corresponding increase in supportive hospital policies. Pediatricians may, however, overestimate baby-friendly aspirations, given that merely 7% of hospitals were actually designated at the time of the 2014 survey.[17] Pediatricians may believe they are affiliated with hospitals seeking baby-friendly designation because the affiliated hospital has implemented 1 or more of the ten steps.

The percent of primary care pediatricians who, in their own counseling, recommend exclusive breastfeeding has increased from 65% to 76% over this time, and nearly all now recommend a postnatal visit within 5 days for breastfed infants. Pediatricians may be receiving additional education about breastfeeding because the baby-friendly designation process itself requires mandatory physician education. There are now also multiple opportunities for in-person, online, and remote, web-based learning about breastfeeding.[18]

Even with these expanded educational opportunities, this analysis indicates that gaps remain in pediatricians' awareness about breastfeeding best practices, such as only 47% reporting that they

refer to community support groups and just 47% recommending to avoid pacifiers until breastfeeding is established. Furthermore, 17% of pediatricians do not make any recommendation regarding infant feeding for the first month of life. These gaps may indicate that pediatricians may not fully understand policies supportive of breastfeeding.[19]

With this analysis, we showed that the area of most significant improvement is the recommendation to initiate breastfeeding within the first hour of delivery; the PV increased 48 percentage points from 1995 to 2014, from 44% to 92% ($P < .05$). Breastfeeding in the first hour is now part of the fourth step of the Ten Steps to Successful Breastfeeding, which now states that all healthy newborns should be placed immediately skin-to-skin regardless of feeding decision.[20] The finding that 92% of the respondents in 2014 supported this recommendation is somewhat surprising given the backlash of concerns that have been raised about safety during skin-to-skin care.[21] In response to these concerns and other safety issues related to the ten steps, the AAP issued guidelines for implementation.[22]

Additional areas of promise include the increase in pediatricians recommending exclusive versus supplemented breastfeeding during the first month (9 percentage points from 1995 to 2014) and a dramatic rise in pediatricians recommending all newborns return for a postnatal office visit within 5 days of birth. Given that it is not uncommon for problems to arise in the establishment of breastfeeding, to fully support avoidance of supplementation, early follow-up by providers capable of managing breastfeeding is necessary to monitor the maternal transition to lactogenesis II as well as infant weight trajectories.[2,23,24]

Pediatricians' attitudes about breastfeeding have become modestly more positive on some issues; For example, fewer pediatricians believe formula-fed infants are as healthy as breastfed infants. However, on other issues pediatrician's attitudes have declined. For example, the percent of pediatricians that believe a mother can be successful at breastfeeding if she keeps trying declined by 12 percentage points to 57%, and the share that believe that the benefits of breastfeeding outweigh the difficulties or inconveniences encountered fell by 15 percentage points to 53%. These attitudinal changes from 1995 to 2014 indicate that even while noting the health benefits of breastfeeding relative to formula feeding, there is a growing awareness among pediatricians of the challenges that breastfeeding can present for mothers. Pediatricians may be increasingly wary of the fragmented and insufficient support system available to breastfeeding mothers. Despite evidence that individual-level support for women that spans from the prenatal to postpartum period and includes both professionals and peers can increase the duration of any breastfeeding and exclusive breastfeeding,[4] these support systems are not yet widespread.[25] These declining attitudes may contribute to the precipitous decline in exclusive breastfeeding over the first few months and may adversely affect pediatricians' willingness to provide support.

Although confidence in breastfeeding management has remained steady across survey years, younger respondents are less confident in this area. This finding may seem paradoxical given that more pediatricians in recent years are females who have had personal experience with breastfeeding, a factor known to be associated with greater confidence in managing breastfeeding problems.[5] However, it is possible that our findings reflect a greater awareness of the potential problems that exist. Researchers

conducting future studies could examine the relationship between type of personal experience (positive or negative) and confidence in managing breastfeeding problems. The AAP has a role in enhancing pediatricians' attitudes about breastfeeding, including supporting personal breastfeeding experiences. Lack of resident support for breastfeeding is apparent among many programs and may set the stage for attitudes about breastfeeding for years to come.[26]

There are several limitations to this study. Our findings are based on self-report data rather than actual counseling practices. Furthermore, respondents may have given answers they perceived to be more acceptable to themselves, their peers, their employer, or the AAP. This social desirability bias may have resulted in overestimations or underestimations of perception-based questions. Given that the survey only included AAP member primary care pediatricians, the responses may not be generalizable to non-AAP members or subspecialists. However, the AAP estimates that 60% of board-certified pediatricians in the United States between the ages of 27 and 70 were AAP members in 2016, indicating that AAP members represent the majority of board-certified pediatricians.

Survey response rates declined in recent decades,[27] and the PS is no exception to this trend. However, response rates for the PS compared favorably with other physician-based surveys, and the broader literature indicates that there is no conclusive link between a survey's response rate and response bias,[28] a conclusion that was also reached by a peer-reviewed study of response rates from 50 AAP pediatrician surveys.[29] Although it is conceivable that there are unmeasured factors (eg, interest in breastfeeding issues) that are shaping response rates to this survey, our nonresponse bias

analysis finds that there are no substantial differences in age, sex, or regional characteristics between respondents and nonrespondents. Additionally, sex and age were included as controls in all the multivariable logistic regression models shown here.

Finally, pediatricians were asked whether their hospitals had applied to become baby-friendly, not whether their hospital was already designated. Because the initial application is at the beginning of the process involved in baby-friendly designation, there may be wide variability of hospital policies and practices among pediatricians responding affirmatively to this question. Pediatricians may also be affiliated with >1 hospital and may be reporting if any of their affiliated hospitals have applied to become baby-friendly.

CONCLUSIONS

Pediatricians continue to improve on breastfeeding recommendations over time, concurrent with the upswing of the Baby-Friendly Hospital Initiative in the United States. However, pediatricians have demonstrated a modest decline in attitudes about the potential for breastfeeding success. There are continued opportunities to enhance training in breastfeeding and participate in breastfeeding management and support.

ACKNOWLEDGMENT

We thank the PS respondents for their time and participation.

ABBREVIATIONS

AAP: American Academy of Pediatrics
PS: Periodic Survey
PV: predicted value

DOI: https://doi.org/10.1542/peds.2017-1229

Accepted for publication Jun 27, 2017

Address correspondence to Lori Feldman-Winter, MD, MPH, FAAP, Department of Pediatrics, Children's Regional Hospital at Cooper University Hospital, Three Cooper Plaza Suite 309, Camden, NJ 08103. E-mail: winter-lori@cooperhealth.edu

PEDIATRICS (ISSN Numbers: Print, 0031-4005; Online, 1098-4275).

FINANCIAL DISCLOSURE: The authors have indicated they have no financial relationships relevant to this article to disclose.

FUNDING: Funded by the American Academy of Pediatrics and the Maternal and Child Health Bureau, Health Resources and Services Administration, Department of Health and Human Services, Cooperative Agreement UC4MC21534.

POTENTIAL CONFLICT OF INTEREST: The authors have indicated they have no potential conflicts of interest to disclose.

COMPANION PAPER: A companion to this article can be found online at www.pediatrics.org/cgi/doi/10.1542/peds.2017-2509.

REFERENCES

1. Gartner LM, Morton J, Lawrence RA, et al; American Academy of Pediatrics Section on Breastfeeding. Breastfeeding and the use of human milk. *Pediatrics.* 2005;115(2):496–506

2. Eidelman AI, Schanler RJ, Johnston M, et al; American Academy of Pediatrics Section on Breastfeeding. Breastfeeding and the use of human milk. *Pediatrics.* 2012;129(3). Available at: www.pediatrics.org/cgi/content/full/129/3/e827

3. Schanler RJ, O'Connor KG, Lawrence RA. Pediatricians' practices and attitudes regarding breastfeeding promotion. *Pediatrics.* 1999;103(3). Available at: www.pediatrics.org/cgi/content/full/103/3/e35

4. Patnode CD, Henninger ML, Senger CA, Perdue LA, Whitlock EP. Primary care interventions to support breastfeeding: updated evidence report and systematic review for the US Preventive Services Task Force. *JAMA.* 2016;316(16):1694–1705

5. Feldman-Winter LB, Schanler RJ, O'Connor KG, Lawrence RA. Pediatricians and the promotion and support of breastfeeding. *Arch Pediatr Adolesc Med.* 2008;162(12):1142–1149

6. Whitacre PT, Moats S. *Updating the USDA National Breastfeeding Campaign: Workshop Summary.* Washington, DC: National Academies Press; 2011

7. Feldman-Winter L, Barone L, Milcarek B, et al. Residency curriculum improves breastfeeding care. *Pediatrics.* 2010;126(2):289–297

8. Tayloe D; AAP Endorsement of the WHO/UNICEF Ten Steps to Successful Breastfeeding. August 2009. Available at: http://www.aap.org/breastfeeding/files/pdf/TenStepswosig.pdf. Accessed May 1, 2011

9. Bonuck K, Stuebe A, Barnett J, Labbok MH, Fletcher J, Bernstein PS. Effect of primary care intervention on breastfeeding duration and intensity. *Am J Public Health.* 2014;104(suppl 1):S119–S127

10. Neifert M, Bunik M. Overcoming clinical barriers to exclusive breastfeeding. *Pediatr Clin North Am.* 2013;60(1):115–145

11. Feldman-Winter L. Evidence-based interventions to support breastfeeding. *Pediatr Clin North Am.* 2013;60(1):169–187

12. Wagner EA, Chantry CJ, Dewey KG, Nommsen-Rivers LA. Breastfeeding concerns at 3 and 7 days postpartum and feeding status at 2 months. *Pediatrics.* 2013;132(4). Available at: www.pediatrics.org/cgi/content/full/132/4/e865

13. Centers for Disease Control. Breastfeeding report card: progressing toward national breastfeeding goals. 2016. Available at: https://www.cdc.gov/breastfeeding/pdf/2016breastfeedingreportcard.pdf. Accessed August 27, 2016

14. Perrine CG, Galuska DA, Dohack JL, et al; MLIS. Vital signs: improvements in maternity care policies and practices that support breastfeeding - United States, 2007-2013. *MMWR Morb Mortal Wkly Rep.* 2015;64(39):1112–1117

15. Grummer-Strawn LM, Shealy KR, Perrine CG, et al. Maternity care practices that support breastfeeding: CDC efforts to encourage quality improvement. *J Womens Health (Larchmt).* 2013;22(2):107–112

16. Long JS, Freese J. *Regression Models for Categorical Dependent Variables Using Stata.* College Station, TX: Stata Press; 2006

17. Feldman-Winter L, Ustianov J, Anastasio J, et al. Best fed beginnings: a nationwide quality improvement initiative to increase breastfeeding. *Pediatrics.* 2017;140(1):e20163121

18. Edwards RA, Colchamiro R, Tolan E, et al. Online continuing education for expanding clinicians' roles in breastfeeding support. *J Hum Lact.* 2015;31(4):582–586

19. Feldman-Winter L, Ustianov J. Lessons learned from hospital leaders who participated in a national effort to improve maternity care practices and breastfeeding. *Breastfeed Med.* 2016;11(4):166–172

20. World Health Organization; UNICEF. Baby-friendly hospital initiative: revised, updated and expanded for integrated care. 2009. Available at: http://apps.who.int/iris/bitstream/10665/43593/7/9789241594998_eng.pdf. Accessed February 18, 2017

21. Goldsmith JP. Hospitals should balance skin-to-skin contact with safe sleep policies. *AAP News.* 2013;34(11):22

22. Feldman-Winter L, Goldsmith JP; Committee on Fetus and Newborn; Task Force on Sudden Infant Death Syndrome. Safe sleep and skin-to-skin care in the neonatal period for

healthy term newborns. *Pediatrics*. 2016;138(3):e20161889

23. Flaherman VJ, Schaefer EW, Kuzniewicz MW, Li SX, Walsh EM, Paul IM. Early weight loss nomograms for exclusively breastfed newborns. *Pediatrics*. 2015;135(1). Available at: www.pediatrics.org/cgi/content/full/135/1/e16

24. Grossman X, Chaudhuri JH, Feldman-Winter L, Merewood A. Neonatal weight loss at a US Baby-Friendly Hospital. *J Acad Nutr Diet*. 2012;112(3):410–413

25. Dennison BA, Nguyen TQ, Gregg DJ, Fan W, Xu C. The impact of hospital resources and availability of professional lactation support on maternity care: results of breastfeeding surveys 2009-2014. *Breastfeed Med*. 2016;11(9):479–486

26. Dixit A, Feldman-Winter L, Szucs KA. "Frustrated," "depressed," and "devastated" pediatric trainees: US academic medical centers fail to provide adequate workplace breastfeeding support. *J Hum Lact*. 2015;31(2):240–248

27. Brick JM, Williams D. Explaining rising nonresponse rates in cross-sectional surveys. *Ann Am Acad Pol Soc Sci*. 2013;645(1):36–59

28. Groves RM, Peytcheva E. The impact of nonresponse rates on nonresponse bias: a meta-analysis. *Public Opin Q*. 2008;72(2):167–189

29. Cull WL, O'Connor KG, Sharp S, Tang SF. Response rates and response bias for 50 surveys of pediatricians. *Health Serv Res*. 2005;40(1):213–226

Measuring Breastfeeding Success

Dr Lydia Furman, MD, Associate Editor, *Pediatrics*

In *Pediatrics* (10.1542/peds.2017-0142), Dr. Trang Nguyen and colleagues looked at a very interesting and clinically important question: what is the prevalence of formula supplementation among breastfed infants in maternity hospitals, and what factors impact this? The authors focused on their home state of New York (NY) because NY has the second highest rate of formula supplementation (26.1%) in the US, which is meaningfully higher than the national average (17.1%), and almost double the Healthy People 2020 Maternal, Infant and Child Health goal of 14.2% (https://www.healthypeople.gov/2020/topics-objectives/topic/maternal-infant-and-child-health/objectives). Solid evidence supports the urgency of reducing in-hospital not medically indicated formula supplementation of breastfed infants: although previously viewed as a benign practice that "helped" mothers, we now know that the impact of this practice is measurably negative. Chantry and colleagues demonstrated that among first time mothers who intended to breastfeed, those whose infants received formula in the hospital were 1.8 times less likely to be exclusively breastfeeding by 60 days postpartum and were 2.7 times more likely to have stopped breastfeeding than those whose infants were not supplemented.[1] Nguyen et al used 2014 enhanced birth certificate data for all eligible infants from the 126 birthing hospitals in NY (n=160,911 infants); a major strength of this study is the completeness and size of their sample. They found that observed formula supplementation rates varied widely across NY, and their analytical approach, which adjusts for confounding factors, is clear, well explained and easy to read.

A couple of points bear comment. Although we can and should consider enhanced birth certificate data to be as close an approximation to "the truth" as we have, challenges to data collection and accuracy are also important to consider. I am not suggesting that these issues invalidate the results of Dr. Nguyen and colleagues' excellent work, but rather that being well informed about data collection difficulties is good background. States including NY and my home state of Ohio (OH) have struggled both to collect accurate data on exclusive breastfeeding (and supplementation) and to improve maternity care practices. In 2008, NY reported a range of 0-99% for supplementation of breastfed infants among all NY hospitals (excluding NY City); it is unlikely that this data fully and accurately represented practice, and multiple initiatives to improve practice and data collection were begun.[2] In OH, until 2014, information at the state level on the virtual birth certificate (IPHIS- integrated perinatal health information system) was not collected separately regarding exclusive breastfeeding and formula supplementation of breastfed infants– only lumped data on "any breastfeeding" was gathered. Trainings by the Ohio Perinatal Quality Collaborative at the level of individual hospitals and data collectors were conducted over a period of a year, and additional web-based and reminder trainings are ongoing (https://opqc.net/announcements/04042016/new-iphis-training-dates). To complicate matters further (and after the data for Nguyen et al's study was collected) the Joint Commission retired Perinatal Core Measure PC-05a and replaced it with PC-05: this meant that the mother's preference to not breastfeed was no longer recorded, and maternal exclusions were discontinued (https://manual.jointcommission.org/releases/TJC2015B/MIF0170.html). This change led to another round of trainings for those tasked with collecting the actual chart data, and IPHIS data accuracy and completeness were again at some risk.

A final point to consider: while Nguyen et al did not find that Baby-Friendly Hospital designation ensured low rates of formula supplementation, this should not be discouraging or considered a lack of endorsement of Baby-Friendly designation. Another article in *Pediatrics* by Dr. Lori Feldman-Winter and colleagues (10.1542/peds.2016-3121) describe the Best Fed Beginnings program, a quality improvement initiative which supported Baby-Friendly designation of more than 70 participating hospitals. Selection for participation was based upon "low breastfeeding rates…sociodemographics of the population served, geographic locations (with preference for regions with low breastfeeding rates)…" in addition to hospital readiness factors. Thus for hospitals participating in this type of major initiative, even huge improvements in their individual rates of exclusive breastfeeding may not translate directly into the highest breastfeeding or lowest supplementation rates in comparison to birthing hospitals in the same state with more favorable demographics.

All in all, I find this subject fascinating, and hope I have been able to share a bit of my enthusiasm for the facts and figures and measurement of breastfeeding rates and promotion efforts with you!

REFERENCES

1. Chantry CJ, Dewey KG, Peerson JM, Wagner EA, Nommsen-Rivers LA. In-hospital formula use increases early breastfeeding cessation among first-time mothers intending to exclusively breastfeed. *J Pediatr*. 2014 Jun; 164(6):1339-45.e5.
2. DNPAO State Program Highlights Maternity Care Practices. Centers for Disease Control and Prevention. https://www.cdc.gov/obesity/downloads/CDC_MaternityCarePractices.pdf. Accessed 6/13/2017.

Variation in Formula Supplementation of Breastfed Newborn Infants in New York Hospitals

Trang Nguyen, MD, DrPH,[a,b] Barbara A. Dennison, MD,[a,b] Wei Fan, PhD,[a] Changning Xu, MPH,[a] Guthrie S. Birkhead, MD, MPH[b]

OBJECTIVES: We examined the variation between 126 New York hospitals in formula supplementation among breastfed infants after adjusting for socioeconomic, maternal, and infant factors and stratifying by level of perinatal care.

METHODS: We used 2014 birth certificate data for 160 911 breastfed infants to calculate hospital-specific formula supplementation percentages by using multivariable hierarchical logistic regression models.

RESULTS: Formula supplementation percentages varied widely among hospitals, from 2.3% to 98.3%, and was lower among level 1 hospitals (18.2%) than higher-level hospitals (50.6%–57.0%). Significant disparities in supplementation were noted for race and ethnicity (adjusted odds ratios [aORs] were 1.54–2.05 for African Americans, 1.85–2.74 for Asian Americans, and 1.25–2.16 for Hispanics, compared with whites), maternal education (aORs were 2.01–2.95 for ≤12th grade, 1.74–1.85 for high school or general education development, and 1.18–1.28 for some college or a college degree, compared with a Master's degree), and insurance coverage (aOR was 1.27–1.60 for Medicaid insurance versus other). Formula supplementation was higher among mothers who smoked, had a cesarean delivery, or diabetes. At all 4 levels of perinatal care, there were exemplar hospitals that met the HealthyPeople 2020 supplementation goal of ≤14.2%. After adjusting for individual risk factors, the hospital-specific, risk-adjusted supplemental formula percentages still revealed a wide variation.

CONCLUSIONS: A better understanding of the exemplar hospitals could inform future efforts to improve maternity care practices and breastfeeding support to reduce unnecessary formula supplementation, reduce disparities, increase exclusive breastfeeding and breastfeeding duration, and improve maternal and child health outcomes.

aNew York State Department of Health, Albany, New York; and bSchool of Public Health, University at Albany, State University of New York, Rensselaer, New York

Dr Nguyen conceptualized and designed the study, conducted statistical analyses, interpreted the data, and drafted the manuscript; Dr Dennison conceptualized and designed the study, interpreted the data, and drafted the manuscript; Dr Fan and Mr Xu contributed to statistical analyses, interpretation of the findings, and revision of the manuscript; Dr Birkhead critically reviewed and revised the manuscript for important intellectual content; and all authors approved the final manuscript as submitted.

DOI: https://doi.org/10.1542/peds.2017-0142

Accepted for publication Apr 20, 2017

Address correspondence to Trang Nguyen, MD, DrPH, Office of Public Health Practice, New York State Department of Health, Room 913 Corning Tower at ESP, Albany, NY 12237. E-mail: trang. nguyen@health.ny.gov

WHAT'S KNOWN ON THIS SUBJECT: Nonmedically indicated formula supplementation has been shown to adversely impact exclusive breastfeeding and is associated with shorter duration of breastfeeding. A number of maternal and infant factors are associated with formula supplementation; their prevalence varies across hospitals in New York.

WHAT THIS STUDY ADDS: Formula supplementation of breastfed infants varies across hospitals. Much of this variation persists even after adjusting for maternal and infant factors. Hospital breastfeeding policies and supplementation practices contribute to this variation. Improving hospital practices could lead to improved breastfeeding outcomes.

To cite: Nguyen T, Dennison BA , Fan W, et al. Variation in Formula Supplementation of Breastfed Newborn Infants in New York Hospitals. *Pediatrics.* 2017;140(1):e20170142

ARTICLE

Exclusive breastfeeding for the first 6 months, with continued human breast milk feeding through 12 months or longer, is recommended to provide optimal infant and maternal health benefits.[1,2] Maternity care provided during birth hospitalization has been shown to directly impact breastfeeding success. The Ten Steps to Successful Breastfeeding (Ten Steps), individually or combined, have been associated with reduced formula supplementation, increased exclusive breastfeeding, and longer breastfeeding duration through at least 8 weeks of age.[3] Implementation of the Ten Steps by hospital maternity services is widely recommended,[2,4] and forms the basis for the Baby-Friendly Hospital initiative.[5] Step 6 (not providing supplemental formula to healthy breastfed infants unless medically indicated) is the step most predictive of breastfeeding success.[6] However, only 26% of US hospitals report having implemented Step 6.[7] Although there is no US benchmark for formula supplementation of breastfed infants during birth hospitalization, the HealthyPeople 2020 (HP2020) objective MICH-23, which is to reduce the proportion of breastfed newborns who receive formula supplementation within the first 2 days of life to no more than 14.2%, seems applicable.[8] Because US insurance carriers are required to cover 48 hours of newborn care, most infants spend the first 2 days in the hospital. Whether this objective is met is highly dependent on the hospital's maternity care policies and practices.[7,9] New York, compared with other US states, has the second-highest proportion of mothers who report that their breastfed infant received formula before 2 days of age (26.1%). This is much higher than the national average (17.1%).[10] It is unlikely that infants in New York are at increased medical risk and have a medical indication for formula supplementation.

Many women (68%) report not meeting their own breastfeeding goals during birth hospitalization or after discharge.[11] One of the most common disappointments expressed by new mothers is their inability to exclusively breastfeed during birth hospitalization because their newborn was fed formula.[12] Maternal factors, infant health status, and hospital maternity care, including timing and duration of mother-infant skin-to-skin bonding, timing of the first breastfeeding, and duration of mother-infant rooming-in, are important determinants in whether the newborn receives supplemental formula.[13] Disparities in breastfeeding by race, ethnicity, and socioeconomic status (SES) have also been reported.[14] Although variation among hospitals in formula supplementation of breastfed newborn infants has been reported in New York and California,[15,16] there is no formal, published study in which the researchers evaluate the variation across hospitals in formula supplementation or control for individual factors known to impact breastfeeding, such as SES or maternal or infant risk factors.

Our purpose in this study is to measure (1) the variation across hospitals in formula supplementation of breastfed newborn infants; (2) the impact of socioeconomic, maternal, and infant factors on formula supplementation; and (3) the variation in formula supplementation across hospitals after adjustment for these risk factors.

METHODS

Study Population

All infants born alive during 2014 in 126 New York hospitals that provide maternity services were eligible to be included in the study. Infants were excluded for the following reasons: (1) they were admitted to the NICU, (2) transferred between hospitals, (3) received an unknown method of feeding, (4) were not fed any breast milk during birth hospitalization, (5) had a gestational age that was unknown or <37 weeks' gestation, (6) had an unknown or low birth weight (ie, <2500 g), or (7) were the product of a multiple birth (Fig 1; N = 160 911).

Data Source

The 2014 enhanced birth certificate data, collected via the New York Statewide Perinatal Data System, were used. Self-reported maternal socioeconomic and health status variables included race, ethnicity, educational attainment, and smoking history. Hospital staff reported maternal prepregnancy weight and height, infant birth weight, gestational age, NICU admission, hospital transfer, birth order, delivery method, prenatal care, gravida, parity, maternal risk factors (prepregnancy diabetes, gestational diabetes, prepregnancy hypertension, and gestational hypertension), infant feeding method (breast milk only, formula only, both breast milk and formula, or other [ie, not fed breast milk or formula]), and payer source (Medicaid versus others). New York Public Health Law § 4130 requires that birth data be reported within 5 days of birth; thus, infant feeding data are truncated for infants hospitalized longer than 5 days.

Study Variables

The outcome of interest (dependent variable) was defined as an infant who was fed both breast milk and formula (formula supplementation). Independent variables included maternal SES and maternal and infant risk factors such as race and ethnicity, educational attainment, marital status, primary payer, maternal age group, prepregnancy weight status, prepregnancy or gestation hypertension, prepregnancy or gestational diabetes, smoking before or during pregnancy, late care or no perinatal

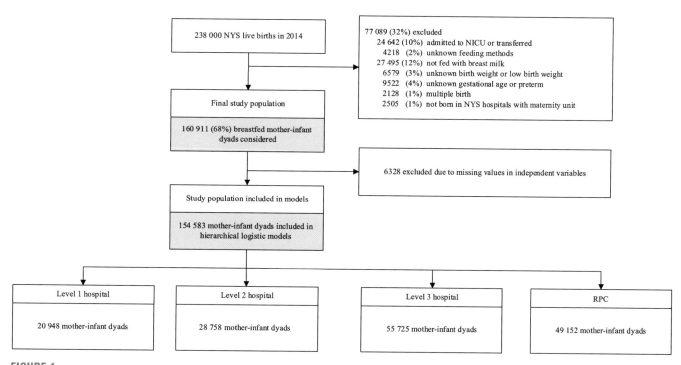

FIGURE 1

Determination of study population, New York state (NYS), 2014. The flow diagram illustrates the selection of the final population and the study population in models. Excluded mother-infant dyads may have met more than 1 exclusion criterion. (Data Source: 2014 New York Statewide Perinatal Data System).

care, first live birth, and cesarean delivery. Maternal prepregnancy BMI was calculated on the basis of prepregnancy weight and height.

In New York, perinatal care is regionalized to provide the full range of perinatal services in a geographic area. There are 4 hierarchical levels of perinatal care. Level 1 hospitals provide care to low-risk pregnant women and newborns; they do not operate NICUs. Level 2 hospitals provide care to moderate-risk women and newborns. Level 3 hospitals provide complex care. The regional perinatal center (RPC) hospitals provide the most sophisticated care in the region for specialized consultation on complicated cases. Each RPC also provides support, training, and quality improvement services to the affiliated hospitals within their region, and ensures timely transfer of patients to higher-level perinatal hospitals within the region. For level 2, level 3, and RPC hospitals, the number of births and intensity of neonatal care must meet minimum

volume standards during each calendar year.[17]

Statistical Analysis

Bivariate analysis: We determined the formula supplementation percentages for the total study population and each independent variable. χ^2 tests were conducted to assess the unadjusted association of formula supplementation with each of the independent variables.

We conducted multivariable hierarchical logistic regression modeling separately for each level of perinatal care to account for any unmeasured differences in hospital policies or practices at each level. Independent variables for mother-infant dyads were entered as fixed-effect components, and the hospital identifier was entered as a random intercept component.[18]

A full model was fit with all independent variables described above. Model selection for the fixed effects were performed by using backward elimination with

preference given to models with lower Akaike information criterion.[19] For each perinatal level, the final model with the lowest Akaike information criterion was used to estimate the adjusted odds ratios (aORs) (95% confidence intervals [CIs]) for formula supplementation. The final models only included variables with a *P* value <.2.

We calculated the observed percentage of formula supplementation for each hospital and each perinatal care level. Hospital-specific predicted and expected formula supplementation percentages were determined from the final model for each perinatal care level.[18] The risk-adjusted formula supplementation percentage for each hospital was calculated by multiplying the hospital-specific ratio for formula supplementation (predicted percentage divided by expected percentage) by the observed formula supplementation percentage for the corresponding perinatal care level.[18]

TABLE 1 Distribution of Study Variables by Formula Supplementation, New York State, 2014

	Final Study Population ($N = 160\,911$)		
	Births	Formula Supplementation	P^a
	No. (%)	No. (%)	
Total	160 911 (100.0)	78 003 (48.5)	
Hospital			
Level of perinatal care			<.001
Level 1 hospitals	22 004 (13.7)	4005 (18.2)	
Level 2 hospitals	30 275 (18.8)	15 320 (50.6)	
Level 3 hospitals	56 964 (35.4)	29 248 (51.3)	
RPC	51 668 (32.1)	29 430 (57.0)	
Maternal SES			
Race and ethnicity			<.001
White, non-Hispanic	78 854 (49.0)	26 753 (33.9)	
African American, non-Hispanic	22 090 (13.7)	13 495 (61.1)	
Asian American, non-Hispanic	17 301 (10.8)	10 621 (61.4)	
Other race, non-Hispanic	3082 (1.9)	1316 (42.7)	
Any race, Hispanic	39 536 (24.6)	25 786 (65.2)	
Educational attainment			<.001
Twelfth grade or less	24 545 (15.3)	16 703 (68.1)	
High school graduate or GED	33 288 (20.8)	18 422 (55.3)	
Some college to bachelor's degree	72 367 (45.1)	31 921 (44.1)	
Master's or doctoral degree	30 165 (18.8)	10 619 (35.2)	
Marital status			<.001
Married	101 566 (63.1)	44 606 (43.9)	
Single	59 345 (36.9)	33 397 (56.3)	
Primary payer			<.001
Not Medicaid	80 371 (50.0)	29 484 (36.7)	
Medicaid	80 324 (50.0)	48 394 (60.2)	
Maternal and infant health conditions			
Age (y)			<.001
13–19	6052 (3.8)	3486 (57.6)	
20–24	27 583 (17.1)	14 612 (53.0)	
25–39	120 633 (75.0)	56 446 (46.8)	
40 or older	6641 (4.1)	3458 (52.1)	
Prepregnancy weight status (BMI)			<.001
Underweight (<18.5)	6518 (4.2)	3299 (50.6)	
Normal (18.5–<25)	79 358 (50.6)	36 867 (46.5)	
Overweight (25–<30)	40 550 (25.9)	20 421 (50.4)	
Obese (30–<40)	25 847 (16.5)	13 295 (51.4)	
Severely obese (≥40)	4470 (2.9)	2216 (49.6)	
Prepregnancy or gestational hypertension			<.001
No	153 568 (95.4)	74 599 (48.6)	
Yes	7343 (4.6)	3404 (46.4)	
Prepregnancy or gestational diabetes			<.001
No	150 781 (93.7)	72 385 (48.0)	
Yes	10 130 (6.3)	5618 (55.5)	
Smoking before or during pregnancy			<.001
No	151 078 (94.2)	74 551 (49.3)	
Yes	9258 (5.8)	3327 (35.9)	
Late (third trimester) care or no perinatal care			<.001
No	150 203 (94.7)	72 108 (48.0)	
Yes	8487 (5.3)	4980 (58.7)	
First live birth			<.001
No	91 879 (57.1)	46 723 (50.9)	
Yes	69 021 (42.9)	31 271 (45.3)	
Cesarean delivery			<.001
No	112 434 (70.1)	52 219 (46.4)	
Yes	47 977 (29.9)	25 736 (53.6)	

GED, general educational development.

[a] P value for χ^2 test.

We compared the between-hospital variances for models of supplemental feeding before and after risk adjustment and calculated the IntraClass coefficient and the proportional change in variances.[20,21] The predictive accuracy of the models was assessed by the area under receiver operating characteristic curve. SAS version 9.4 was used for all analyses. P values <.05 were considered statistically significant.

The study was approved by the New York State Department of Health Institutional Review Board.

RESULTS

Sixty-eight percent ($N = 160\,911$) of infants met the study inclusion criteria (Fig 1). Approximately half (48.5%) of the infants who were fed breast milk were also supplemented with formula (Table 1). The mean formula supplementation percentages differed by perinatal level of care; formula supplementation was much lower at level 1 hospitals (18.2%) compared with higher-level hospitals (50.6%–57%).

Before adjustment, all independent variables were statistically associated with formula supplementation (Table 1, all P values <.001). Of note, infants whose mother did not smoke before or during pregnancy, compared with mothers who smoked, were more likely to be supplemented with formula.

We show in Table 2 the aORs for the associations between formula supplementation with the independent variables from the final model for each perinatal care level. Newborn infants whose mothers were non-Hispanic African American, Asian American, or Hispanic were more likely to receive formula supplementation compared with non-Hispanic white mothers. Asian American infants were at the highest

TABLE 2 Odds of Formula Supplementation by Hospital Level of Perinatal Care, Adjusted for Sociodemographic, Health, and Other Factors, New York State, 2014 (N = 154 583)

Independent Variable	Level 1 (N = 20 948) aOR (95% CI)	Level 2 (N = 28 758) aOR (95% CI)	Level 3 (N = 55 725) aOR (95% CI)	RPC (N = 49 152) aOR (95% CI)
Maternal SES				
Race and ethnicity				
White, non-Hispanic[a]	1.00	1.00	1.00	1.00
African American, non-Hispanic	2.05 (1.75–2.40)	2.00 (1.79–2.24)	1.67 (1.55–1.79)	1.54 (1.43–1.66)
Asian American, non-Hispanic	2.74 (2.21–3.40)	2.63 (2.35–2.95)	1.99 (1.85–2.15)	1.85 (1.72–1.99)
Other race, non-Hispanic	1.76 (1.41–2.19)	1.50 (1.25–1.81)	1.26 (1.06–1.49)	1.12 (0.96–1.32)
Any race, Hispanic	2.16 (1.88–2.48)	2.01 (1.85–2.18)	1.60 (1.50–1.71)	1.25 (1.17–1.34)
Educational attainment				
Twelfth grade or less	2.95 (2.47–3.52)	2.74 (2.41–3.10)	2.01 (1.83–2.19)	2.09 (1.91–2.30)
High school graduate or GED	1.76 (1.51–2.05)	1.85 (1.66–2.07)	1.78 (1.64–1.93)	1.74 (1.61–1.89)
Some college to bachelor's degree	1.19 (1.04–1.35)	1.28 (1.18–1.40)	1.24 (1.17–1.33)	1.18 (1.12–1.25)
Master's or doctoral degree[a]	1.00	1.00	1.00	1.00
Marital status				
Married[a]	1.00	1.00	1.00	1.00
Single	1.29 (1.17–1.42)	1.19 (1.11–1.29)	1.08 (1.03–1.14)	1.17 (1.10–1.24)
Primary payer				
Not Medicaid[a]	1.00	1.00	1.00	1.00
Medicaid	1.27 (1.15–1.41)	1.32 (1.22–1.43)	1.42 (1.34–1.50)	1.60 (1.51–1.71)
Maternal and infant health conditions				
Age (y)				
13–24[b]	0.99 (0.90–1.10)	1.06 (0.97–1.15)	1.13 (1.06–1.20)	1.20 (1.13–1.29)
25–39[a]	1.00	1.00	1.00	1.00
40 or older	1.38 (1.08–1.77)	1.16 (0.98–1.36)	1.15 (1.04–1.28)	1.06 (0.96–1.17)
Prepregnancy weight status (BMI)				
Underweight (<18.5)	1.09 (0.86–1.38)	0.90 (0.77–1.05)	1.00 (0.90–1.11)	0.98 (0.88–1.09)
Normal (18.5–<25)[a]	1.00	1.00	1.00	1.00
Overweight (25–<30)	1.23 (1.11–1.35)	1.15 (1.07–1.23)	1.15 (1.09–1.21)	1.12 (1.06–1.18)
Obese (30–<40)	1.53 (1.38–1.69)	1.24 (1.14–1.35)	1.17 (1.10–1.25)	1.26 (1.18–1.35)
Severely obese (≥40)	1.63 (1.37–1.94)	1.41 (1.18–1.69)	1.36 (1.18–1.56)	1.39 (1.20–1.62)
Prepregnancy or gestational hypertension				
No[a]	1.00	1.00	1.00	1.00
Yes	1.43 (1.23–1.67)	1.16 (0.99–1.35)	1.11 (0.99–1.25)	1.22 (1.09–1.36)
Prepregnancy or gestational diabetes				
No[a]	1.00	1.00	1.00	1.00
Yes	1.33 (1.14–1.55)	1.42 (1.25–1.61)	1.34 (1.22–1.47)	1.50 (1.36–1.65)
Smoking before or during pregnancy				—
No[a]	1.00	1.00	1.00	
Yes	1.33 (1.20–1.48)	1.20 (1.04–1.38)	1.11 (0.98–1.25)	
Late (third trimester) care or no perinatal care			—	—
No[a]	1.00	1.00		
Yes	1.18 (0.94–1.47)	1.15 (1.00–1.33)		
First live birth	—			
No		1.18 (1.10–1.26)	1.24 (1.18–1.29)	1.17 (1.12–1.23)
Yes[a]		1.00	1.00	1.00
Cesarean delivery				
No[a]	1.00	1.00	1.00	1.00
Yes	1.65 (1.52–1.80)	1.54 (1.44–1.65)	1.39 (1.33–1.46)	1.57 (1.49–1.65)

GED, general educational development; —, variable was not included in the final model because of elimination.

[a] Reference group.

[b] Two maternal age groups (13–19 and 20–24) that had a similar association with the study outcome were combined into 1 age group.

risk of receiving supplemental formula at all perinatal care levels. The aORs for mothers who were non-Hispanic other race were also significantly higher at level 1, 2, or 3 hospitals. The strength of associations for race and ethnicity varied by the level of perinatal care, with stronger associations seen at lower-level hospitals. There was a strong, consistent inverse relationship with maternal educational attainment and formula supplementation at all 4 perinatal care levels (Table 2). The aORs were also higher for mothers with Medicaid insurance (a marker for low income) and who were not married.

At all perinatal levels, increasing maternal weight status was

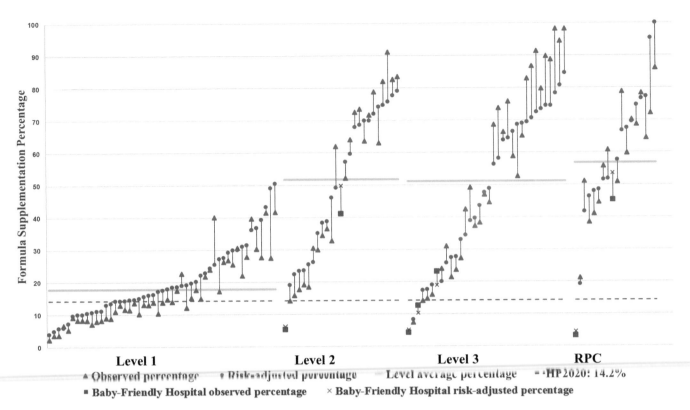

Level 1   Level 2   Level 3   RPC

▲ Observed percentage   ● Risk-adjusted percentage   — Level average percentage   - - HP 2020: 14.2%
■ Baby-Friendly Hospital observed percentage   × Baby-Friendly Hospital risk-adjusted percentage

FIGURE 2

Hospital observed and adjusted formula supplementation percentage by level of perinatal care, New York state, 2014. Each square represents the observed percentage of formula supplementation for a Baby-Friendly hospital, and the cross represents the hospital's corresponding risk-adjusted percentage of formula supplementation. Each triangle represents the observed percentage of formula supplementation for a specific hospital (not Baby-Friendly hospital) and the circle represents the hospital's corresponding risk-adjusted percentage of formula supplementation. The pink horizontal line shows the average percentage of formula supplementation for each perinatal care level, and the green dash line shows the HP2020 objective of formula supplementation rate.

associated with increasing odds that the infant received formula supplementation after adjusting for socioeconomic, maternal, and infant risk factors, a finding that was not observed in the unadjusted results (Table 1). Newborns whose mothers smoked were at higher odds for formula supplementation, which is opposite from the unadjusted results. Newborns whose mothers had diabetes or hypertension were more likely to receive supplemental formula compared with newborns whose mothers did not have these conditions. Infants born by cesarean delivery or were not the first child also had higher odds for formula supplementation at all levels of perinatal care.

The observed (unadjusted) formula supplementation percentages varied widely across hospitals, from 2.3% to 98.3% (Fig 2). The average

supplementation percentages for level 1, level 2, level 3, and RPC hospitals were 17.7%, 51.7%, 51.2%, and 56.7%, respectively (Fig 2). At each perinatal care level, there were exemplar hospitals that met the HP2020 target of ≤14.2%. The proportion of hospitals meeting this objective, however, was much higher among level 1 hospitals (55%, N = 27) compared with level 2 (4%, N = 1), level 3 (12%, N = 4), or RPC hospitals (6%, N = 1). In 2014, 7 New York hospitals were designated as Baby-Friendly. Among the higher-level perinatal hospitals, 4 of the 6 exemplar hospitals were designated as Baby-Friendly (level 2 [1 out of 1], level 3 [2 out of 4], and RPC hospitals [1 out of 1]), but none of the exemplar level 1 hospitals were designated as Baby-Friendly (0 out of 27) (Fig 2).

We show in Table 3 the between-hospital variance results, which are consistent with the patterns seen in Fig 2. Before statistical adjustment for any risk factors, level 3 hospitals had the largest variation in formula supplementation (48%), followed by level 2, RPC, and level 1 hospitals (34%, 28%, and 15%, respectively). Risk adjustment had the greatest impact in reducing the variance in level 2 hospitals (by ~18%), primarily because of socioeconomic factors.

DISCUSSION

In this study, we confirm previous findings that formula supplementation varies by multiple sociodemographic and maternal and infant risk factors, and that race and/or ethnicity and low educational

TABLE 3 Between-Hospital Variance of Formula Supplementation in the Null Model, SES Model, and the Final Model

Level of Perinatal Care	Null Model		SES Model	Final Model	Proportional Change in Variance (SES Model to Null Model), %	Proportional Change in Variance (Final Model to Null Model), %
	Variance (SE)[a]	ICC	Variance (SE)	Variance (SE)		
Level 1 hospitals	0.57 (0.12)	0.15	0.56 (0.12)	0.58 (0.13)	−0.7	2.7
Level 2 hospitals	1.68 (0.48)	0.34	1.35 (0.39)	1.38 (0.40)	−19.9	−17.7
Level 3 hospitals	3.02 (0.74)	0.48	2.54 (0.62)	2.62 (0.64)	−15.8	−13.1
RPC	1.28 (0.43)	0.28	1.31 (0.44)	1.32 (0.43)	2.7	3.5

Null models contained only hospital-specific random intercepts and no independent variables. SES models contained hospital-specific random intercepts and race and/or ethnicity, educational attainment, marital status, and primary payer as fixed effects. Final models contained hospital-specific random intercepts and independent variables as fixed effects specified in Table 2. ICC, intraclass coefficient; SE, standard error.

[a] Variance and SE were estimated by the random intercepts in hierarchical models.

attainment are 2 of the strongest determiants.[12,22–24] Researchers in an earlier study found a large variation among hospitals in the percentages of newborn infants who were exclusively breastfed, after adjusting for some mother and infant characteristics.[25] We are the first, however, to risk-adjust hospital-specific rates of formula supplementation for the many socioeconomic and patient factors known to impact breastfeeding. After doing so, we found that most of the hospital variation in formula supplementation of breastfed infants persisted. Researchers in previous studies have found that breastfeeding initiation and exclusive breastfeeding rates differed between hospitals, and that these percentages were related in a dose-response manner with the number of recommended hospital maternity practices (ie, Ten Steps) received by the mother.[13]

Most women decide whether to breastfeed before delivery,[26] and these planned intentions to breastfeed are associated with both initiation and duration of breastfeeding.[27–29] Intention to breastfeed by itself, however, is only one factor. Researchers conducting a study of mothers found that social support and subjective norms were important enabling factors that determined continued breastfeeding at 1 month.[30] Among women who intended to exclusively breastfeed for several months, 68% reported they did not meet their own breastfeeding goals.[11]

Formula supplementation during birth hospitalization can be a contributing factor, interfering with exclusive breastfeeding as well as being associated with shorter duration of breastfeeding. The provision of supplemental formula (when not medically indicated) may undermine a mother's intention to exclusively breastfeed, leading to feelings of frustration, powerlessness, and a sense of failure.[31] It can provide a conflicting message that may be interpreted as the hospital staff or providers promoting formula feeding for healthy infants.[32]

Hospital staff report that one of the most common reasons for in-hospital formula supplementation is the mother's request.[33] Whether the variation in formula supplementation by race and/or ethnicity or income reflects variation in maternal requests for formula by race and/or ethnicity or SES factors is not known. Increased formula supplementation of breastfed infants was observed among families on Medicaid, with higher odds at higher-care level perinatal hospitals. The reasons for this are not known, but researchers in other studies suggest that factors such as not participating in prenatal classes or distributing gift bags with free formula at discharge increase formula supplementation.[34] A mother's request for formula is often due to inadequate preparation for newborn care, lack of knowledge about breastfeeding, or a belief that formula was the solution for perceived breastfeeding problems.[33,34]

Researchers of a previous study in New York showed that the ratio of professional lactation consultants per 1000 births was lower at higher-level perinatal hospitals.[35] Therefore, on-site lactation support for new mothers may be less in higher-level hospitals. In addition, the authors of a study of African American women found that they were more likely to encounter unsupportive cultural norms, such as perceptions that breastfeeding is inferior to formula feeding and lack of partner support.[36] The levels of social support, cultural norms, and beliefs around breastfeeding may contribute to the high supplementation rate and disparities in breastfeeding.[37]

Researchers in numerous studies have found that the specific hospital maternity care a woman receives is related to her breastfeeding success,[38,39] and that the numbers of the recommended policies and practices present correlates with hospital-specific breastfeeding initiation and exclusivity rates.[13] Women who deliver at hospitals that implement Baby-Friendly policies and become designated as Baby-Friendly have higher breastfeeding initiation rates and longer breastfeeding duration.[40,41]

In New York, no level 1 hospitals were designated as Baby-Friendly (ie, none met the certification criteria that they have implemented the Ten Steps[42] and the International Code of Marketing of Breast-milk Substitutes[43]).[44] However, 55% (N = 27) of level 1 hospitals had low supplementation rates. In contrast, among the higher-level perinatal hospitals, in which the average supplementation rate is higher and the variability greater, there were exemplar hospitals, and 4 of the 6 exemplar hospitals were designated as Baby-Friendly. However, among the 7 Baby-Friendly designated hospitals, 3 did not have low supplementation rates (ie, ≤14.2%). Thus, being designated Baby-Friendly is not sufficient to ensure that a hospital has a low supplementation rate. Prenatal breastfeeding education, health care provider and staff training, lactation support, social support, and peer counseling are also related to breastfeeding outcomes.[45–47]

Research into these exemplar hospitals by using community-based participatory methodology and/or a positive deviance approach might provide insight into important but hitherto undocumented maternal behaviors, family characteristics, staff or community attitudes, and cultural determinants (beyond the recognized hospital policies and practices and socioeconomic, infant, and maternal factors) that are contributing to their better breastfeeding outcomes.[48,49] Recent community-based efforts, sensitive to the cultural determinants and focused on changing social norms, are proving to be successful in improving breastfeeding rates, particularly in disadvantaged communities.[50,51]

The finding that formula supplementation is much lower (30%–40%) at level 1 hospitals compared with level 2, level 3, or RPC hospitals is striking. A notable difference between level 1 hospitals and the higher-level hospitals is that level 1 hospitals do not have an NICU. This might contribute to differences in the hospital breastfeeding culture, such that formula feeding, which is more prevalent at higher-level perinatal hospitals, is viewed as more acceptable by hospital staff

and/or providers. Alternatively, the "healthy" infants might be sicker or have more complicated health needs that are not measured by the maternal health conditions or infant factors included in the current risk adjustment. (Note that infants admitted to the NICU and those born at <37 weeks or <2500 g are excluded from this study.)

The level 1 hospitals had less variation in formula supplementation, which remained unchanged after risk adjustment, suggesting that the maternity care practices and the hospital breastfeeding culture at level 1 hospitals may be more consistent, more supportive, and/or better at deterring unnecessary, nonmedically indicated formula supplementation. Level 1 hospitals tend to be smaller community hospitals with fewer deliveries per year. They are rarely teaching hospitals and are less likely to have residents or medical or nursing students. As such, mother-infant dyads tend to have fewer interruptions or separations for resident or student teaching, and mother-infant dyads spend more time rooming-in.[52,53] The number of interruptions has been negatively correlated with the frequency of breastfeeding, maternal perceptions of breastfeeding success, and maternal satisfaction.[52,53] Because of these concerns and the recognition that separating mothers and infants can adversely impact breastfeeding success, recent recommendations call for providers to conduct newborn examinations and screening tests in the patient's room to reduce maternal-infant separation time,[54] and to limit visiting hours except for the mother's primary support person.

This study has some limitations. Maternal demographic information is self-reported; however, authors of a previous study found that birth records include good quality maternal demographic data.[55]

Information was not available concerning the mother's planned feeding intentions, her requests for formula, or the reasons why the infant was supplemented with formula. Information concerning maternal health conditions before and during pregnancy were provided, but information about the mother's clinical course after birth was not available. Information about the infant was limited to his or her birth size, gestation, and admission to the NICU. Clinical conditions among term infants not admitted to the NICU that might require formula supplementation are limited and should be no more than 14.2%. Unless their prevalence differed significantly between hospitals within the same perinatal care level, clinical conditions would not impact the variation or relative ranking of hospitals.

This study, however, has many strengths. First, we used a large data set that includes the entire newborn population of a large, diverse state. Much of the information was reported on the birth certificate by hospital staff, including infant feeding and breastfeeding. The maternal demographic information is self-reported on the birth record, which has been shown to be of good quality maternal demographic data.[55] Each mother also self-reported her race and ethnicity, which is more accurate than staff observations and is the recommended method for collecting racial and ethnic data.[56] The analyses included many known risk factors for formula supplementation. The analyses were stratified by hospital level of perinatal care, which resulted in more homogeneous populations regarding maternal and infant clinical risk factors and hospital characteristics within each stratum. We designed the hierarchical modeling method to adjust for random effects at the hospital level, and the final models were a good fit in predicting the data with area under the curve ~0.80.

Additional research is needed to understand why healthy breastfed newborns are supplemented with formula, and whether maternal requests for formula and how they are handled differ across hospitals or among patient populations. A better understanding of why level 1 hospitals are more likely to have low percentages of formula supplementation than higher-level perinatal hospitals is needed. The factors (eg, maternal, family or community characteristics, hospital leadership or staff knowledge, attitudes or behaviors, or hospital breastfeeding culture) that contribute to less formula supplementation at exemplar hospitals need to be identified by using positive deviance or other approaches. In addition, once best practices or strategies are identified, translational research is needed to increase their adoption to help reduce nonmedically indicated supplemental formula feeding, increase exclusive breastfeeding, support longer breastfeeding duration, and improve maternal and infant health outcomes.

CONCLUSIONS

We have found a wide variation in hospital-specific formula supplementation percentages, even when hospitals are stratified by level of perinatal care. There were hospitals at each of the 4 levels of perinatal care that met the HP2020 objective for limiting early formula supplementation (ie, ≤14.2%). Most of the variation in formula supplementation across hospitals was not accounted for by patient characteristics known to affect breastfeeding, such as SES or maternal or infant risk factors. To improve public health breastfeeding outcomes, a better understanding of the hospital, maternal, or community factors contributing to the disparities in formula supplementation is needed.

ABBREVIATIONS

aOR: adjusted odds ratio
CI: confidence interval
HP2020: HealthyPeople 2020
RPC: regional perinatal center
SES: socioeconomic status
Ten Steps: Ten Steps to Successful Breastfeeding

PEDIATRICS (ISSN Numbers: Print, 0031-4005; Online, 1098-4275).

Copyright © 2017 by the American Academy of Pediatrics

FINANCIAL DISCLOSURE: The authors have indicated they have no financial relationships relevant to this article to disclose.

FUNDING: Support for this project was provided by the Robert Wood Johnson Foundation's Public Health Law Research program (grant 12-069) and the New York State Department of Health. These findings do not necessarily represent the views of the funders.

POTENTIAL CONFLICT OF INTEREST: The authors have indicated they have no potential conflicts of interest to disclose.

COMPANION PAPER: A companion to this article can be found online at www.pediatrics.org/cgi/doi/10.1542/peds.2017-0946.

REFERENCES

1. Ip S, Chung M, Raman G, et al. Breastfeeding and maternal and infant health outcomes in developed countries. *Evid Rep Technol Assess (Full Rep)*. 2007;(153):1–186

2. Section on Breastfeeding. Breastfeeding and the use of human milk. *Pediatrics*. 2012;129(3). Available at: www.pediatrics.org/cgi/content/full/129/3/e827

3. World Health Organization. *Evidence for the ten steps to successful breastfeeding*. Geneva, Switzerland: World Health Organization; 1998. Report No.: WHO/CHD/98.9

4. American College of Obstetricians and Gynecologists' Committee on Obstetric Practice; Breastfeeding Expert Work Group. Committee opinion no. 658: optimizing support for breastfeeding as part of obstetric practice. *Obstet Gynecol*. 2016;127(2):e86–e92

5. Baby-Friendly USA. The ten steps to successful breastfeeding. Available at: https://www.babyfriendlyusa. org/about-us/baby-friendly-hospital-initiative/the-ten-steps. Accessed March 20, 2017

6. World Health Organization; UNICEF. *Acceptable medical reasons for use of breast-milk substitutes*. Geneva, Switzerland: World Health Organization; 2009. Report No.: WHO/NMH/NHD/09.01

7. Perrine CG, Galuska DA, Dohack JL, et al. Vital signs: improvements in maternity care policies and practices that support breastfeeding - United States, 2007-2013. *MMWR Morb Mortal Wkly Rep*. 2015;64(39):1112–1117

8. U.S. Department of Health and Human Services, Office of Disease Prevention and Health Promotion. 2020 topics and objectives: maternal, infant, and child health. Health People 2020. Available at: https://www.healthypeople.gov/2020/topics-objectives/topic/maternal-infant-and-child-health/objectives. Accessed February 17, 2016

9. Centers for Disease Control and Prevention. Vital Signs: Hospital Actions Affect Breastfeeding. Available at: www.cdc.gov/vitalsigns/pdf/2015-10-vitalsigns.pdf. Accessed February 17, 2016

10. Centers for Disease Control and Prevention. Breastfeeding Report Card - United States. Available at: www.cdc.gov/breastfeeding/data/reportcard.htm. Accessed March 13, 2017

11. Perrine CG, Scanlon KS, Li R, Odom E, Grummer-Strawn LM. Baby-Friendly hospital practices and meeting exclusive breastfeeding intention. *Pediatrics*. 2012;130(1):54–60

12. Chantry CJ, Dewey KG, Peerson JM, Wagner EA, Nommsen-Rivers LA. In-hospital formula use increases early breastfeeding cessation among first-time mothers intending to exclusively breastfeed. *J Pediatr*. 2014;164(6):1339–1345.e5

13. Declercq E, Labbok MH, Sakala C, O'Hara M. Hospital practices and women's likelihood of fulfilling their intention to exclusively breastfeed. *Am J Public Health*. 2009;99(5):929–935

14. Li R, Grummer-Strawn L. Racial and ethnic disparities in breastfeeding among United States infants: Third National Health and Nutrition Examination Survey, 1988-1994. *Birth*. 2002;29(4):251–257

15. NYS Hospital Profile. Breast Fed Infants Supplemented With Formula. Available at: https://profiles.health.ny.gov/measures/all_state/16543. Accessed March 10, 2017

16. The California WIC Association and the UC Davis Human Lactation Center. One hospital at a time - overcoming barriers to breastfeeding. Available at: www.breastfeedingor.org/wp-content/uploads/2012/10/2011ca_bf_ratereport.pdf. Accessed March 18, 2017

17. New York State Department of Health. New York Codes, Rules and Regulations, Title 10, SubChapter C – State Hospital Code, Article 3 – Hospital Operation, Part 721 – Perinatal Regionalization, Section 721.3 - Perinatal Designation of Hospitals. Available at: https://regs.health.ny.gov/content/section-7213-perinatal-designation-hospitals. Accessed March 20, 2017

18. Rothberg MB, Pekow PS, Priya A, Lindenauer PK. Variation in diagnostic coding of patients with pneumonia and its association with hospital risk-standardized mortality rates: a cross-sectional analysis. *Ann Intern Med*. 2014;160(6):380–388

19. Burnham KP, Anderson DR. *Model Selection and Multimodel Inference: A Practical Information-Theoretic Approach*. New York, NY: Springer Science & Business Media; 2003

20. Merlo J, Chaix B, Ohlsson H, et al. A brief conceptual tutorial of multilevel analysis in social epidemiology: using measures of clustering in multilevel logistic regression to investigate contextual phenomena. *J Epidemiol Community Health*. 2006;60(4):290–297

21. Sebastião YV, Womack L, Vamos CA, et al. Hospital variation in cesarean delivery rates: contribution of individual and hospital factors in Florida. *Am J Obstet Gynecol*. 2016;214(1):123.e1–123.e18

22. Holmes AV, Auinger P, Howard CR. Combination feeding of breast milk and formula: evidence for shorter breast-feeding duration from the National Health and Nutrition Examination Survey. *J Pediatr*. 2011;159(2):186–191

23. Biro MA, Sutherland GA, Yelland JS, Hardy P, Brown SJ. In-hospital formula supplementation of breastfed babies: a population-based survey. *Birth*. 2011;38(4):302–310

24. Parry JE, Ip DKM, Chau PYK, Wu KM, Tarrant M. Predictors and consequences of in-hospital formula supplementation for healthy breastfeeding newborns. *J Hum Lact*. 2013;29(4):527–536

25. Kruse L, Denk CE, Feldman-Winter L, Rotondo FM. Comparing sociodemographic and hospital influences on breastfeeding initiation. *Birth*. 2005;32(2):81–85

26. Gurka KK, Hornsby PP, Drake E, et al. Exploring intended infant feeding decisions among low-income women. *Breastfeed Med*. 2014;9(8):377–384

27. DiGirolamo A, Thompson N, Martorell R, Fein S, Grummer-Strawn L. Intention or experience? Predictors of continued breastfeeding. *Health Educ Behav*. 2005;32(2):208–226

28. Marrone S, Vogeltanz-Holm N, Holm J. Attitudes, knowledge, and intentions related to breastfeeding among university undergraduate women and men. *J Hum Lact*. 2008;24(2):186–192

29. Wojcicki JM, Gugig R, Tran C, Kathiravan S, Holbrook K, Heyman MB. Early exclusive breastfeeding and maternal attitudes towards infant feeding in a population of new mothers in San Francisco, California. *Breastfeed Med*. 2010;5(1):9–15

30. Göksen F. Normative vs. attitudinal considerations in breastfeeding behavior: multifaceted social influences in a developing country context. *Soc Sci Med*. 2002;54(12):1743–1753

31. Braimoh J, Davies L. When 'breast' is no longer 'best': post-partum constructions of infant-feeding in the hospital. *Soc Sci Med*. 2014;123:82–89

32. Rosenberg KD, Eastham CA, Kasehagen LJ, Sandoval AP. Marketing infant formula through hospitals: the impact of commercial hospital discharge packs on breastfeeding. *Am J Public Health*. 2008;98(2):290–295

33. Nelson JM, Perrine CG, Scanlon KS, Li R. Provision of non-breast milk supplements to healthy breastfed newborns in U.S. hospitals, 2009 to 2013. *Matern Child Health J*. 2016;20(11):2228–2232

34. Tender JA, Janakiram J, Arce E, et al. Reasons for in-hospital formula supplementation of breastfed infants from low-income families. *J Hum Lact*. 2009;25(1):11–17

35. Dennison BA, Nguyen TQ, Gregg DJ, Fan W, Xu C. The impact of hospital resources and availability of professional lactation support on maternity care: results of breastfeeding surveys 2009-2014. *Breastfeed Med*. 2016;11(9):479–486

36. Ludington-Hoe SM, McDonald PE, Satyshur R. Breastfeeding in African-American women. *J Natl Black Nurses Assoc*. 2002;13(1):56–64

37. Centers for Disease Control and Prevention (CDC). Progress in increasing breastfeeding and reducing racial/ethnic differences - United States, 2000-2008 births. *MMWR Morb Mortal Wkly Rep*. 2013;62(5):77–80

38. DiGirolamo AM, Grummer-Strawn LM, Fein SB. Effect of maternity-care practices on breastfeeding. *Pediatrics*. 2008;122(Suppl 2):S43-S49

39. McKinney CO, Hahn-Holbrook J, Chase-Lansdale PL, et al; Community Child Health Research Network. Racial and ethnic differences in breastfeeding. *Pediatrics*. 2016;138(2):e20152388

40. Philipp BL, Merewood A, Miller LW, et al. Baby-friendly hospital initiative improves breastfeeding initiation rates in a US hospital setting. *Pediatrics.* 2001;108(3):677–681

41. Merewood A, Philipp BL, Chawla N, Cimo S. The baby-friendly hospital initiative increases breastfeeding rates in a US neonatal intensive care unit. *J Hum Lact.* 2003;19(2):166–171

42. World Health Organization/UNICEF Joint Statement. Ten Steps to Successful Breast-feeding. In: *Protecting, Promoting and Supporting Breast-Feeding: The Special Role of Maternity Services.* Geneva, Switzerland: World Health Organization; 1989

43. World Health Organization. *International Code of Marketing of Breast-milk Substitutes.* Geneva, Switzerland: World Health Organization; 1981

44. Baby-Friendly Hospital Initiative. Baby-friendly USA. Available at: www.babyfriendlyusa.org/about-us/baby-friendly-hospital-initiative. Accessed March 20, 2017

45. Britton C, McCormick FM, Renfrew MJ, Wade A, King SE. Support for breastfeeding mothers. *Cochrane Database Syst Rev.* 2007;(1):CD001141

46. Bartick M, Stuebe A, Shealy KR, Walker M, Grummer-Strawn LM. Closing the quality gap: promoting evidence-based breastfeeding care in the hospital. *Pediatrics.* 2009;124(4). Available at: www.pediatrics.org/cgi/content/full/124/4/e793

47. Chapman DJ, Morel K, Anderson AK, Damio G, Pérez-Escamilla R. Breastfeeding peer counseling: from efficacy through scale-up. *J Hum Lact.* 2010;26(3):314–326

48. Lapping K, Marsh DR, Rosenbaum J, et al. The positive deviance approach: challenges and opportunities for the future. *Food Nutr Bull.* 2002;23(suppl 4):130–137

49. Marsh DR, Schroeder DG. The positive deviance approach to improve health outcomes: experience and evidence from the field. Introduction. *Food Nutr Bull.* 2002;23(suppl 4):5–8

50. Pierre J, Noyes P, Marshall-Taylor S, Srivastava K, Maybank A. *Feeding Our Future: Breastfeeding Realities Among North and Central Brooklyn Women and Their Babies.* New York, NY: Center for Health Equity, New York City Department of Health and Mental Hygiene; 2016

51. Gregg DJ, Dennison BA, Restina K. Breastfeeding-friendly erie county: establishing a baby café network. *J Hum Lact.* 2015;31(4):592–594

52. Morrison B, Ludington-Hoe S. Interruptions to breastfeeding Dyads in an DRP Unit. *MCN Am J Matern Child Nurs.* 2012;37(1):36–41

53. Morrison B, Ludington-Hoe S, Anderson GC. Interruptions to breastfeeding dyads on postpartum day 1 in a university hospital. *J Obstet Gynecol Neonatal Nurs.* 2006;35(6):709–716

54. Holmes AV, McLeod AY, Bunik M. ABM Clinical Protocol #5: peripartum breastfeeding management for the healthy mother and infant at term, revision 2013. *Breastfeed Med.* 2013;8(6):469–473

55. Reichman NE, Hade EM. Validation of birth certificate data. A study of women in New Jersey's HealthStart program. *Ann Epidemiol.* 2001;11(3):186–193

56. Hasnain-Wynia R, Baker DW. Obtaining data on patient race, ethnicity, and primary language in health care organizations: current challenges and proposed solutions. *Health Serv Res.* 2006;41(4 pt 1):1501–1518

Fathers, Coparenting, and Breastfeeding

Investigators from Toronto studied the effect of a coparenting breastfeeding support intervention on breastfeeding rates. Mothers were recruited from a teaching hospital within their first 2 days postpartum and were eligible if they were primiparous, ≥18 years old, English-speaking, planning to breastfeed for >12 weeks, living with a male partner who could participate in the study, and had delivered a healthy singleton infant at ≥37 weeks' gestation. Couples were randomized to receive either usual care or a coparenting breastfeeding support intervention. Usual care consisted of standard in-hospital breastfeeding support and any breastfeeding assistance that was proactively sought in the community. The coparenting intervention included both parents and involved a 15 minute in hospital discussion, a video, a workbook, a breastfeeding booklet, access to a secure study website, 2 follow-up emails, and 1 telephone call.

The primary study outcomes were exclusive breastfeeding and continuation of breastfeeding assessed at 6 and 12 weeks postpartum. Secondary outcomes included maternal satisfaction with their partner's involvement with breastfeeding, maternal perception of the coparenting relationship as measured by the Coparenting Relationship Scale at 12 weeks, and maternal perception of breastfeeding support from their partner as measured by the Postpartum Partner Support Scale at 6 and 12 weeks. Also, paternal breastfeeding confidence was measured by the Breastfeeding Self-Efficacy Scale at birth and 6 weeks and paternal attitude towards breastfeeding was measured by the Iowa Infant Attitude Scale at birth and 6 weeks.

There were 107 couples in the control group and 107 in the intervention group. Significantly more mothers in the intervention group than the control group continued to breastfeed at 12 weeks postpartum (96% vs 88%, $P = .02$). There were no significant differences in breastfeeding rates at 6 weeks nor in exclusive breastfeeding rates at 6 and 12 weeks. There were no significant differences between groups with regard to maternal perception of the coparenting relationship, maternal perception of support, or paternal infant feeding attitude. Fathers in the intervention group had a significantly greater increase in breastfeeding self-efficacy scores from baseline to 6 weeks postpartum compared with fathers in the control group ($P = .03$). In addition, significantly more mothers in the intervention group than in the control group reported that their partners provided them with breastfeeding help in the first 6 weeks (71% vs 52%, $P = .02$) and that they were satisfied with their partners' involvement with breastfeeding (89% vs 78%, $P = .04$).

The authors conclude that including fathers in a coparenting breastfeeding support intervention may have a beneficial effect for first-time parents.

Source: *Abbass-Dick J, Stern SB, Nelson LE, et al. Coparenting breastfeeding support and exclusive breastfeeding: a randomized controlled trial. Pediatrics. 2015; 135(1): 102– 110; doi:10.1542/peds.2014-1416*

COMMENTARY

Lawrence M. Noble, MD, FAAP,
Elmhurst, NY

Dr Noble has disclosed no financial relationship relevant to this commentary. This commentary does not contain a discussion of an unapproved/investigative use of a commercial product/device.

This study confirms the importance of coparenting interventions for new parents. Coparenting aims for more cooperative and supportive teamwork between parents by teaching effective communication, problem solving, and conflict resolution. For instance, in a recently published study, a brief coparenting intervention was shown to positively affect family relationships and decrease maternal stress.[1] The present study shows that a coparenting intervention may increase breastfeeding.

This study also adds to the growing literature demonstrating that including fathers in breastfeeding interventions increases breastfeeding rates.[2] In reality, most breastfeeding interventions are designed exclusively for mothers. Most new fathers report being ignored by or having a negative experience with postpartum nurses.[3] A recent study revealed that fathers often felt helpless to support their partner, as they were excluded from antenatal breastfeeding education and postnatal support.[4] Fathers wanted more information about breastfeeding to be directed towards them as well as ideas about how they could practically support their partner. Without paternal breastfeeding interventions, fathers may feel that breastfeeding excludes them and continues the exclusive relationship that the mother and infant experienced during pregnancy.

A limitation of this current study is that it measured a multifaceted intervention. Therefore, it is not possible to ascertain which specific components of the intervention (ie, the discussion, video, workbook, booklet, website, emails, or telephone call) were responsible for the increased breastfeeding duration.

We also cannot measure whether the improvement was related to coparenting education, breastfeeding education, or paternal involvement in breastfeeding. Nevertheless, the results of this study suggest that a relatively simple intervention combining support of coparenting and breastfeeding could be effective. If further studies confirm these results, this could be a simple but effective method to improve parenting and breastfeeding.

REFERENCES

1. Doss DB, et al. J Fam Psychol. 2014;28(4):483–494; doi:10.1037/a0037311
2. Maycock B, et al. J Hum Lact. 2013;29(4):484–490; doi:10.1177/0890334413484387
3. de Montigny F, et al. J Obstet Gynecol Neonatal Nurs. 2004;33(3):328–339; doi:10.1177/0884217504266012
4. Brown A, et al. Matern Child Nutr. 2014;10(4):510–526; doi:10.1111/mcn.12129

Coparenting Breastfeeding Support and Exclusive Breastfeeding: A Randomized Controlled Trial

Jennifer Abbass-Dick, PhD[a], Susan B. Stern, PhD[b], LaRon E. Nelson, PhD[c], William Watson, MD[d], Cindy-Lee Dennis, PhD[e,f]

abstract

OBJECTIVE: To evaluate the effectiveness of a coparenting intervention on exclusive breastfeeding among primiparous mothers and fathers.

METHODS: A randomized controlled trial was conducted in a large teaching hospital in Toronto, Canada. Couples were randomized to receive either usual care ($n = 107$) or a coparenting breastfeeding support intervention ($n = 107$). Follow-up of exclusive breastfeeding and diverse secondary outcomes was conducted at 6 and 12 weeks postpartum.

RESULTS: Significantly more mothers in the intervention group than in the control group continued to breastfeed at 12 weeks postpartum (96.2% vs 87.6%, $P = .02$). Although proportionately more mothers in the intervention group were exclusively breastfeeding at 6 and 12 weeks, these differences were not significant. Fathers in the intervention group had a significantly greater increase in breastfeeding self-efficacy scores from baseline to 6 weeks postpartum compared with fathers in the control group ($P = .03$). In addition, significantly more mothers in the intervention group than in the control group reported that their partners provided them with breastfeeding help in the first 6 weeks (71% vs 52%, $P = .02$) and that they were satisfied with their partners' involvement with breastfeeding (89% vs 78.1%, $P = .04$). Mothers in the intervention group were also more satisfied with the breastfeeding information they received (81% vs 62.5%, $P < .001$).

CONCLUSIONS: The significant improvements in breastfeeding duration, paternal breastfeeding self-efficacy, and maternal perceptions of paternal involvement and assistance with breastfeeding suggest that a coparenting intervention involving fathers warrants additional investigation.

WHAT'S KNOWN ON THIS SUBJECT: Fathers' attitude and support affects breastfeeding outcomes. Fathers are currently not targeted in breastfeeding support and care provided by health care professionals. Breastfeeding interventions delivered to fathers have been shown to increase breastfeeding exclusivity and duration.

WHAT THIS STUDY ADDS: A coparenting breastfeeding support intervention delivered to mothers and fathers in the postpartum period showed beneficial effects on breastfeeding duration, paternal breastfeeding confidence, breastfeeding help provided by fathers, and mothers' satisfaction with fathers' involvement with breastfeeding.

[a]Faculty of Health Sciences, University of Ontario Institute of Technology, Oshawa, Ontario, Canada; [b]Factor-Inwentash Faculty of Social Work, [d]Department of Family and Community Medicine, [e]Perinatal Community Health, [f]Women's College Research Institute, University of Toronto, Toronto, Ontario, Canada; and [c]School of Nursing, University of Rochester, Rochester, New York

Dr Abbass-Dick conceptualized and designed the study, collected and analyzed data, and drafted the initial manuscript; Drs Stern, Nelson, and Watson were consulted throughout all phases of study completion and reviewed the manuscript; Dr Dennis supervised all elements of the study, including the conceptualization and design of the study and data analysis, and reviewed and revised the manuscript; and all authors approved the final manuscript as submitted.

This trial has been registered at www.clinicaltrials.gov (identifier NCT01536119).

www.pediatrics.org/cgi/doi/10.1542/peds.2014-1416

DOI: 10.1542/peds.2014-1416

Accepted for publication Oct 9, 2014

Address correspondence to Jennifer Abbass-Dick, PhD, Faculty of Health Sciences, University of Ontario Institute of Technology, 2000 Simcoe St North, Oshawa, Ontario, Canada, L1H 7K4. E-mail: jennifer.abbassdick@uoit.ca

PEDIATRICS (ISSN Numbers: Print, 0031-4005; Online, 1098-4275).

ARTICLE

All leading health authorities recommend that infants be exclusively breastfed for the first 6 months of life[1-3] because of the well-documented health-promoting and disease-preventing effects for both infants and mothers.[4] Despite this recommendation, North American breastfeeding rates are suboptimal.[5-7] The reasons for these poor breastfeeding outcomes are multifaceted and include demographic, biologic, psychosocial, and social factors.[8,9] To address this long-standing clinical issue, effective interventions that target modifiable risk factors for the premature discontinuation of breastfeeding are needed, and 1 such modifiable factor that has not been sufficiently examined is partner support for breastfeeding.[10,11]

Fathers' attitude and support for breastfeeding have consistently been found to positively or negatively affect maternal infant feeding intentions[12-15] and breastfeeding initiation,[16-19] duration,[14,20-24] and exclusivity rates.[25-27] This research highlights the importance of fathers in improving breastfeeding outcomes. Fathers are in an ideal position to assist breastfeeding mothers, with qualitative research indicating they also want to be involved and often feel ignored.[28,29] However, to date little is known about how best to include fathers in improving breastfeeding outcomes because few studies have incorporated them in breastfeeding support interventions.[24-27] Four studies have evaluated breastfeeding interventions with fathers and found positive breastfeeding outcomes. In a study conducted in Italy ($N = 280$), the mothers who had partners that received education and printed material about breastfeeding had significantly higher rates of exclusive breastfeeding at 6 months postpartum than those in the control group (25% vs 15%; $P < .05$).[25] In a Brazilian study ($N = 586$), mothers

and fathers who received education about breastfeeding had a significantly higher rate of exclusive breastfeeding at 16 weeks (16.4%) compared with the mother-only group (11.1%) and the control group (5.7%, $P < .00$) and a lower risk of discontinuing exclusive breastfeeding before 24 weeks.[26] In another study ($N = 492$), Vietnamese fathers who received breastfeeding education, materials, and professional support had partners who had significantly higher exclusive breastfeeding rates at 4 (20.6% vs 11.3%, $P = .006$) and 6 ($n = 16$, 6.7% vs $n = 2$, 0.9%; $P = .001$) months compared with those in the control group.[27] Lastly, in an Australian randomized controlled trial ($N = 699$) that evaluated the effects of an antenatal breastfeeding session and postpartum support provided to fathers, the rate of any breastfeeding at 6 weeks was significantly higher in the intervention group (81.6%) than the control group (75.2%).[24]

These studies together provide preliminary evidence that the inclusion of fathers in breastfeeding interventions may improve breastfeeding outcomes; however, all studies were atheoretical, and none specifically evaluated the effect of coparenting breastfeeding support. Coparenting refers to the manner in which parents worked together to achieve their parenting and child health goals.[30] It consists of 4 elements: jointly determined goals, coparenting support, joint parental involvement, and fair division of labor.[30] The core skills for effective coparenting consist of effective communication, problem solving, and conflict resolution.[31] Coparenting has been previously shown to positively affect family relationships and emotional well-being,[31] so it is hypothesized that teaching couples about coparenting may also be effective in improving breastfeeding outcomes. The purpose of this trial was to evaluate the effect of a coparenting breastfeeding support

intervention on exclusive breastfeeding among primiparous mothers and fathers. We hypothesized that among couples who received the multicomponent coparenting intervention, mothers would have increased breastfeed duration and exclusivity rates and be more satisfied with the support and assistance received from their partner than mothers who did not receive the intervention.

METHODS

Participants

Participants were recruited from a large teaching hospital in Toronto, Canada between March and July 2012. The hospital has >6000 deliveries a year and provides services to a culturally and economically diverse population. Eligible women were all primiparous mothers in the first 2 days postpartum who had a singleton birth and were ≥18 years old, ≥37 weeks' gestation at delivery, able to speak and read English, and living with a male partner. Women were excluded if they shared a hospital room with a current study participant, had a medical problem that could interfere with breastfeeding, had an infant who would not be discharged from the hospital with them, did not have access to the Internet or a telephone, were planning to breastfeed <12 weeks, and had a partner who would not be available to participate in the study.

Design and Procedure

A randomized controlled trial was conducted (Fig 1) after ethics approval was obtained from both the University of Toronto and the North York General Hospital. Eligible and consenting couples were provided with a detailed trial description. After informed consent procedures were completed, baseline data were collected and couples were randomly assigned to either a control group or

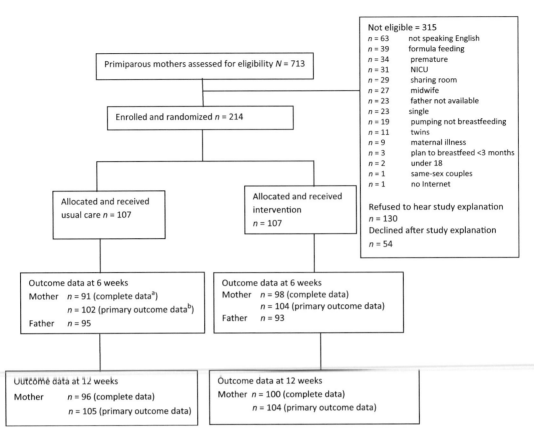

Primiparous mothers assessed for eligibility *N* = 713

Not eligible = 315
n = 63   not speaking English
n = 39   formula feeding
n = 34   premature
n = 31   NICU
n = 29   sharing room
n = 27   midwife
n = 23   father not available
n = 23   single
n = 19   pumping not breastfeeding
n = 11   twins
n = 9   maternal illness
n = 3   plan to breastfeed <3 months
n = 2   under 18
n = 1   same-sex couples
n = 1   no Internet

Refused to hear study explanation
n = 130
Declined after study explanation
n = 54

Enrolled and randomized *n* = 214

Allocated and received usual care *n* = 107

Allocated and received intervention *n* = 107

Outcome data at 6 weeks
Mother   *n* = 91 (complete data[a])
      n = 102 (primary outcome data[b])
Father   *n* = 95

Outcome data at 6 weeks
Mother   *n* = 98 (complete data)
      n = 104 (primary outcome data)
Father   *n* = 93

Outcome data at 12 weeks
Mother   *n* = 96 (complete data)
      n = 105 (primary outcome data)

Outcome data at 12 weeks
Mother *n* = 100 (complete data)
      n = 104 (primary outcome data)

FIGURE 1
Participant flowchart. [a] Mothers completed all follow-up data questionnaires. [b] Mothers provided only information on infant feeding (duration and exclusivity).

an intervention group by sequentially numbered, sealed, opaque envelopes containing randomly generated numbers. These envelopes were constructed by a research assistant who was not involved in any other trial procedure. Couples assigned to the control group received usual care, which included standard in-hospital breastfeeding support and any breastfeeding assistance that was proactively sought in the community. Couples allocated to the intervention group also had access to usual care, in addition to receiving the coparenting breastfeeding support intervention. Follow-up data were collected from mothers and fathers at 6 weeks postpartum and mothers at 12 weeks postpartum via a self-report web-based questionnaire or a telephone interview conducted by a trained research assistant blinded to group allocation. The method of follow-up was determined by participant preference.

Intervention

The trial intervention was a multifaceted coparenting breastfeeding support intervention (Table 1). The intervention was provided face to face on the postpartum unit, at which time the couples were provided with breastfeeding information, the information package was reviewed, and couples were given the option of watching the video. The session took ~15 min in the majority of cases. The couples were followed up at home with e-mails at 1 and 3 weeks postpartum and a telephone call at 2 weeks postpartum. A coparenting workbook, video, and Web site were developed by the first author and contained extensive information on breastfeeding and coparenting. The intervention was adapted from a previous coparenting intervention trial that evaluated the effects of coparenting on the parental

relationship, parental mental health, the parent–child relationship, and infant emotional and physiologic regulation.[31] The elements included in the coparenting breastfeeding support intervention were designed to help couples work cooperatively toward meeting their jointly determined child health outcomes. The intervention was piloted with 10 couples, and slight modifications were made based on maternal and paternal feedback. For example, the in-hospital viewing of the video was often rushed or interrupted, and so couples were given the option of watching the video in the hospital, and they were provided with a copy to view at home.

Outcome Measures

Baseline Demographic Variables

All participants completed a baseline questionnaire before randomization that included demographic,

TABLE 1 Intervention Components

Component	Description
In-hospital discussion	A 15-min discussion with a lactation specialist to review the intervention information package and discuss how breastfeeding works, how fathers can assist breastfeeding mothers, and where to get breastfeeding help in the community
Coparenting booklet	A take-home booklet that included activities for couples to complete and covered the elements and skills of coparenting
Breastfeeding booklet	A take-home breastfeeding booklet, developed by Best Start: Ontario's Maternal, Newborn and Early Child Development Resource Centre[39]
Video	An 11-min coparenting and breastfeeding video that provided information on coparenting and breastfeeding and showed scenarios of couples working as coparents to achieve their breastfeeding goals
Web site	Access to a secure study Web site that consisted of extensive information on breastfeeding and coparenting and contained links to related information and resources on the Internet
E-mails	Follow-up e-mails to each parent at 1 and 3 wk postpartum, designed to assist the couples in navigating through the intervention information package and serve as a reminder of the resources provided
Telephone call	A telephone call made to the mother at 2 wk postpartum to answer any questions or concerns about the information provided

breastfeeding, and delivery variables such as age, ethnicity, educational status, income, paternal employment, breastfeeding intentions, breastfeeding self-efficacy, prenatal education, mode of delivery, and in-hospital infant feeding.

Exclusive Breastfeeding

The primary outcome for this trial was exclusive breastfeeding, defined as no food or liquid other than breast milk given to the infant in the last 24 hours and included feeding expressed breast milk and undiluted drops or syrups consisting of vitamins, minerals, supplements, or medicines.[32,33] Exclusive breastfeeding was assessed in hospital and at 6 and 12 weeks postpartum.

Breastfeeding Duration

A secondary outcome for this trial was breastfeeding duration, defined as the infant receiving any breast milk in the past 24 hours. Breastfeeding duration was assessed at 6 and 12 weeks postpartum and included

questions about frequency of breast milk feeds and the quantity of formula fed.

Maternal Perception of the Coparenting Relationship

We assessed this outcome at 12 weeks postpartum by using the Coparenting Relationship Scale (CRS), a 35-item self-report instrument.[34] This scale was developed to assess the elements of coparenting, which include jointly determined goals, coparenting support, joint parental involvement, and fair division of labor. Items are rated on a 7-point scale to produce a summative score ranging from 0 to 210, with higher scores indicating higher degrees of positive coparenting. The CRS was developed based on exploratory and confirmatory factor analysis and established reliability and validity with mothers and fathers.[34] For this trial the Cronbach's α was .94. At baseline and at 6 weeks postpartum the Brief CRS was used to reduce participant burden. This scale has 14 items, and the total score ranges from

0 to 84.[34] For this trial the Cronbach's α ranged from .73 to .88.

Maternal Perceptions of Breastfeeding Support

We assessed this outcome at 6 and 12 weeks postpartum by using the Postpartum Partner Support Scale, a 25-item self-report instrument designed to assess partner postpartum-specific perceptions of support. Items are rated on a 4-point scale to produce a summative score ranging from 25 to 100, with higher scores indicating higher levels of postpartum-specific partner support. This measure has been used with postpartum women and has good reliability and validity.[35,36] The Cronbach's α for this trial ranged from .95 to .97.

Paternal Breastfeeding Self-Efficacy

We assessed this outcome at baseline and at 6 weeks postpartum by using an adapted version of the Breastfeeding Self-Efficacy Scale–Short Form (BSES-SF).[36] The BSES-SF is a 14-item self-report instrument designed to assess maternal breastfeeding self-efficacy, defined as a mother's confidence in her ability to breastfeed her infant. Paternal breastfeeding self-efficacy was defined as the father's confidence in his ability to assist the mother with breastfeeding. Items were reworded to capture the father's role in assisting the breastfeeding mother. Items were rated on a 5-point scale to produce a summative score ranging from 14 to 70, with higher scores indicating higher levels of breastfeeding self-efficacy. Although this scale has not been used with fathers before, it has well-established reliability and validity in maternal populations.[37] The Cronbach's α for this trial was .90 for mothers and ranged from .91 to .92 for fathers.

Paternal Infant Feeding Attitude

We assessed this outcome at baseline and 6 weeks postpartum by using the Iowa Infant Feeding Attitude Scale, a 17-item self-report instrument.[38] This scale was developed to assess attitudes toward various dimensions of infant feeding. Items were rated on a 5-point scale to produce a summative score ranging from 17 to 85, with lower scores reflecting a preference for formula feeding and higher scores reflecting a preference for breastfeeding. This measure has been used postpartum, has well-established reliability and validity,[38] and has previously been used with fathers.[17] The Cronbach's α in this study ranged from .55 at baseline to .72 at 6 weeks postpartum.

Intervention Use

Among couples randomly assigned to the intervention group, use of the intervention materials (eg, coparenting workbook, breastfeeding book, coparenting video, Web site, and e-mails) was assessed at 6 weeks with both mothers and fathers and at 12 weeks among mothers only in the intervention group. Couples were asked to indicate the degree to which they had used the intervention components over the previous 6 weeks, and the items were rated on a 4-point scale that ranged from "I used the resource frequently" to "I was not interested in using the resource."

Maternal Breastfeeding Support

This outcome was assessed at 6 and 12 weeks. Mothers were asked to identify individuals (both professional and lay) who supported

their breastfeeding and the frequency with which the support was provided. Overall satisfaction with breastfeeding supports such as the breastfeeding information received and partner's involvement with breastfeeding was measured on a 5-point scale ranging from dissatisfied to satisfied.

Data Analysis

A sample size of 214 couples (107 per study group) was needed at 80% power and a 2-tailed error of .05 to detect a 15% difference in breastfeeding exclusivity at 12 weeks postpartum between groups, with a 25% attrition rate. Local health professionals were consulted and indicated that a 15% increase in breastfeeding exclusivity rates would warrant implementing this intervention in a practice setting. We analyzed data with SPSS version 21 (IBM SPSS Statistics, IBM Corporation) by using an intention-to-treat approach. A 2-sided significant level of .05 was used for all study outcomes. For dichotomous data, the frequencies and percentages were calculated and differences between groups examined using Pearson χ^2 tests, supplemented where necessary by Fisher exact test. Relative risks and corresponding 95% confidence intervals were estimated. For continuous data, means and SDs were calculated, and differences between groups were examined with independent 2-sample t tests and Mann–Whitney U tests as

appropriate. One-way repeated-measures analysis of variance were conducted to assess group differences in mean scores over time.

RESULTS

Participant Characteristics

Of the 713 primiparous mothers screened, 315 (44.2%) were ineligible (Fig 1). Of the 398 potentially eligible mothers, 130 (32.7%) declined to hear a detailed study explanation. Of the 268 mothers who heard a detailed explanation, 54 (20.1%) declined participation. The most common reason for declining was not interested (n = 43, 79.6%). Overall, 53.8% of eligible mothers agreed to trial participation, representing 79.9% of those who received a detailed explanation. The majority of mothers and fathers were married, had some university education, were born outside Canada, had an annual household income >$60 000, and planned to exclusively breastfeed for 6 months (Table 2).

There were no significant differences in baseline characteristics between the groups except for prenatal education. In particular, more couples in the intervention group than in the control group attended a prenatal class (n = 74, 69.2% compared with n = 57, 53.3%). However, there was no significant difference between the 2 groups in attendance at a prenatal breastfeeding class (n = 43, 40.2% vs n = 41, 38.1%).

TABLE 2 Demographic Characteristics

Demographics	Maternal Data			Paternal Data		
	Intervention (n = 107), n (%)	Control (n = 107), n (%)	P	Intervention (n = 107), n (%)	Control (n = 107), n (%)	P
Age, y	Mean 30.4 (SD 3.7)	Mean 30.7 (SD 3.8)	.60	Mean 33 (SD 5.2)	Mean 33 (SD 5.5)	.51
≥30 y	62 (57.9)	68 (63.5)	.40	85 (79.4)	85 (79.4)	.99
Born in Canada	37 (34.6)	40 (37.5)	.67	38 (35.5)	34 (31.8)	.56
Attended university	78 (72.9)	78 (72.9)	1.0	79 (73.8)	69 (64.4)	.14
Plan to exclusively breastfeed	95 (88.8)	95 (88.8)	1.0	75 (70.1)	76 (71)	.88
Plan to exclusively breastfeed >6 mo	75 (70.1)	65 (60.7)	.15	57 (53.3)	61 (57)	.58
Married	98 (91.6)	94 (87.9)	.37	98 (91.6)	94 (87.9)	.37
Annual household income >$60 000	87 (81.3)	77 (72.0)	.13	87 (81.3)	77 (72.0)	.13
Employed				103 (96.3)	98 (91.6)	.15

Complete follow-up data were collected from 87.9% (*n* = 188) of fathers at 6 weeks and 88.3% (*n* = 189) of mothers at 6 weeks and 91.6% (*n* = 196) at 12 weeks. No differences were found between those who were lost to follow-up and those for whom outcome data were collected.

Intervention Details

The coparenting intervention was delivered to all of the 107 couples randomly assigned to the intervention group. In the majority of cases (*n* = 104, 97.2%), both mothers and fathers were present for the in-hospital discussion, at which time the information package was explained. Of the 3 fathers who were not present for the in-hospital discussion, 1 reviewed the information package at home, resulting in 105 (98%) fathers receiving a portion of the intervention. All mothers were present for the in-hospital discussion, and 98 (98%) of the mothers indicated at follow-up that they had reviewed the intervention package at home.

Outcomes

More mothers in the intervention group (*n* = 102, 98.1%) were practicing any breastfeeding at 6 weeks compared with those in the control group (*n* = 94, 92.2%); however, these differences were not statistically significant (*P* = .06). Similarly, more mothers in the intervention group (*n* = 75, 72.1%) were exclusively breastfeeding than in the control group (*n* = 62, 60.8%), yet the 11% difference was not statistically significant (*P* = .09). At 12 weeks, significantly more women in the intervention group (*n* = 100, 96.2%) were breastfeeding than in the control group (*n* = 92, 87.6%; *P* = .02). Although more mothers in the intervention group (*n* = 70, 67.3%) were exclusively breastfeeding than in the control group (*n* = 63, 60.0%), this 7% difference was not statistically significant (*P* = .27). Table 3 shows the differences in formula

supplementation of breastfed infants between the 2 groups.

Table 4 shows the mean scores related to secondary outcomes at 6 and 12 weeks postpartum. Although there were no significant differences between groups in maternal perception of the coparenting relationship, maternal perception of support, paternal breastfeeding self-efficacy, or paternal infant feeding attitude, all mean scores were higher for the intervention group than for the control group. When group differences in mean paternal breastfeeding self-efficacy scores were examined over time, there was a significantly greater increase over the first 6 weeks postpartum in mean BSES-SF scores in the intervention group compared with the control group (*P* = .03). Additionally, significantly more mothers in the intervention group (*n* = 76, 71%) than in the control group (*n* = 56, 52%) reported receiving help from their partners in the first 6 weeks postpartum (*P* = .02). When asked to rate their overall satisfaction with their breastfeeding support received, significantly more mothers in the intervention group (*n* = 89, 89%) than the control group (*n* = 75, 78.1%) were satisfied with their partners' involvement with breastfeeding (*P* = .04) and with the breastfeeding information they received (*n* = 81, 81% vs *n* = 60, 62.5%; *P* < .001).

DISCUSSION

The purpose of this randomized controlled trial was to evaluate the effect of a coparenting intervention on

breastfeeding outcomes among primiparous mothers and fathers. Overall, the coparenting intervention increased breastfeeding duration rates by ~9% at 12 weeks. The breastfeeding duration rate at 6 weeks postpartum and exclusivity rates at 6 weeks and at 12 weeks postpartum were higher for mothers in the intervention group compared with the control group, but these differences were not statistically significant. There was significantly greater improvement in paternal breastfeeding self-efficacy over the first 6 weeks postpartum in the intervention group than in the control group. Furthermore, significantly more mothers in the intervention group compared with the control group received breastfeeding help from the fathers in the first 6 weeks and were satisfied with the fathers' involvement with breastfeeding and the breastfeeding information they received. These research findings suggest that including fathers in a coparenting breastfeeding support intervention may have a potential beneficial effect for first-time mothers and fathers and warrants additional investigation.

The increase in exclusive breastfeeding rates among mothers in the intervention group is consistent with previous studies. For example, Pisacane et al,[25] Susin and Giugliani,[26] and Bich et al[27] found that the inclusion of fathers in the breastfeeding interventions increased exclusive breastfeeding at 16[26,27] and 24[25,27] weeks. These studies measured their outcomes at a later time point, and it is possible that we measured the outcome too early to

TABLE 3 Differences in Quantity of Formula Supplementation Between Groups at 6 and 12 Weeks

Quantity of Formula Supplementation	Control Group, n (%)		Intervention Group, n (%)	
	6 Wk (n = 91)	12 Wk (n = 97)	6 Wk (n = 98)	12 Wk (n = 101)
More than half of the feeds	8 (7.5)	3 (2.8)	6 (5.6)	11 (10.3)
Half of the feeds	8 (7.5)	5 (4.7)	3 (2.8)	4 (3.7)
Less than half of the feeds	8 (7.5)	10 (9.3)	8 (7.5)	4 (3.7)
1 time per day	5 (4.7)	5 (4.7)	5 (4.7)	5 (4.7)
≥1 time per week	4 (3.7)	3 (2.8)	3 (2.8)	4 (3.7)
<1 time per week	0	1 (0.9)	0	1 (0.9)

TABLE 4 Secondary Outcomes

Secondary Outcome	Measure	Time	Intervention Group, Mean (SD)	Control Group, Mean (SD)	P
Coparenting relationship	Brief CRS	Baseline (*n* = 214)	75.1 (7.9)	75. 5 (7.3)	.78[a]
		6 wk (*n* = 189)	73.01 (9.8)	71.3 (10.6)	.25[b]
		12 wk (*n* = 196)	72.4 (11.2)	71.1 (12.2)	.64[b]
	CRS	12 wk (*n* = 196)	179.9 (27.4)	174.93 (27.4)	.29[b]
Partner support	Postpartum Partner Support Scale	6 wk (*n* = 189)	88.0 (10.9)	85.6 (10.5)	.12[a]
		12 wk (*n* = 196)	86.6 (11.7)	83.6 (14.4)	.21[b]
Paternal breastfeeding self-efficacy	Paternal BSES-SF	Baseline (*n* = 214)	48.5 (9.7)	49.5 (9.9)	.46[a]
		6 wk[c] (*n* = 173)	55.9 (8.4)	53.1 (11.2)	.06[a]
Paternal infant feeding attitude	Paternal Iowa Infant Feeding Attitude Scale	Baseline (*n* = 214)	61.4 (5.9)	61.1 (6.0)	.70[a]
		6 wk (*n* = 188)	62.1 (8.1)	61.2 (6.7)	.43[a]

[a] 2-sided independent *t* test.
[b] Mann–Whitney *U* test.
[c] Paternal BSES-SF: fathers who had infants being breastfed at 6 wk (intervention group *n* = 87, control group *n* = 86).

detect a significant difference in exclusive breastfeeding between our study groups. Unfortunately, in our trial the sample was highly motivated to breastfeed, and the exclusive breastfeeding rates in both groups was higher than the national breastfeeding exclusivity rate of 51.7%[5] at 3 months postpartum.

More mothers in the intervention group than in the control group continued to breastfeed to 12 weeks postpartum, suggesting that the intervention helped couples work together as coparents to meet their breastfeeding goals and to overcome breastfeeding challenges. This finding is consistent with the randomized controlled trial conducted by Maycock et al,[24] who found that the inclusion of fathers in a breastfeeding intervention increased breastfeeding duration at 6 weeks postpartum, and Pisacane et al,[25] who found that significantly fewer mothers in the intervention group stopped breastfeeding because they experienced problems.

For both groups, paternal breastfeeding self-efficacy levels increased over time from baseline to 6 weeks postpartum, with greater increases found among those who received the coparenting intervention. This self-efficacy finding suggests the intervention may have a potential beneficial effect for first-time fathers. The fathers in the intervention group were provided

with support and detailed information about how they could be involved with breastfeeding. These fathers indicated that the information was very helpful and that they particularly enjoyed the in-hospital discussion. This finding is noteworthy because fathers are often not targeted and included in breastfeeding support programs. The high follow-up rate with fathers in both groups (*n* = 188, 87.9%) also indicates they valued being involved and having an opportunity to share their experiences in the postpartum period.

There are numerous strengths of this trial. A power analysis was included to determine the sample size, and data were analyzed using an intention-to-treat approach. The trial incorporated randomized procedures, and sequentially numbered, sealed, opaque envelopes were used to determine group allocation. Attrition was low, and no differences were found between those who were lost to follow-up and those for whom outcome data were collected. The web-based questionnaire was an effective means of collecting follow-up data from mothers and fathers during the postpartum period, and 96.7% (*n* = 557) of participant surveys were completed online. Finally, the sample was multicultural, with less than half of the population born in Canada.

Despite these strengths, the sample was highly motivated to breastfeed. The mothers in both groups were

committed to breastfeeding and to doing so exclusively, which limited the variability and decreased our ability to detect differences. The enrollment rate of potentially eligible mothers may have added selection bias. The intervention package was provided in the postpartum period, and this may have limited the time parents had available to review the information. The intervention was also multifaceted, with materials provided to the couple in a variety of formats. Therefore, it is not known which specific component of the intervention was related to the increased breastfeeding duration or paternal breastfeeding self-efficacy.

CONCLUSIONS

The coparenting intervention increased breastfeeding duration rates by 9% at 12 weeks. The improvement in paternal breastfeeding self-efficacy and maternal perceptions of paternal involvement and assistance indicate that coparenting breastfeeding support programs may be beneficial for fathers as well as mothers. Although not all outcomes were statistically different between study groups, the numerous positive trends favoring the intervention group in relation to breastfeeding duration and exclusivity, as well as higher mean scores on outcome measures, may indicate the coparenting intervention has clinical importance. Although this study adds to the literature on the effectiveness of including fathers in breastfeeding interventions, additional research is warranted. Future studies should be conducted with more vulnerable couples, in multiple sites, and the intervention should be delivered over the prenatal and postnatal period to allow couples sufficient time to review the coparenting and breastfeeding material.

FINANCIAL DISCLOSURE: The authors have indicated they have no financial relationships relevant to this article to disclose.

FUNDING: Partial funding for this project was received from the Canadian Institutes of Health Research, Canada Research Chair Program.

POTENTIAL CONFLICT OF INTEREST: The authors have indicated they have no potential conflicts of interest to disclose.

REFERENCES

1. American Academy of Pediatrics. Policy statement: breastfeeding and the use of human milk. *Pediatrics.* 2012;129(3). Available at: www.pediatrics.org/cgi/content/full/129/3/e827

2. World Health Organization. The optimal duration of exclusive breastfeeding: report of an expert consultation. 2002. Available at: http://whqlibdoc.who.int/hq/2001/WHO_NHD_01.09.pdf. Accessed January 30, 2009

3. Health Canada. Exclusive breastfeeding duration: 2004 Health Canada recommendations. 2004. Available at: www.hc-sc.gc.ca/fn-an/nutrition/child-enfant/infant-nourisson/excl_bf_dur-dur_am_excl-eng.php. Accessed January 7, 2009

4. Bartick M, Reinhold A. The burden of suboptimal breastfeeding in the United States: a pediatric cost analysis. *Pediatrics.* 2010;125(5). Available at: www.pediatrics.org/cgi/content/full/125/5/e1048

5. Public Health Agency of Canada. What mothers say, the Canadian Maternity Experiences Survey. 2011. Available at: www.phac-aspc.gc.ca/rhs-ssg/pdf/survey-eng.pdf. Accessed January 10, 2012

6. Gionet L. Breastfeeding trends in Canada. 2013. Available at: www.statcan.gc.ca/pub/82-624-x/2013001/article/11879-eng.htm#a1. Accessed April 2, 2014

7. Centers for Disease Control and Prevention. Breastfeeding report card 2013. 2013. Available at: www.cdc.gov/breastfeeding/pdf/2013BreastfeedingReportCard.pdf. Accessed October 25, 2013

8. Thulier D, Mercer J. Variables associated with breastfeeding duration. *J Obstet Gynecol Neonatal Nurs.* 2009;38(3):259–268

9. Dennis C-L. Breastfeeding initiation and duration: a 1990–2000 literature review. *J Obstet Gynecol Neonatal Nurs.* 2002;31(1):12–32

10. Renfrew MJ, McCormick FM, Wade A, Quinn B, Dowswell T. Support for healthy breastfeeding mothers with healthy term babies. *Cochrane Database Syst Rev.* 2012;5:CD001141

11. Chung M, Raman G, Trikalinos T, Lau J, Ip S. Interventions in primary care to promote breastfeeding: an evidence review for the U.S. Preventive Services Task Force. *Ann Intern Med.* 2008;149(8):565–582

12. Bar-Yam NB, Darby L. Fathers and breastfeeding: a review of the literature. *J Hum Lact.* 1997;13(1):45–50

13. Nelson AM. A metasynthesis of qualitative breastfeeding studies. *J Midwifery Womens Health.* 2006;51(2):e13–e20

14. Rempel L, Rempel J. Partner influence on health behaviour decision-making: increasing breastfeeding duration. *J Soc Pers Relat.* 2004;21(1):92–111

15. Kessler LA, Gielen AC, Diener-West M, Paige DM. The effect of a woman's significant other on her breastfeeding decision. *J Hum Lact.* 1995;11(2):103–109

16. Scott JA, Binns CW, Aroni RA. The influence of reported paternal attitudes on the decision to breast-feed. *J Paediatr Child Health.* 1997;33(4):305–307

17. Shaker I, Scott JA, Reid M. Infant feeding attitudes of expectant parents: breastfeeding and formula feeding. *J Adv Nurs.* 2004;45(3):260–268

18. Giugliani ER, Caiaffa WT, Vogelhut J, Witter FR, Perman JA. Effect of breastfeeding support from different sources on mothers' decisions to breastfeed. *J Hum Lact.* 1994;10(3):157–161

19. Littman H, Medendorp SV, Goldfarb J. The decision to breastfeed. The importance of father's approval. *Clin Pediatr (Phila).* 1994;33(4):214–219

20. Kong SK, Lee DT. Factors influencing decision to breastfeed. *J Adv Nurs.* 2004;46(4):369–379

21. Scott JA, Landers MC, Hughes RM, Binns CW. Factors associated with breastfeeding at discharge and duration of breastfeeding. *J Paediatr Child Health.* 2001;37(3):254–261

22. Sullivan ML, Leathers SJ, Kelley MA. Family characteristics associated with duration of breastfeeding during early infancy among primiparas. *J Hum Lact.* 2004;20(2):196–205

23. Swanson V, Power KG. Initiation and continuation of breastfeeding: theory of planned behaviour. *J Adv Nurs.* 2005;50(3):272–282

24. Maycock B, Binns CW, Dhaliwal S, et al. Education and support for fathers improves breastfeeding rates: a randomized controlled trial. *J Hum Lact.* 2013;29(4):484–490

25. Pisacane A, Continisio GI, Aldinucci M, D'Amora S, Continisio P. A controlled trial of the father's role in breastfeeding promotion. *Pediatrics.* 2005;116(4). Available at: www.pediatrics.org/cgi/content/full/116/4/e494

26. Susin LR, Giugliani ER. Inclusion of fathers in an intervention to promote breastfeeding: impact on breastfeeding rates. *J Hum Lact.* 2008;24(4):386–392, quiz 451–453

27. Bich TH, Hoa DT, Mälqvist M. Fathers as supporters for improved exclusive

breastfeeding in Vietnam. *Matern Child Health J.* 2014;18(6):1444–1453

28. Tohotoa J, Maycock B, Hauck YL, Howat P, Burns S, Binns CW. Dads make a difference: an exploratory study of paternal support for breastfeeding in Perth, Western Australia. *Int Breastfeed J.* 2009;4(15):15

29. Goodman JH. Becoming an involved father of an infant. *J Obstet Gynecol Neonatal Nurs.* 2005;34(2):190–200

30. Feinberg ME. The internal structure and ecological context of coparenting: a framework for research and intervention. *Parent Sci Pract.* 2003;3(2):95–131

31. Feinberg ME, Kan ML. Establishing family foundations: intervention effects on coparenting, parent/infant well-being, and parent–child relations. *J Fam Psychol.* 2008;22(2):253–263

32. Labbok M, Krasovec K. Toward consistency in breastfeeding definitions. *Stud Fam Plann.* 1990;21(4):226–230

33. World Health Organization. Indicators for assessing infant and child feeding practices: part two: measurement. 2010. Available at: http://unicef.org/nutrition/files/IYCF_Indicators_part_III_country_profiles.pdf. Accessed January 3, 2011

34. Feinberg ME, Brown LD, Kan ML. A multi-domain self-report measure of coparenting. *Parent Sci Pract.* 2012;12(1):1–21

35. Will T, Shina O. Measuring received and perceived social support. In: Cohen S, Underwood L, Gottlieb B, eds. *Social Support Measurement and Intervention: A Guide for Health and Social Scientist.* New York, NY: Oxford University Press; 2000:86–135

36. Dennis C-L, Ross L. Women's perceptions of partner support and conflict in the development of postpartum depressive symptoms. *J Adv Nurs.* 2006;56(6):588–599

37. Dennis C-L. The breastfeeding self-efficacy scale: psychometric assessment of the short form. *J Obstet Gynecol Neonatal Nurs.* 2003;32(6):734–744

38. de la Mora A, Russell DW, Dungy CI, Losch M, Dusdieker L. The Iowa Infant Feeding Attitude Scale: analysis of reliability and validity. *J Appl Soc Psychol.* 1999;29(11):2362–2380

39. Best Start: Ontario's Maternal, Newborn and Early Child Development Resource Centre. Breastfeeding Matters: An Important Guide for Breastfeeding for Women and Their Families. 2011. Available at: www.beststart.org/resources/breastfeeding/index.html. Accessed January 1, 2014

New Ways of Understanding Disparities in Rates of Breastfeeding

Dr Lydia Furman, MD, Associate Editor, *Pediatrics*

In a study released in *Pediatrics*, "Racial and Ethnic Differences in Breastfeeding", Dr. Chelsea McKinney et al. (peds.2015-2388) examine and untangle the interconnected factors that underlie racial and ethnic differences in breastfeeding rates in the United States (US).[1] Generalists and breastfeeding medicine specialists alike will be fascinated (I think) because this article is a welcome reprieve from the mainstream in 2 ways. First, rather than (metaphorically) heaping risk factors for not breastfeeding into a giant pile and walking away, the authors elucidate and explore distinct contributing risk factors not routinely considered. Second, their methodology is clearly explained and makes sense even to those of us who lack statistical sophistication. The authors include familiar demographic factors such as poverty, education and marital status, but also examine non-demographic factors including "family history of breastfeeding" (meaning whether the mother herself was breastfed) and hospital introduction of formula. The study results are nuanced and severalhelp explain significant disparities in rates of breastfeeding in the US. Please read to find your own "ah-ha" moment(s) since there are so many in this article!

Two results stand out for me. Black mothers as compared to those of all other races and ethnicities were less likely to initiate breastfeeding (BF) and to plan to BF postnatally (postnatal BF intent), and had shorter durations of BF. No surprise, unfortunately. But when comparing BF initiation and postnatal BF intent between black and white mothers, the triad of poverty, marital status and education fully mediated (explained) the differences in rates.

Wow. This was the first result that grabbed me. At face value, this might also not seem surprising since we are used to seeing these demographic factors as increasing risk for *not* breastfeeding. But what a wake-up call that demographics fully explain the racial differences in these BF rates. What is the collective sociocultural power of marriage, education and money?

After all, breastfeeding is essentially free and formula is expensive (setting aside WIC- the Special Supplemental Nutrition Program for Women Infants and Children- for a moment), so there must be historical, cultural, personal and perhaps neighborhood contexts that are more meaningful and explanatory than poverty alone.[2] And while we can easily agree that it would be a ludicrous strategy to urge all black mothers into matrimony in order to increase BF rates, I wonder - what is the elusive and complex melding of financial, emotional and perhaps even housing stability that marriage possibly contributes to BF choice beyond "partner support?" And how can a high school or college degree impact what is basically a parenting decision? That the difference between black and white mothers' BF initiation and postnatal BF intent can essentially be fully explained by poverty, educational level and marital status opens a Pandora's box of very uncomfortable societal questions that I believe ultimately demand answers.

The second result that I found interesting is one that also intrigued the authors. In-hospital formula introduction was the biggest predictor of the shorter duration of BF among black as compared with white mothers. The authors appropriately note that this is a variable that can be impacted, and as increasing numbers of birthing hospitals become designated "Baby Friendly," in-hospital formula supplementation for all infants and especially for minority infants may decrease, in compliance with Baby Friendly Step 6 ("Give infants no food or drink other than breast-milk, unless medically indicated" - https://www.babyfriendlyusa. org/about-us/baby-friendly-hospital-initiative/the-ten-steps). In-hospital formula supplementation is a visible risk factor for early BF cessation,[3] targeted and measured by both the Department of Health and Human Services (DHHS) Healthy People 2020 goals (MICH-23, https://www.healthypeople.gov/2020/topics-objectives/topic/maternal-infant-and-child-health/objectives) and the Centers for Disease Control mPINC survey (maternity Practices in Infant Care & Nutrition, https://www.cdc.gov/breastfeeding/data/mpinc/results-tables.htm). McKinney and colleagues give us evidence that providing early or limited or any formula that is not medically necessary contributes to racial disparities in breastfeeding duration, and should therefore be avoided.

In summary, "Racial and Ethnic Differences in Breastfeeding" has so much "first food" for thought that I am confident you will enjoy reading it from beginning to end for yourself!

REFERENCES

1. McKinney CO, Hahn-Holbrook J, Chase-Lansdale PL, et al. Racial and Ethnic Differences in Breastfeeding. *Pediatrics* 2016; 138(2): e20152388.
2. Gross TT, Powell R, Anderson AK, et al "WIC peer counselors' perceptions of breastfeeding in African American women with lower incomes." *J Hum Lact* 2015; 31: 99-110.
3. Chantry CJ, Dewey KG, Peerson JM et al. "In-Hospital Formula Use increases Early Breastfeeding Cessation among First-time Mothers Intending to Exclusively Breastfeed." *J Pediatr* 2014; 164: 1339-1345.

Racial and Ethnic Differences in Breastfeeding

Chelsea O. McKinney, PhD, MPH,[a] Jennifer Hahn-Holbrook, PhD,[b] P. Lindsay Chase-Lansdale, PhD,[c] Sharon L. Ramey, PhD,[d] Julie Krohn, MS, RDN, LDN,[e] Maxine Reed-Vance, RN, MS,[f] Tonse N.K. Raju, MD, DCH,[g] Madeleine U. Shalowitz, MD, MBA,[a,h] on behalf of the Community Child Health Research Network

OBJECTIVES: Breastfeeding rates differ among racial/ethnic groups in the United States. Our aim was to test whether racial/ethnic disparities in demographic characteristics, hospital use of infant formula, and family history of breastfeeding mediated racial/ethnic gaps in breastfeeding outcomes.

METHODS: We analyzed data from the Community and Child Health Network study (N = 1636). Breastfeeding initiation, postnatal intent to breastfeed, and breastfeeding duration were assessed postpartum. Hierarchical linear modeling was used to estimate relative odds of breastfeeding initiation, postnatal intent, and duration among racial/ethnic groups and to test the candidate mediators of maternal age, income, household composition, employment, marital status, postpartum depression, preterm birth, smoking, belief that "breast is best," family history of breastfeeding, in-hospital formula introduction, and WIC participation.

RESULTS: Spanish-speaking Hispanic mothers were most likely to initiate (91%), intend (92%), and maintain (mean duration, 17.1 weeks) breastfeeding, followed by English-speaking Hispanic mothers (initiation 90%, intent 88%; mean duration, 10.4 weeks) and white mothers (initiation 78%, intent 77%; mean duration, 16.5 weeks); black mothers were least likely to initiate (61%), intend (57%), and maintain breastfeeding (mean duration, 6.4 weeks). Demographic variables fully mediated disparities between black and white mothers in intent and initiation, whereas demographic characteristics and in-hospital formula feeding fully mediated breastfeeding duration. Family breastfeeding history and demographic characteristics helped explain the higher breastfeeding rates of Hispanic mothers relative to white and black mothers.

CONCLUSIONS: Hospitals and policy makers should limit in-hospital formula feeding and consider family history of breastfeeding and demographic characteristics to reduce racial/ethnic breastfeeding disparities.

WHAT'S KNOWN ON THIS SUBJECT: Breastfeeding rates differ between racial/ethnic groups in the United States, resulting in considerable health disparities for infants. Black infants are breastfed for substantially shorter periods compared with white infants, and Hispanic infants are breastfed for significantly longer periods.

WHAT THIS STUDY ADDS: We show that demographic characteristics and in-hospital formula feeding explain breastfeeding gaps between black and white mothers, whereas demographic characteristics and family history of breastfeeding help explain higher rates of breastfeeding in Hispanic mothers compared with white and black mothers.

To cite: McKinney CO, Hahn-Holbrook J, Chase-Lansdale PL, et al. Racial and Ethnic Differences in Breastfeeding. *Pediatrics.* 2016;138(2):e20152388

[a]NorthShore University HealthSystem Department of Pediatrics and Research Institute, Evanston, Illinois; [b]Crean College of Health and Behavioral Sciences, Chapman University, Orange, California; [c]Institute for Policy Research, Northwestern University, Evanston, Illinois; [d]Virginia Tech Carilion Research Institute, Virginia Tech, Roanoke, Virginia; [e]Lake County Health Department and Community Health Center, Waukegan, Illinois; [f]Baltimore Healthy Start, Inc, Baltimore, Maryland; [g]Pregnancy and Perinatology Branch, Eunice Kennedy Shriver National Institute of Child Health and Human Development, National Institutes of Health, Rockville, Maryland; and [h]Department of Pediatrics, University of Chicago, Pritzker School of Medicine, Chicago, Illinois

Dr McKinney conceptualized the research questions, helped design the data collection instruments, conducted data collection, helped conduct the analyses, and drafted the initial and revised manuscripts; Dr Hahn-Holbrook helped conceptualize the research questions, draft the initial and revised manuscripts, and conduct the analyses; Dr Chase-Lansdale critically reviewed the initial manuscript; Dr Ramey helped design the data collection instruments, coordinated and supervised data collection, and critically reviewed the initial and revised manuscripts; Mrs Krohn helped design the data collection instruments and critically reviewed the initial manuscript; Mrs

Substantial research shows that breastfeeding benefits the neurologic, immunologic, digestive, and physical development of children.[1] The American Academy of Pediatrics recommends exclusive breastfeeding for the first 6 months of life, with continued breastfeeding and complementary foods at least until the child's first birthday. Despite this recommendation, approximately one-half of children in the United States are no longer breastfed by 6 months, with only a small percentage breastfed for the recommended period of 12 months.[2] Suboptimal levels of breastfeeding cost the US economy billions of dollars annually[3,4] and contribute to an estimated 911 (predominantly infant) deaths each year.[4] Importantly, the social, health, and economic burdens of low breastfeeding rates are not shared equally across racial and ethnic groups.

In the most recent US National Immunization Survey, only 66.4% of black mothers initiated breastfeeding in 2012, compared with 83% of white mothers and 82.4% of Hispanic mothers.[2] Racial/ethnic gaps in breastfeeding remained significant at 6 months, with only 35.3% of black mothers still breastfeeding, compared with 55.8% of white mothers and 51.4% of Hispanic mothers. Black women consistently remain at the bottom on all breastfeeding indices, although the gap between black mothers and other ethnic groups has narrowed by a few percentage points since 2000, suggesting breastfeeding promotion efforts have helped.

Many factors have been proposed to explain these racial/ethnic breastfeeding disparities. Black mothers, for example, tend to be younger, unmarried, and of lower income and education compared with white mothers, all factors linked to lower breastfeeding rates.[5] Interestingly, although Hispanic mothers share many of these demographic characteristics with black mothers, they have higher rates of breastfeeding than white mothers. Moreover, accounting for income and maternal education differences between black and white mothers does not eliminate disparities in breastfeeding.[6,7] To address the persistent large gap in breastfeeding rates between black mothers and mothers of other groups, the current article includes these demographic factors, but it also considers other causes.

The goal of the current study was to identify key nondemographic factors that might explain disparities in breastfeeding among black, white, and Hispanic mothers in the United States. We considered racial/ethnic differences in attitudes toward breastfeeding, family history of breastfeeding, in-hospital formula introduction, and participation in the Special Supplemental Nutrition Program for Women, Infants, and Children. Our objective was to determine whether racial/ethnic disparities in breastfeeding initiation, postnatal intent, and duration could be more fully explained by using statistical mediation techniques that included these hypothesized new factors.

METHODS

Study Sample

The sample consisted of 1636 mothers from the Community and Child Health Network, an National Institutes of Health multisite, community-based participatory research project designed to examine how community, family, and individual factors contribute to racial/ethnic health disparities for mothers and infants. The current study uses data from sites in Baltimore, Maryland, Washington, DC, and Lake County, Illinois. Each site sought to include mothers of low socioeconomic status (SES) from the 3 race/ethnicity groups, reflecting the local population; oversampling was included when needed. Data were obtained when mothers enrolled between 2008 and 2010 during their postpartum hospital stay and from in-home interviews 1 and 6 months' postpartum. Mothers included in this study provided infant feeding data (regardless of feeding method) for at least 2 time points. Overall, <1% of initiation and postnatal intent data were missing, although 12% of mothers did not provide breastfeeding duration data and 30% lacked information on family breastfeeding history. We attempted to address this missing data issue by using the multiple imputation function in Stata,[8] generating 10 possible data sets from which estimates were pooled.

Measures

Independent Variables

Racial/ethnic identification was based on mothers' self-report as either non-Hispanic white (hereafter referred to as white), non-Hispanic black (hereafter referred to as black), or Hispanic. The Community Child Health Research Network was designed to recruit mothers with these primary racial/ethnic identities (irrespective of legal status); thus, <1% also identified as other or mixed race. Participants who designated mixed race were placed in either the Hispanic or the black group to which they partially self-identified. Hispanic participants were further categorized as primarily English- or Spanish-speaking because markers of acculturation, including language spoken at home,[8] have been shown to have a large impact on breastfeeding outcomes.[9]

Potential Mediators

Candidate mediators were chosen based on known associations with breastfeeding as rereported in the literature. We tested these factors for their ability to mediate or explain a significant proportion of the variance in racial/ethnic disparities in breastfeeding outcomes. Demographic factors included maternal age,[10] education, employment at 1 month postpartum,[11] poverty status[10] (adjusted for family size by using federal guidelines[12]), relationship status[13] (single, in a relationship, or married [mutually exclusive categories]), coresident father,[14] and coresident grandparent.[15] Health-related variables included 1 month postpartum depression,[16] according to the Edinburgh Postnatal Depression Scale[17] (scores ≥ 9 were categorized as depressed); smoking at 1 month[18]; and infant preterm birth[19] (via medical records, gestation <37 weeks). We also collected maternal and paternal family history of breastfeeding[20] (determined by asking mothers and fathers "Did the woman who raised you breastfeed any children?") and the mother's belief[21] that "breast is best" (assessed by asking "Which of the following do you think is the best way to feed a baby—breastfeeding, a mix of breast milk and formula, only formula, or either breast milk or formula?"). Mothers who indicated breastfeeding was the best feeding method were compared with those who did not. Mothers were asked during their in-hospital stay whether they had participated in the Special Supplemental Nutrition Program for Women, Infants, and Children[22] at any time during the past year. Finally, patient medical records indicated whether formula was introduced during the hospital stay[23] after birth.

Outcome Variables

Primary outcomes of interest were breastfeeding initiation, postnatal breastfeeding intent, and breastfeeding duration. Breastfeeding initiation was measured at 1 month postpartum with the question "Have you ever breastfed your baby?" Mothers were categorized as having initiated breastfeeding if they breastfed at least once. Postnatal

breastfeeding intent was assessed during the in-hospital interview and derived from the question "How do you plan to feed your baby?" Mothers were categorized as intending to breastfeed if they planned to provide any amount of breast milk or not intending to breastfeed if they planned to provide only infant formula. Breastfeeding duration was defined as the number of weeks that the infant had been breastfed by the 6-month interview. Women who did not initiate breastfeeding were included in our duration measure and coded as 0. If the mother was no longer breastfeeding at the 1- or 6-month interviews, mothers were asked "How old was the child in weeks when you stopped breastfeeding?" to extrapolate total duration.

Statistical Analysis

Hierarchical linear modeling offers advantages over other statistical tools in evaluating nested data, which, in this case, adjusts for shared variance that participants (level 1) may have if they are from the same site and allows for heterogeneity of effect sizes for different sites (level 2).[24] All analyses were performed by using multilevel analysis, with study site added to the level 2 regression equation as a random factor, and independent and mediator variables included in univariate and multivariate models in the regression equation at level 1. Comparisons with Hispanic participants excluded the Baltimore site because only 4 Hispanic subjects were recruited, precluding good estimates at level 2. All analyses were conducted by using Stata version 14 (Stata Corp, College Station, TX).

Mediation Analysis

A mediator is a variable, or set of variables, hypothesized to explain or cause the observed association between an independent variable (ie, race/ethnicity) and a dependent

variable (eg, breastfeeding outcome). Using classic mediation criteria,[25] a variable can be said to mediate the relationship between an independent and dependent variable (Path C) if: (1) the independent variable significantly accounts for variation in the mediator (Path A); (2) the mediator significantly accounts for variation in the outcome variable (Path B); and (3) both the mediator and the independent variable are included in a multivariate model, and the relationship between the independent variable and the outcome variable is significantly reduced or no longer statistically significant (Path C′), while the mediator continues to predict significant variation in the outcome variable (Fig 1). There are often multiple mediators or causes of an association between an independent and dependent variable.[26] The same mediation criteria are used to test multiple mediators; however, all mediators must be added simultaneously to equations testing Path A, Path B, and Path C′ to ensure that each mediator accounts for a unique proportion of the variance shared between the independent and dependent variable.

Mediation analysis was performed to test whether the candidate mediators helped to explain racial/ethnic breastfeeding disparities (Figs 1 and 2). First, hierarchical linear modeling was used to obtain estimates of racial/ethnic gaps in breastfeeding outcomes (Path C). Racial/ethnic differences in potential mediators were next tested (Path A). The association between these potential mediators and breastfeeding outcomes was then assessed (Path B). Only variables that were significant at Paths C, A, and B, respectively, were considered further. To avoid introducing reverse causality when assessing mediators of racial/ethnic disparities in breastfeeding initiation and postnatal intent, we did not consider variables that occurred

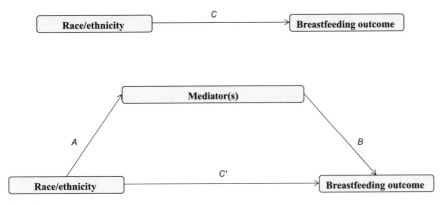

FIGURE 1

Mediation model pathways. Path C and C′ differ in that path C is the raw association between the independent and outcome variables, and path C′ is the residual association between the independent and outcome variables after the indirect effect of the mediator(s) is included in the model. Only racial/ethnic contrasts significant at Path C were pursued. Of those, mediation analysis was discontinued if Path A was not significant.

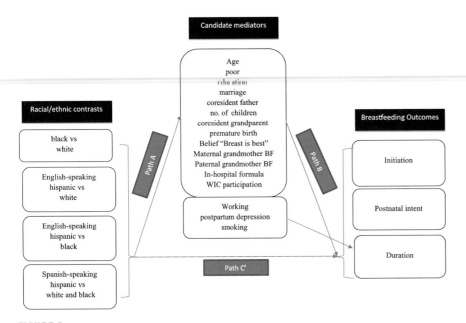

FIGURE 2

Summary of possible mediation relationships. Working, postpartum depression, and smoking were only tested with duration because they were measured at 1 month postpartum, which occurs after breastfeeding initiation and postnatal intent were measured in the hospital. BF, breastfed; WIC, Special Supplemental Nutrition Program for Women, Infants, and Children.

after the hospital stay (ie, working at 1 month, postpartum depression, smoking). Smoking, for instance, was measured at 1 month postpartum, which occurs after breastfeeding initiation and thus carries no predictive power.

The fourth and final step regressed significant mediator(s) on a breastfeeding outcome, with race/ethnicity included in the model to estimate the indirect effect (Path C′).

Sobel tests were performed (data not shown) to ensure that mediators had significant indirect effects ($P < .05$) when the aforementioned mediation criteria were met. Once mediators are included in the model, a racial/ethnic gap in breastfeeding can be said to be partially mediated if the association between race/ethnicity and breastfeeding was reduced and C′ is still statistically significant, and it is fully mediated

if C′, representing the racial/ethnic disparity in breastfeeding, is no longer statistically significant.[25] Unstandardized betas (β) and confidence intervals are reported.

RESULTS

Consistent with previous findings, black mothers had significantly lower rates of breastfeeding initiation, postnatal intent, and duration compared with other racial/ethnic groups, whereas Spanish-speaking Hispanic mothers tended to have the highest breastfeeding indicators (Table 1). Many other significant differences emerged between racial/ethnic groups among our candidate mediator variables (Table 2), and candidate variables that did not differ (Path A) were not considered further. Tables 3, 4, 5, 6, and 7 report regression coefficients for all significant mediation pathways, which are summarized in Fig 1.

Disparities Between Black and White Mothers

Initiation

Black mothers were less likely to initiate breastfeeding than white mothers (Table 3, Path C). Black women also experienced higher rates of poverty and were less likely to have a college degree or be married compared with white women, all of which predicted less breastfeeding initiation (Table 3, Paths A and B). Together, poverty, college education, and marital status fully mediated the gap in breastfeeding initiation (Table 3, Path C′).

Postnatal Intent

Black mothers were less likely to intend to breastfeed than white mothers (Table 3, Path C). Again, poverty, a college degree, and being married fully mediated the gap in postnatal breastfeeding intent (Table 3, Path C′).

TABLE 1 Breastfeeding Outcomes According to Race/Ethnicity

Outcome	Total (*N* = 1632)	White (*n* = 310)	Black (*n* = 907)	Hispanic-Spanish (*n* = 268)	Hispanic-English (*n* = 147)
Initiation	72	78[a]	61[b]	91[c]	90[c]
Postnatal intent	70	77[a]	57[b]	92[c]	88[c]
Duration, mean ± SD, wk	10.29 ± 13.13	16.51[a] ± 15.88	6.40[b] ± 9.86	17.09[a] ± 14.66	10.44[c] ± 12.50

Data are presented as the percent mean unless otherwise indicated. Values that differ in superscripts within the same row indicate that there is a significant difference ($P < .05$) between racial/ethnic groups. (For example: A value with *a* is significantly different from values with *b, c,* or *d* in the same row but not different from other values with *a* in the same row.)

TABLE 2 Differences in Potential Mediators as a Function of Race/Ethnicity

Variable	Total (*N* = 1632)	White (*n* = 310)	Black (*n* = 907)	Hispanic-Spanish (*n* = 268)	Hispanic-English (*n* = 147)
Mother's mean age, y	25.15	29.19[a]	23.82[a,b]	25.93[a]	23.38[c]
Poor	40	15[a]	49[b]	40[a,b]	36[a,b]
Working	24	25	24	24	26
Coresident father	62	86[a]	44[b]	87[a]	78[a]
Mean total no. of children	1.93	1.71[a]	197[b]	2.07[a]	1.87[a]
Coresident grandparent	34	16[a]	42[b]	20[a,b,c]	49[a,b]
Postpartum depression	17	14	18	19	17
Smoker	16	24[a]	17[b]	2[c]	17[b]
Premature birth	14	15	14	14	18
Maternal grandmother breastfed	57	62[a]	39[a]	93[b]	77[b]
Paternal grandmother breastfed	60	63[a]	43[a]	91[b]	76[b]
Mother: "Breastfeeding best for baby"	41	51	37	46	36
WIC participant	69	30[a]	75[b]	89[c]	76[b]
Fed formula at hospital	66	39[a]	76[b]	68[a,b]	58[a,b]
Education					
Less than high school	21	5[a]	18[a,b]	46[c]	26[b,c]
(High school or GED)	41	23	48	40	44
Some higher education	24	21[a]	28[a]	11[b]	23[a]
College or beyond	14	51[a]	6[b]	3[c]	8[b]
Relationship status					
Single	15	6[a]	22[b]	6[b]	9[a,b]
In relationship	56	28[a]	65[b]	58[a,b]	52[a,b]
(Married)	29	66[a]	13[b]	36[a,b]	38[c]

Data are presented as the percent mean unless otherwise indicated. Means represent raw data, without imputation. Parentheses indicate reference category. Values that differ in superscripts within the same row indicate that there is a significant difference ($P < .05$) between racial/ethnic groups. (For example: A value with *a* is significantly different from values with *b, c,* or *d* in the same row but not different from other values with *a* in the same row.) GED, General Educational Development; WIC, Special Supplemental Nutrition Program for Women, Infants, and Children.

Duration

Black mothers weaned their infants 10.3 weeks earlier than did white mothers (Table 3, Path C). College education and marital status differed between groups and predicted shorter breastfeeding durations (Table 3, Paths A and B). In addition, white mothers were significantly less likely to experience in-hospital formula introduction than black mothers, which was the biggest predictor of breastfeeding duration, even in models controlling for racial/ethnic disparities in initiation and postnatal intent. Together, these factors fully mediated the disparity in breastfeeding duration (Table 3, Path C'). Poverty was not a unique predictor of breastfeeding duration.

Disparities Between White and Spanish-speaking Hispanic Mothers

Initiation

Spanish-speaking Hispanic mothers were more likely to initiate breastfeeding compared with white mothers (Table 4, Path C). Spanish-speaking mothers were more likely to have had their own mothers breastfeed children, which predicted higher breastfeeding initiation (Table 4, Paths A and B). Maternal family history of breastfeeding fully mediated the initiation gap between white and Spanish-speaking Hispanic mothers (Table 4, Path C').

Postnatal Intent

Spanish-speaking Hispanic mothers were significantly more likely to intend to breastfeed than were white mothers (Table 4, Path C). However, no variables met mediation criteria.

Duration

Spanish-speaking Hispanic and white mothers had comparable durations for breastfeeding. Mediation analysis was therefore not pursued.

Disparities Between White and English-speaking Hispanic Mothers

Initiation

English-speaking Hispanic mothers exhibited significantly higher rates of initiation than did white mothers (Table 5, Path C). English-speaking mothers were more likely to have had their own mothers breastfeed children, which predicted higher breastfeeding initiation (Table 5, Paths A and B). Maternal family history of breastfeeding fully mediated the initiation gap between white and English-speaking Hispanic mothers (Table 5, Path C').

Postnatal Intent

English-speaking Hispanic mothers were more likely to intend to breastfeed than were white mothers (Table 5, Path C), although no variables met mediation criteria.

Duration

White mothers breastfed ~6.9 weeks longer than did English-speaking Hispanic mothers (Table 5, Path C); the latter group tended to be younger and lack a college degree (Table 5, Path A), both of which fully mediated the gap in duration (Table 5, Path C').

Disparities Between Black and Spanish-speaking Hispanic Mothers

Initiation

Spanish-speaking Hispanic mothers had significantly higher rates of initiation than did black mothers (Table 6, Path C). Spanish-speakers were also more likely to have a mother who had breastfed (Table 6, Path A), which predicted greater breastfeeding initiation in the next generation (Table 6, Path B) and partially mediated this racial/ethnic disparity (Table 6, Path C').

Postnatal Intent

Black mothers were less likely to intend to breastfeed after leaving the hospital than were Spanish-speaking mothers (Table 6, Path C). Having a

TABLE 3 Mediation of Differences in Breastfeeding Initiation, Postnatal Intent, and Duration Between White and Black Mothers

Variable	β	95% Confidence Interval
Breastfeeding initiation		
Path C		
Black	−0.81	−1.15 to 0.46
Path A		
Poor	1.14	0.71 to 1.57
College	−1.64	−2.15 to −1.14
Married	−1.52	−1.94 to −1.10
Path B and Path C'		
Poor	−0.44	−0.71 to −0.17
College	1.64	1.00 to 2.28
Married	0.99	0.56 to 1.41
Black	0.26	−0.17 to 0.69
Breastfeeding postnatal intent		
Path C		
Black	−1.02	−1.35 to −0.68
Path A		
Poor	1.14	0.71 to 1.57
College	−1.64	−2.15 to −1.14
Married	−1.52	−1.94 to −1.10
Path B and Path C'		
Poor	−0.56	−0.83 to −0.29
College	1.73	1.09 to 2.37
Married	1.02	0.61 to 1.44
Black	0.13	−0.29 to 0.55
Breastfeeding duration		
Path C		
Black	−10.31	−12.04 to −8.58
Path A		
College	−0.29	−0.35 to −0.23
Married	−0.24	−0.30 to −0.19
Hospital formula	−0.08	−0.03 to −0.12
Path B and Path C'		
College	6.54	4.26 to 8.81
Married	4.34	2.52 to 6.17
Hospital formula	−9.79	−11.43 to −8.16
Black	−1.51	−3.36 to 0.34

In these models, white mothers were coded as 0, and black mothers were coded as 1.

TABLE 4 Mediation of Differences in Breastfeeding Initiation, Postnatal Intent, and Duration Between White and Spanish-speaking Hispanic Mothers

Variable	β	95% Confidence Interval
Breastfeeding initiation		
Path C		
Hispanic, Spanish-speaking	0.84	0.23 to 1.44
Path A		
Maternal grandmother breastfed	1.66	1.04 to 2.27
Path B and Path C'		
Maternal grandmother breastfed	0.75	0.09 to 1.42
Hispanic, Spanish-speaking	0.55	−0.09 to 1.19
Breastfeeding postnatal intent		
Path C[a]		
Hispanic, Spanish-speaking	0.94	0.33 to 1.52
Breastfeeding duration		
Path C[a]		
Hispanic, Spanish-speaking	−2.08	−4.91 to 0.75

In these models, white mothers were coded as 0, and Spanish-speaking Hispanic mothers were coded as 1.
[a] Denotes contrasts in which no mediators were identified.

mother who breastfed also partially mediated the difference in postnatal intent (Table 6, Path C').

Duration

Black mothers nursed an estimated 10.3 weeks less than did Spanish-speaking Hispanic mothers (Table 6, Path C). Again, black mothers were less likely to have a family history of breastfeeding but were also less likely to live with the infant's father (Table 6, Path A). Together, these 2 variables partially explained the large gap in duration (Table 6, Path C').

Disparities Between Black and English-speaking Hispanic Motherse

Initiation

English-speaking Hispanic mothers initiated breastfeeding more often than did black mothers (Table 7, Path C). Mothers whose own mothers had breastfed were more prevalent among English-speakers than black mothers (Table 7, Path A), which partially mediated the initiation gap (Table 7, Path C').

Postnatal Intent

English-speaking Hispanic mothers were more likely to intend to breastfeed than were black mothers (Table 7, Path C). English-speaking Hispanic mothers were also more likely to have maternal and paternal mothers who had breastfed (Table 7, Path A). In this model, both family history variables predicted unique variations in postnatal intent and partially mediated the racial/ethnic gap in intent (Table 7, Paths B and C').

Duration:

Black women weaned their infants ~3.0 weeks earlier than English-speaking Hispanic women (Table 7, Path C). Black mothers were less likely to be married or have a maternal history of breastfeeding than English-speaking Hispanic

mothers (Table 7, Path A). Both variables fully mediated the disparity in duration (Table 7, Path C').

TABLE 5 Mediation of Differences in Breastfeeding Initiation, Postnatal Intent, and Duration Between White and English-speaking Hispanic Mothers

Variable	β	95% Confidence Interval
Breastfeeding initiation		
Path C		
Hispanic, English-speaking	0.77	0.11 to 1.42
Path A		
Maternal grandmother breastfed	0.60	0.02 to 0.06
Path B and Path C'		
Maternal grandmother breastfed	0.71	0.02 to 1.41
Hispanic, English-speaking	0.66	−0.01 to 1.32
Breastfeeding postnatal intent		
Path Cª		
Hispanic, English-speaking	0.66	0.04 to 1.27
Breastfeeding duration		
Path C		
Hispanic, English-speaking	−6.89	−9.99 to −3.79
Path A		
College	−0.28	−0.41 to −0.16
Age	−0.02	−0.03 to −0.01
Path B and Path C'		
College	5.57	1.61 to 9.53
Age	0.84	0.53 to 1.14
Hispanic, English-speaking	−0.03	−3.36 to 3.29

In these models, white mothers were coded as 0, and English-speaking Hispanic mothers were coded as 1.
ª Denotes contrasts in which no mediators were identified.

TABLE 6 Mediation of Differences in Breastfeeding Initiation, Postnatal Intent, and Duration Between Black and Spanish-speaking Hispanic Mothers

Variable	β	95% Confidence Interval
Breastfeeding initiation		
Path C		
Black	−1.57	−2.04 to −1.10
Path A		
Maternal grandmother breastfed	−2.84	−3.56 to −2.11
Path B and Path C'		
Maternal grandmother breastfed	0.90	0.37 to 1.43
Black	−1.12	−1.66 to −0.57
Breastfeeding postnatal intent		
Path C		
Black	−1.64	−2.11 to −1.16
Path A		
Maternal grandmother breastfed	−2.84	−3.56 to −2.11
Path B and Path C'		
Maternal grandmother breastfed	1.21	0.60 to 1.82
Black	−1.04	−1.60 to −0.48
Breastfeeding duration		
Path C		
Black	−10.25	−12.30 to −8.21
Path A		
Coresident father	−0.27	−0.33 to −0.21
Maternal grandmother breastfed	−0.36	−0.43 to −0.29
Path B and Path C'		
Coresident father	4.07	2.09 to 6.04
Maternal grandmother breastfed	4.68	2.55 to 6.81
Black	−6.07	−8.49 to −3.65

In these models, black mothers were coded as 0, and Spanish-speaking Hispanic mothers were coded as 1.

DISCUSSION

In line with previous reports,[2,5] black mothers in the current sample

TABLE 7 Mediation of Differences in Breastfeeding Initiation, Postnatal Intent, and Duration Between Black and English-speaking Hispanic Mothers

Variable	β	95% Confidence Interval
Breastfeeding initiation		
Path C		
Black	−1.45	−2.04 to −0.87
Path A		
Maternal grandmother breastfed	−1.66	−2.36 to −0.96
Path B and Path C′		
Maternal grandmother breastfed	0.88	0.36 to 1.39
Black	−1.19	−1.80 to −0.58
Breastfeeding postnatal intent		
Path C		
Black	−1.26	−1.80 to −0.71
Path A		
Maternal grandmother breastfed	−1.32	−2.04 to −0.59
Paternal grandmother breastfed	−1.14	−1.81 to −0.47
Path B and Path C′		
Maternal grandmother breastfed	1.06	0.43 to 1.69
Paternal grandmother breastfed	0.72	0.19 to 1.24
Black	−0.78	−1.37 to −0.19
Breastfeeding duration		
Path C		
Black	−3.03	−5.16 to −0.90
Path A		
Married	−0.08	−0.15 to −0.02
Maternal grandmother breastfed	−0.17	−0.24 to −0.11
Path B and Path C′		
Married	7.25	4.92 to 9.58
Maternal grandmother breastfed	4.47	2.50 to 6.43
Black	0.11	−2.02 to 2.25

In these models, black mothers were coded as 0, and English-speaking Hispanic mothers were coded as 1.

intended, initiated, and maintained breastfeeding to a lesser degree than white mothers. Lower levels of breastfeeding initiation and postnatal intent among black mothers compared with white mothers were fully mediated by demographic factors. This finding is not surprising given that black women had higher rates of poverty and lower levels of education and marriage, variables that predicted lower rates of breastfeeding initiation and postnatal intent in the overall sample. Breastfeeding duration disparities between black and white women, however, were not fully explained by using demographic factors.

Poverty did not significantly mediate differences in duration between black and white mothers as it did for initiation and postnatal intent. Poverty may act as a proxy for in-hospital formula introduction, which more often occurs in predominately black communities that may also be low-income.[27] In fact, the use of in-hospital formula feeding played the most important role for duration. Black mothers' newborns were much more likely to be fed formula in the hospital than newborns of white mothers. This difference was not explained by higher rates of breastfeeding intent and initiation in white mothers. Our finding echoes reports from the Centers for Disease Control and Prevention that documented higher rates of supplemental feeding in hospitals serving black communities. In-hospital supplementation of formula prohibits establishing a pattern of exclusive breastfeeding early on, which has been shown to hinder breastfeeding outcomes postdischarge.[28] Our study suggests that if only hospital formula introduction were eliminated, the black/white gap in breastfeeding duration could be reduced by

~1.8 weeks or 20% of the overall difference.

Consistent with notions that cultural norms regarding breastfeeding practices drive the effect of acculturation/immigrant status on breastfeeding outcomes, Spanish-speaking Hispanic women were more likely to have a family history of breastfeeding compared with white and English-speaking Hispanic women. Maternal family history of breastfeeding fully mediated the initiation disparity between white and both Spanish-and English-speaking Hispanic mothers. Racial/ethnic differences in maternal age and education fully explained disparities in duration between white and English-speaking Hispanic mothers. No mediators were found for postnatal intent or duration among Spanish-speaking Hispanic and white mothers, which speaks to previous evidence of the Hispanic paradox in US breastfeeding rates.[29] This paradox is a phenomenon in which Hispanic people in the United States experience good health outcomes despite low SES and common risk factors, particularly among recent immigrants.[30] Comparable duration of breastsfeeding between white and Spanish-speaking Hispanic women in our sample suggests that breastfeeding norms of Spanish speakers' native countries[31] may overcome adverse effects of low SES that characterizes this less acculturated group in the United States. It is also notable that no significant racial/ethnic differences were found in the belief that "breast is best" or maternal employment at 1 month postpartum, because both factors have been hypothesized to mediate racial/ethnic breastfeeding.[32] It is possible, however, that the oversampling of low SES participants of all racial/ethnic groups in this study restricted variability on these factors, leading to null results.

Family history of breastfeeding, especially from the mother's side, bolsters breastfeeding outcomes, and this intergenerational factor mediates racial/ethnic breastfeeding disparities. This finding complements previous research which found that markers of acculturation, such as language spoken at home,[8] predict substantial differences in breastfeeding behavior.[9,33] In addition to family history of breastfeeding, higher rates of coresident fathers and marriage among Hispanic women accounted for some of the breastfeeding disparities between black and both English- and Spanish-speaking Hispanic women. This finding supports previous research showing the important role that the infant's father can play in fostering positive breastfeeding outcomes.[34]

The current study had several limitations. We cannot establish causality; interventions are needed to test whether decreasing the introduction of formula in hospitals serving black communities, for example, would reduce disparities between black and white women in breastfeeding duration. Second, this study included an overrepresentation of mothers of low SES, and the results may not be generalizable to understanding racial/ethnic disparities in breastfeeding rates between white, black, and Hispanic mothers among the middle- or upper-class. Finally, future research is needed to explore additional potential mediators because many racial/ethnic disparities in breastfeeding were not fully explained by our analyses.

CONCLUSIONS

Large ethnic/racial gaps in breastfeeding rates exist in the United States among black, white, and Hispanic infants and their mothers. In line with previous speculations, intergenerational experience with breastfeeding seems to be an important predictor of infant feeding behaviors and helps explain why Hispanic women have better breastfeeding outcomes. Just as importantly, the negative impact of hospital infant formula feeding practices on black women warrants strong consideration.[35] Changing hospital relationships with formula companies that relinquish fiscal dependency on free formula is a notorious challenge for many hospitals that strive to improve breastfeeding outcomes.[36] Change is possible, however, as evidenced by the emergence of "baby-friendly hospitals," some of which serve areas with largely low-income and minority patient populations.[37] This active inquiry into functional variables that can yield healthier outcomes for infants and mothers has produced new findings and may support planned interventions at the levels of individual families and health care providers.

ABBREVIATION

SES: socioeconomic status

Vance helped design the data collection instruments, coordinated and supervised data collection, and critically reviewed the initial manuscript; Dr Raju provided *Eunice Kennedy Shriver* National Institute of Child Health and Human Development leadership for the Community and Child Health Network and critically reviewed the initial manuscript; Dr Shalowitz helped conceptualize the study, helped design data collection instruments, coordinated and supervised data collection, and critically reviewed and gave feedback on the initial and revised manuscripts; and all authors approved the final manuscript as submitted.

DOI: 10.1542/peds.2015-2388

Accepted for publication May 11, 2016

Address correspondence to Chelsea O. McKinney, PhD, MPH, NorthShore University HealthSystem Department of Pediatrics and Research Institute, 1001 University Place, Suite 348, Evanston, IL 60201. E-mail: chelseaomckinney@gmail.com

PEDIATRICS (ISSN Numbers: Print, 0031-4005; Online, 1098-4275).

FINANCIAL DISCLOSURE: The authors have indicated they have no financial relationships relevant to this article to disclose.

FUNDING: All phases of this study were supported by grants to the Community and Child Health Network through cooperative agreements with the *Eunice Kennedy Shriver* National Institute of Child Health and Human Development (UHD44207, U HD44219, UHD44226, U HD44245, U HD44253, U HD54791, U HD54019, UHD44226-05S1, U HD44245-06S1, and R03 HD59584) and the National Institute for Nursing Research (U NR008929). Funded by the National Institutes of Health (NIH).

POTENTIAL CONFLICT OF INTEREST: The authors have indicated they have no potential conflicts of interest to disclose.

REFERENCES

1. American Academy of Pediatrics Section on Breastfeeding. Policy statement: breastfeeding and the use of human milk. *Pediatrics*. 2012;129(3). Available at: www.pediatrics.org/cgi/content/full/129/3/e827

2. Centers for Disease Control and Prevention. Breastfeeding among US children born 2002–2012, national immunization surveys. Available at: www.cdc.gov/breastfeeding/data/nis_data/ rates-any-exclusive-bf-socio-dem-2012.htm

3. Bartick M, Reinhold A. The burden of suboptimal breastfeeding in the United States: a pediatric cost analysis.

Pediatrics. 2010;125(5). Available at: www.pediatrics.org/cgi/content/full/125/5/e1048

4. Bartick MC, Stuebe AM, Schwarz EB, Luongo C, Reinhold AG, Foster EM. Cost analysis of maternal disease associated with suboptimal breastfeeding. *Obstet Gynecol.* 2013;122(1):111–119

5. Grummer-Strawn LM, Shealy KR. Progress in protecting, promoting, and supporting breastfeeding: 1984-2009. *Breastfeed Med.* 2009;4(suppl 1):S31–S39

6. Centers for Disease Control and Prevention (CDC). Racial and socioeconomic disparities in breastfeeding—United States, 2004. *MMWR Morb Mortal Wkly Rep.* 2006;55(12):335–339

7. Li R, Grummer-Strawn L. Racial and ethnic disparities in breastfeeding among United States infants: Third National Health and Nutrition Examination Survey, 1988-1994. *Birth.* 2002;29(4):251–257

8. Berry JW. Immigration, acculturation, and adaptation. *Appl Psychol.* 1997;46(1):5–34

9. Singh GK, Kogan MD, Dee DL. Nativity/immigrant status, race/ethnicity, and socioeconomic determinants of breastfeeding initiation and duration in the United States, 2003. *Pediatrics.* 2007;119(suppl 1):S38–S46

10. US Department of Health and Human Services, Health Resources and Services Administration. *Women's Health USA 2011.* Rockville, MD: US Department of Health and Human Services; 2011

11. Ryan AS, Zhou W, Arensberg MB. The effect of employment status on breastfeeding in the United States. *Womens Health Issues.* 2006;16(5):243–251

12. Sebelius K. *Annual Update of the HHS Poverty Guidelines.* Washington, DC: US Department of Health and Human Services; 2011

13. Kiernan K, Pickett KE. Marital status disparities in maternal smoking during pregnancy, breastfeeding and maternal depression. *Soc Sci Med.* 2006;63(2):335–346

14. Jones JR, Kogan MD, Singh GK, Dee DL, Grummer-Strawn LM. Factors associated with exclusive breastfeeding in the United States. *Pediatrics.* 2011;128(6):1117–1125

15. Pilkauskas NV. Breastfeeding initiation and duration in coresident grandparent, mother and infant households. *Matern Child Health J.* 2014;18(8):1955–1963

16. Dennis CL, McQueen K. The relationship between infant-feeding outcomes and postpartum depression: a qualitative systematic review. *Pediatrics.* 2009;123(4). Available at: www.pediatrics.org/cgi/content/full/123/4/e736

17. Cox JL, Holden JM, Sagovsky R. Detection of postnatal depression. Development of the 10-item Edinburgh Postnatal Depression Scale. *Br J Psychiatry.* 1987;150:782–786

18. Liu J, Rosenberg KD, Sandoval AP. Breastfeeding duration and perinatal cigarette smoking in a population-based cohort. *Am J Public Health.* 2006;96(2):309–314

19. Callen J, Pinelli J. A review of the literature examining the benefits and challenges, incidence and duration, and barriers to breastfeeding in preterm infants. *Adv Neonatal Care.* 2005;5(2):72–88, quiz 89–92

20. Bentley ME, Dee DL, Jensen JL. Breastfeeding among low income, African-American women: power, beliefs and decision making. *J Nutr.* 2003;133(1):305S–309S

21. Cox KN, Giglia RC, Binns CW. The influence of infant feeding attitudes on breastfeeding duration: evidence from a cohort study in rural Western Australia. *Int Breastfeed J.* 2015;10(25):25

22. Ryan AS, Zhou W. Lower breastfeeding rates persist among the Special Supplemental Nutrition Program for Women, Infants, and Children participants, 1978-2003. *Pediatrics.* 2006;117(4):1136–1146

23. Centers for Disease Control and Prevention (CDC). Breastfeeding-related maternity practices at hospitals and birth centers—United States, 2007. *MMWR Morb Mortal Wkly Rep.* 2008;57(23):621–625

24. Raudenbush SW, Bryk AS. *Hierarchical Linear Models: Applications and Data Analysis Methods.* Thousand Oaks, CA: Sage Publications; 2002

25. Baron RM, Kenny DA. The moderator-mediator variable distinction in social psychological research: conceptual, strategic, and statistical considerations. *J Pers Soc Psychol.* 1986;51(6):1173–1182

26. Preacher KJ, Hayes AF. Asymptotic and resampling strategies for assessing and comparing indirect effects in multiple mediator models. *Behav Res Methods.* 2008;40(3):879–891

27. Lind JN, Perrine CG, Li R, Scanlon KS, Grummer-Strawn LM; Centers for Disease Control and Prevention (CDC). Racial disparities in access to maternity care practices that support breastfeeding—United States, 2011. *MMWR Morb Mortal Wkly Rep.* 2014;63(33):725–728

28. UNICEF/WHO. Baby-friendly hospital initiative: revised, updated and expanded for integrated care, section 1, background and implementation, preliminary version. Available at: www.who.int/nutrition/topics/BFHI_Revised_Section1.pdf. Accessed May 5, 2008

29. Kimbro RT, Lynch SM, McLanahan S. The influence of acculturation on breastfeeding initiation and duration for Mexican-Americans. *Popul Res Policy Rev.* 2008;27(2):183–199

30. Franzini L, Ribble JC, Keddie AM. Understanding the Hispanic paradox. *Ethn Dis.* 2001;11(3):496–518

31. Lauer JA, Betrán AP, Victora CG, de Onís M, Barros AJ. Breastfeeding patterns and exposure to suboptimal breastfeeding among children in developing countries: review and analysis of nationally representative surveys. *BMC Med.* 2004;2(26):26

32. Centers for Disease Control and Prevention (CDC). Progress in increasing breastfeeding and reducing racial/ethnic differences—United States, 2000-2008 births. *MMWR Morb Mortal Wkly Rep.* 2013;62(5):77–80

33. Topolyan I, Wang Q, Xu X. Peer effects in breastfeeding: evidence from the IFPS II Study. *Review of Economics and Finance*. 2015;5(3):33–44

34. Pisacane A, Continisio GI, Aldinucci M, D'Amora S, Continisio P. A controlled trial of the father's role in breastfeeding promotion. *Pediatrics*. 2005;116(4). Available at: www.pediatrics.org/cgi/content/full/116/4/e494

35. Radford A, Southall DP. Successful application of the baby-friendly hospital initiative contains lessons that must be applied to the control of formula feeding in hospitals in industrialized countries. *Pediatrics*. 2001;108(3):766–768

36. Merewood A, Philipp BL. Becoming baby-friendly: overcoming the issue of accepting free formula. *J Hum Lact*. 2000;16(4): 279–282

37. Merewood A, Philipp BL. Implementing change: becoming baby-friendly in an inner city hospital. *Birth*. 2001;28(1):36–40

Changing Societal and Lifestyle Factors and Breastfeeding Patterns Over Time

Chad Logan, MPH,[a] Tatjana Zittel,[a] Stefanie Striebel,[a] Frank Reister, PD Dr med,[b] Hermann Brenner, Prof Dr med, MPH,[c] Dietrich Rothenbacher, Prof Dr med, MPH,[a] Jon Genuneit, PD Dr med, MSc[a]

BACKGROUND: Breastfeeding is an important determinant of early infant immune function and potentially future health. Although numerous studies have reported rising breastfeeding initiation rates and duration, few longitudinally investigated the impact of shifting societal and lifestyle factors on breastfeeding patterns in developed nations.

METHODS: The Ulm Birth Cohort Study (UBCS) and Ulm SPATZ Health Study (SPATZ) cohorts consist of newborns and their mothers recruited, respectively, from 2000 to 2001 and 2012 to 2013 at the University Medical Center Ulm, Germany. Cox proportional hazards models were used to estimate crude and mutually adjusted hazard ratios for study effect (time trend) and individual risk factors on noninitiation and duration of predominant and total breastfeeding.

RESULTS: Compared with UBCS mothers, SPATZ mothers had lower cessation rates of both predominant breastfeeding by 4 months and total breastfeeding by 6 months: hazard ratio (95% confidence interval) 0.79 (0.67–0.93) and 0.71 (0.60–0.82), respectively. However, this crude time trend was limited to mothers with higher educational achievement. Similar time trend effects were observed among less educated mothers only after adjustment for early cessation risk factors. Mutually adjusted hazard ratios for individual risk factors were similar in both studies: low education, high BMI, smoking within 6 weeks of delivery, and cesarean delivery were associated with early breastfeeding cessation beginning at 6 weeks. In addition, actively abstaining from drinking alcohol was associated with lower rates of early cessation.

CONCLUSIONS: Our results suggest widening socioeconomic disparity in breastfeeding and potentially subsequent child health, which may require new targeted interventions.

[a]Institute of Epidemiology and Medical Biometry, Ulm University, Ulm, Germany; [b]Department of Gynecology and Obstetrics, University Medical Center Ulm, Ulm, Germany; and [c]Division of Clinical Epidemiology and Aging Research, German Cancer Research Center, Heidelberg, Germany

Mr Logan contributed to study design and data collection, conducted the statistical analyses, interpreted the data, and wrote the manuscript; Ms Zittel, Dr Striebel, and Dr Reister contributed to recruitment and data collection and critically reviewed the manuscript; Dr Brenner conceived the Ulm Birth Cohort Study study and critically reviewed and revised the manuscript; Mr Rothenbacher conceived the Ulm Birth Cohort Study and SPATZ studies and critically reviewed and revised the manuscript; Mr Genuneit conceived the SPATZ study and contributed to recruitment and data collection, interpretation of the data, and writing the manuscript; and all authors approval of the final manuscript as submitted.

DOI: 10.1542/peds.2015-4473

Accepted for publication Feb 10, 2016

Address correspondence to Prof. Dr. med. Dietrich Rothenbacher, MPH, Institute of Epidemiology and Medical Biometry, Ulm University, Helmholtzstrasse 22, D-89081 Ulm, Germany. E-mail: dietrich.rothenbacher@uni-ulm.de

WHAT'S KNOWN ON THIS SUBJECT: Early breastfeeding cessation is associated with a number of demographic, lifestyle, and birth factors including maternal education, smoking, and cesarean delivery. Overall rates and duration of predominant and total breastfeeding have improved in most developed countries.

WHAT THIS STUDY ADDS: Socioeconomic disparities in breastfeeding practices have widened between mothers with lower and higher education. Although programs focusing on obesity, smoking, and cesarean delivery would benefit all mothers, programs tailored specifically toward less educated mothers may particularly reach women in need.

To cite: Logan C, Zittel T, Striebel S, et al. Changing Societal and Lifestyle Factors and Breastfeeding Patterns Over Time. *Pediatrics.* 2016;137(5):e20154473

ARTICLE

Breast milk is internationally recognized as the optimal source for infant nutrition,[1] and long-term breastfeeding has been associated with numerous health benefits for both mother and child.[2,3] Therefore, mothers in most developed nations are recommended to exclusively breastfeed for the first 6 months of life, followed by a period of complementary breastfeeding up to 2 years of age.[1] Although initiation rates and average duration are generally increasing, wide variation in breastfeeding behavior is often observed across countries and demographic groups, making it difficult to identify how patterns are affected by changes in societal and lifestyle factors over time.

In Germany, retrospective studies indicate overall breastfeeding rates and duration of exclusive breastfeeding have steadily increased between 1987 and 2000 to become among the highest in Europe.[4] Despite improvement, the most recent data in southern Germany showed that only 41.7% and 51.6% of mothers were meeting minimum German recommendations for exclusive breastfeeding of at least 4 months[5] and feeding any breast milk at 6 months, respectively.[6] In these and other studies, breastfeeding behavior was negatively affected by a number of factors, including maternal education and smoking,[7,8] delivery complications,[9] and social support.[10]

Although these studies shed light on the roles of individual risk factors on early breastfeeding cessation, lack of an appropriate baseline population inhibits their use for time-trend analyses. Furthermore, the impact of health-relevant patterns of behavior related to pregnancy, such as smoking cessation and later resumption, on breastfeeding remain relatively unexplored.

In this study, we compare data obtained from duplicate birth cohorts recruited ~12 years apart to investigate the influence of demographic shifts over time in education, smoking, mode of delivery, maternal BMI, and parity on breastfeeding rates and duration. Another objective was to examine the influence of these factors, as well as alcohol consumption and return-to-work status, on noninitiation and breastfeeding cessation, allowing for time-dependent effects throughout lactation.

METHODS

Study Design and Population

Data were obtained from the Ulm Birth Cohort Study (UBCS) and the Ulm SPATZ Health Study,[11,12] 2 methodologically similar population-based birth cohort studies including newborns and their mothers recruited shortly after delivery in the University Medical Center Ulm, Southern Germany, respectively, from November 2000 to November 2001 and April 2012 to May 2013.[11,12] Exclusion criteria were outpatient delivery, maternal age <18 years, transfer of the newborn or the mother to intensive care immediately after delivery, and/or insufficient knowledge of the German (UBCS and SPATZ), Turkish, or Russian (both UBCS only) language. At baseline, the UBCS and SPATZ cohorts, respectively, included 1090 newborns of 1066 mothers (67% of all 1593 eligible families) and 1006 newborns of 970 mothers (49% of all 1999 eligible families). For the purposes of this analysis, the study populations were restricted to singleton term (gestational age ≥37 weeks) newborns. Ethical approval was obtained from the ethics board of Ulm University (UBCS: #98/2000; SPATZ: #311/11) and of the Physicians' Boards of the states of Baden-Wuerttemberg and Bavaria (both UBCS only). Participation was voluntary, and written informed consent obtained in each case.

Data Collection

Demographic data were collected by self-administered questionnaire at "baseline." Clinical pre- and perinatal data were respectively obtained from routine paper documentation updated at each obstetric appointment during pregnancy and electronic hospital records. Additional data were collected at 6 weeks and 6 months postdelivery by telephone interview or postal self-administered questionnaire (SPATZ only) if subjects could not be reached by telephone or had previously documented breastfeeding cessation. Additional follow-up was conducted at 1 and 2 years postdelivery by self-administered questionnaire.

Breastfeeding Definitions and Assessment

Predominant and any breastfeeding correspond to World Health Organization 2007 definitions.[13] Predominant breastfeeding required breast milk as the primary source of nutrition allowing for supplementation with certain liquids including water. Any breastfeeding required maternal report of breastfeeding regardless of additional foods. Mothers were asked to report if they currently fed their child any breast milk at each follow-up. Furthermore, the number of months and weeks (weeks and days at 6-week follow-up) postdelivery at cessation of predominant and any breastfeeding were assessed. For subjects lost to follow-up or with missing data, duration was censored at the last reported time of breastfeeding.

Covariates and Potential Confounders

The following covariates were selected based on a priori association with breastfeeding duration.

Maternal Age, Education, and Nationality

Maternal age at delivery was categorized as <30, 30 to 35, or >35 years. Maternal education was based on reports of secondary school graduation and translated into years of schooling (≥12 years, <12 years). Maternal nationality was based on country of birth and defined as "German" or "Other" and investigated as a potential confounder.

Smoking and Alcohol Status

Smoking status (yes/no) and frequency (cigarettes per day) in the year before and during pregnancy were assessed at baseline. Current smoking status and frequency were assessed at each follow-up thereafter. Mothers who did not smoke before delivery and up to 6 months thereafter were classified "never smokers." Mothers who smoked before delivery were classified as (1) "abstinent smokers" if they reported not smoking up to 6 months postdelivery, (2) "resumed smoking" if smoking was reported at 6 months but not at 6 weeks, or (3) "continuous smokers" if smoking was reported at 6 weeks. An "undetermined" category was used to account for those whose status was unclear due to missing data.

Alcohol consumption (daily or occasionally) was assessed and defined similarly for SPATZ: (1) never drinkers, (2) abstinent drinkers, (3) resumed between 6 weeks and 6 months, (4) resumed by 6 weeks postdelivery, and (5) undetermined status due to missing data. For UBCS, alcohol consumption was only assessed at baseline.

BMI

BMI was calculated as (mass [kg]/ height [m]^2) based on measurements at the mother's obstetric appointment at which pregnancy was clinically established if the appointment took place within the first 15 weeks of pregnancy (n, mean ± SD in weeks; SPATZ: 794, 9.0 ± 2.3, UBCS: 935, 8.5 ± 2.5) or self-reported weight before pregnancy (SPATZ: n = 35, UBCS: n = 49). BMI was categorized as underweight (<18.5),

normal (18.5 to <25), overweight (25 to <30), or obese (≥30).

Return-to-Work Status

In SPATZ only, maternal working status during each month of life of the newborn was assessed at 6 months and 1 year by asking for the average number of hours per week worked in paid employment. Mothers were considered to have returned to work by the earliest month for which an average of ≥5 hours/week was reported and categorized as (1) not returning to work in the first 12 months or returning between months, (2) 1 and 3, (3) 4 and 6, (4) 7 and 12, or (5) undetermined for those with missing values for all 12 months. Sensitivity analyses were conducted using ≥20 hours per week as the cutoff.

Delivery Mode and Parity

Delivery mode (vaginal spontaneous, elective cesarean, emergency cesarean, or vaginal assisted delivery) and parity (0 or ≥1 birth before the study child) were ascertained from electronic hospital records.

Statistical Analyses

χ^2 and Kruskal-Wallis tests were performed to identify significant differences (α = .05) in breastfeeding proportions and demographic differences across study cohorts. Kaplan-Meier plots and log-rank tests were used to assess predominant and any breastfeeding duration patterns across studies, as well as, bivariate associations with maternal demographic and lifestyle variables. Cox proportional hazards models were used to estimate crude, individually adjusted, and mutually adjusted hazard ratios of study effect on noninitiation and cessation of predominant and/or any breastfeeding at 6 weeks and 3, 4, 6, and 9 months postdelivery. Because of limitations of the proportional hazards model for mediation analysis,[14] models

assessing mediation were checked against an alternative approach of modeling relative risks using a modified Poisson regression with robust variance estimation.[15] These models are not provided here because they did not lead to different conclusions. To assess potential bias resulting from missing data, means or proportions of subject characteristics included in mutually adjusted models were compared with 95% confidence intervals of the mean or proportion of the respective characteristic among the full study population within each study. Approximately 3.4% and 5.0% of subjects were missing data in UBCS and SPATZ, respectively, and no significant differences in characteristics were observed between study and analysis population in either cohort. All statistical analyses were performed by using SAS 9.3 (SAS Institute, Cary, NC).

RESULTS

Demographic characteristics and comparisons between UBCS and SPATZ are provided in Table 1. Notably, interstudy differences were observed for a number of demographic and breastfeeding characteristics. More than 85% and 90% of mothers, respectively, initiated predominant and any breastfeeding in both cohorts. Predominant and any breastfeeding rates appeared similar between cohorts up to 3 weeks postdelivery, after which rates in SPATZ remained higher until 4 months and throughout lactation, respectively (Fig 1A and 1B).

Crude hazard ratios for differences between the 2 studies (study effect/ time trend) on breastfeeding cessation corresponded with the patterns described and were statistically significant at every modeled time point up to 6 months except noninitiation of predominant breastfeeding (see Table 2). In separate models adjusted for single covariates, the association between study effect and breastfeeding behavior was primarily explained by differences in maternal education and partially by differences in smoking behavior and age at delivery (see Supplemental Table 5). In contrast, point estimates were driven away from the null, albeit marginally, when individually adjusted for maternal BMI or cesarean delivery. After mutual adjustment for all maternal demographic and lifestyle factors, estimates were slightly attenuated toward the null but remained significant for all modeled time points except initiation (see Table 2).

To investigate further why the mediating effect of education on time trend was no longer observed in mutually adjusted models, we tested for interaction. Significant *P* values for interaction between study effect and education were observed at every time point except initiation in mutually adjusted predominant and total breastfeeding models (data not shown). Kaplan-Meier plots stratified by study and education showed improvement in breastfeeding patterns between studies among mothers with higher education but nearly identical patterns among less educated mothers who were at greater risk for early cessation throughout lactation (see Fig 2A and 2B). In mutually adjusted models stratified by education, study effects similar to those observed in all-subject models were present for both less and more educated mothers, indicating time trend was confounded among mothers with less education by differences between studies in demographic and lifestyle factors (see Table 3).

In the more recent SPATZ cohort, for which more complete information on potential determinants of breastfeeding was available, the contribution of factors associated with breastfeeding cessation were evaluated in mutually adjusted models (see Table 4). Suboptimal BMI and elective cesarean delivery were independently associated with higher noninitiation and cessation rates, whereas emergency cesarean delivery and maternal education were only associated with higher cessation rates. In particular the strong associations with suboptimal BMI declined over time. The effect of smoking was dependent on smoking behavior or time smoking was resumed. Continuous smoking was associated with higher rates of noninitiation of predominant breastfeeding. Mothers who resumed smoking at 6 weeks postdelivery had significantly higher rates of both predominant and any breastfeeding at 4 and 6 months, respectively. A similar time-dependent association was

TABLE 1 Descriptive Characteristics of the 2000–2001 UBCS and 2012–2013 SPATZ Birth Cohorts

Descriptive Characteristic	2000–2001 UBCS, % (n = 989)	2012–2013 SPATZ, % (n = 856)	P
Education ≥12 y	37.7	60.9	<.001[a]
Alcohol consumed in year before pregnancy	67.8	69.5	.446
Alcohol consumption during lactation			NA
Never drinker	NA	23.1	
Abstinent drinker	NA	26.0	
Resumed at 6 wk to 6 mo	NA	20.5	
Resumed by 6 wk	NA	19.9	
Undetermined drinking	NA	10.5	
Smoked in year before pregnancy	32.5	27.1	.012[a]
Smoking during lactation			<.001[a]
Never smoker	66.4	71.5	
Abstinent smoker	11.7	10.6	
Resumed smoking	2.4	3.4	
Continuous smoker	13.4	6.1	
Undetermined smoker	6.0	8.4	
Prepregnancy BMI			.004[a]
Normal (≤18.5 to <25)	66.7	61.4	
Underweight (<18.5)	3.4	2.2	
Overweight (≤25 to 30)	21.4	23.4	
Obese (≥30)	8.5	13.0	
Delivery mode			<.001[a]
Vaginal spontaneous	80.0	67.1	
Elective cesarean	5.0	12.1	
Emergency cesarean	10.9	12.3	
Vaginal assisted	4.1	8.5	
Age at delivery, y			<.001[a]
<30	37.8	26.6	
30–35	39.3	43.0	
>35	23.0	30.4	
Returned to work after delivery			NA
No	NA	63.7	
Month 1–3	NA	5.3	
Month 4–6	NA	4.4	
Month 7–12	NA	8.3	
Undetermined	NA	18.3	
German nationality	79.8	85.2	.002[a]
Parity ≥1 birth	49.7	48.1	.490
Initiation of predominant breastfeeding	85.2	85.6	.829
Predominant breastfeeding at 4 mo[b]	65.5	64.5	.689
Initiation of any breastfeeding	91.6	94.7	.012[a]
Any breastfeeding at 6 mo[c]	58.6	67.2	<.001[a]

NA, not available.
[a] Significant *P* value.
[b] Restricted to subjects with noncensored data on predominant breastfeeding at 4-month data (UBCS *n* = 829; SPATZ *n* = 673).
[c] Restricted to subjects with noncensored data on any breastfeeding at 6-month data (UBCS *n* = 863; SPATZ *n* = 714).

TABLE 2 Crude and Mutually Adjusted Cox Proportional Hazard Ratios for Study Effect (2000–2001 UBCS vs 2012–2013 SPATZ) on Noninitiation and Cessation of Breastfeeding

Breastfeeding Behavior and Outcome	Hazard Ratio (95% Confidence Interval)	
	Crude	Mutually Adjusted[a]
Predominant		
Noninitiation	1.01 (0.78–1.30)	1.00 (0.76–1.31)
Cessation at 6 wk	0.76 (0.63–0.93)	0.79 (0.64–0.97)
Cessation at 4 mo	0.79 (0.67–0.93)	0.83 (0.69–0.99)
Any	0.68 (0.47–0.99)	0.75 (0.50–1.11)
Noninitiation		
Cessation at 6 wk	0.66 (0.52–0.84)	0.70 (0.54–0.90)
Cessation at 3 mo	0.71 (0.58–0.88)	0.73 (0.59–0.91)
Cessation at 6 mo	0.71 (0.60–0.82)	0.73 (0.62–0.86)
Cessation at 9 mo	0.75 (0.66–0.85)	0.79 (0.70–0.91)

[a] Mutually adjusted for maternal education, smoking, BMI, delivery mode, age, nationality, and first parity.

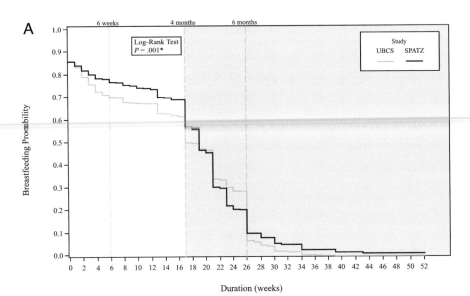

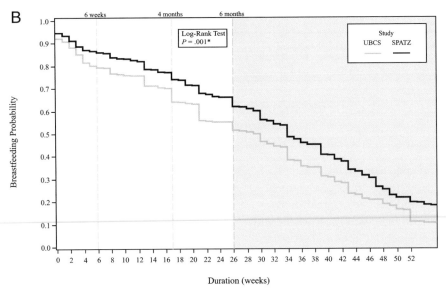

FIGURE 1
A, Duration of predominant breastfeeding in the 2000–2001 UBCS and 2012–2013 SPATZ cohorts. B, Duration of any breastfeeding in the 2000–2001 UBCS and 2012–2013 SPATZ cohorts. *Log-rank statistic for predominant breastfeeding up to 4 months (shaded area not included).

observed for resumption of alcohol consumption. Conversely, abstaining from drinking alcohol throughout lactation was strongly associated with lower risk of breastfeeding cessation. Returning to work did not affect breastfeeding cessation at any time; the significant results for the "undetermined" category are likely attributable to higher proportions of factors associated with breastfeeding cessation observed among mothers who lacked complete data (data not shown).

In the earlier UBCS cohort, in which we were not able to adjust for alcohol consumption or return to work status, we observed some similarities in associations for maternal education, suboptimal BMI, and smoking behavior, but not cesarean delivery (see Supplemental Table 6).

DISCUSSION

In our cohorts, we observed increased rates of initiation and duration of predominant and overall breastfeeding over an 11-year period among mothers with >12 years of education. In contrast, no significant change in breastfeeding behavior was observed among less educated mothers, which was largely explained by corresponding increases in the proportions of smoking, overweight and obesity, and elective cesarean delivery in this group. Of the personal and lifestyle risk factors we examined in both cohorts, none explained the time trend toward more positive breastfeeding patterns. In the latter cohort, actively abstaining from drinking alcohol was significantly associated with lower rates of early cessation, implying the importance of planned behavior in breastfeeding outcomes.

Although at least 1 retrospective study previously identified widening socioeconomic disparity in breastfeeding practices,[16] our study is among the first to investigate the effects of demographic shifts on breastfeeding between 2 population-based cohorts recruited in the same maternity ward using nearly identical methodology thus providing a superior baseline for time-trend analysis. In addition, our study also accounts for time-dependent effects including smoking and alcohol consumption, which may change over the postpartum period thereby reducing misclassification of these risk factors in our models. Still, we did encounter some limitations. Although we were able to control for a number of a priori risk factors, we lacked psychosocial data pertaining to familial attitudes and support, which have also been previously associated with breastfeeding practices.[17] Furthermore, the impact of medical issues related to breastfeeding including lactation issues, counterindicative medications, and mastitis were not assessed.[18-20] It is likely these factors meaningfully contributed to early cessation rates. However, we observed similar patterns of association for individual risk factors in sensitivity analyses restricted to mothers successfully breastfeeding (>6 times/day) at 6 weeks postdelivery (data not shown). This implies validity of our results after any further influence on early breastfeeding cessation. Finally, 67% and 49% of eligible families enrolled in UBCS and SPATZ, respectively. Although these rates are respectable for a population-based study in this setting, some selection bias within each cohort cannot be completely ruled out because characteristics of nonparticipants were not ascertained.

Initial and 6-month breastfeeding rates observed in our cohorts corresponded well with results (89.5% and 51.6%, respectively)

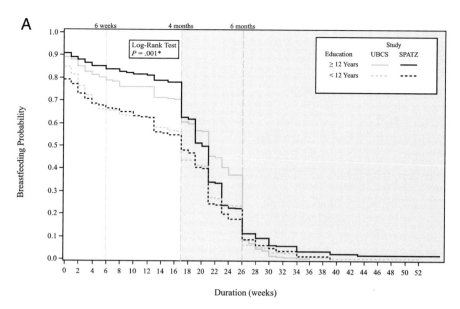

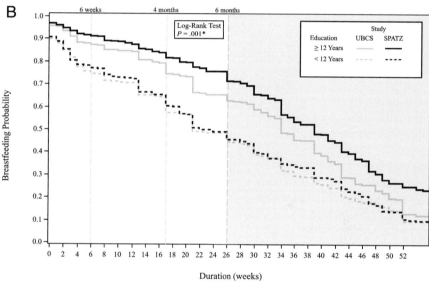

FIGURE 2

A, Duration of predominant breastfeeding in the in 2000–2001 UBCS and 2012–2013 SPATZ cohorts stratified by maternal education. B, Duration of any breastfeeding in the 2000–2001 UBCS and 2012–2013 SPATZ cohorts stratified by maternal education. *Log-rank statistic for predominant breastfeeding up to 4 months (shaded area not included).

reported in 2005 among Bavarian mothers.[6] However, breastfeeding initiation rates and duration were higher than those reported retrospectively and with largely longer recall periods in a nationwide cross-sectional survey conducted in 2003–2006.[4] Predominant breastfeeding patterns compared well between Ulm cohorts, however, were higher than the similarly defined "exclusive breastfeeding"

at 4 months rate (41.7%) and lower than the "fully breastfed for at least 6 months" (~33%), respectively, reported in Bavaria and nationwide.[4,6] Therefore, initial and overall breastfeeding rates in our study may not be representative of areas outside of our study region and predominant rates may not be comparable to those reported using nonanalogous breastfeeding definitions.

The most striking feature of our data were an observed demographic shift marked by an ~60% increase in the proportion of higher educated mothers. This increase is only slightly higher than the 40% to 50% increase derived from statewide census data for Baden-Wurttemberg within women of corresponding age making substantial participation bias unlikely.[21] Furthermore, although we observed an expected decrease in overall smoking rates, the proportion of less educated mothers who smoked increased by 16%. This disparity is analogous to previously reported smoking trends in southern Germany.[22]

Our findings with respect to maternal education are somewhat supported by those of Scott et al, who reported no association between maternal education and initiation of predominant or overall breastfeeding in a similarly designed time-trend analysis of breastfeeding rates at hospital discharge among Australian mothers recruited 10 years apart.[23] They suggested "social inequalities in breastfeeding initiation are less apparent as breastfeeding initiation approaches universality," which may also have been the case in our study. In contrast, they reported no significant difference in total breastfeeding cessation by 6 months over time and no effect of education in the latter cohort.[17] However, the cohorts they examined had much larger proportions of higher educated mothers (86.9% and 96.5%) and no analysis of the effect on time trend was reported.

Differential results between mothers with higher and lower education may be indicative of widening socioeconomic gaps in breastfeeding attitudes, knowledge of the health benefits of long-term breastfeeding, or other unmeasured factors related to general education.[24,25] More educated mothers may also be more likely to seek medical advice and use available health services with regard to breastfeeding.[26] This theory may be supported by differences observed in SPATZ in relation to rates of noninitiation and early cessation associated with elective cesarean delivery, which have also been observed in other studies.[9] Among lower educated mothers, those who chose elective cesarean delivery were at significantly higher risk for noninitiation and early breastfeeding cessation up to 9 months postdelivery (data not shown). In contrast, no significant difference in early breastfeeding behavior was observed among higher educated mothers who had elective cesarean.

Despite overall improvement in breastfeeding patterns, little change was observed in associations between early breastfeeding cessation and individual and lifestyle factors over time. Prepregnancy obesity was independently associated with higher cessation rates by 6 weeks in both cohorts. These results support findings of recent studies conducted in other developed countries associating maternal obesity with higher risk of noninitiation and shorter breastfeeding duration.[27,28] Although reasons for this association remain unclear, some evidence suggests links to psychosocial factors including low self-efficacy among obese mothers.[29] Obese mothers may be more prone to delayed lactogenesis,[30] difficulty positioning the child for breastfeeding, and other issues including fatigue and mastitis.[31] Kohlhuber et al reported that previous breastfeeding experience may mediate this association.[32] Although we did not collect data specifically on previous breastfeeding experience in either cohort, effects were similar after adjustment for parity and within strata of primiparous and multiparous mothers, which may contradict this hypothesis.

Smoking and alcohol consumption during lactation were also associated with higher rates of early cessation but mostly only after resumption of the behavior. Although these associations may be due to reverse causation,[33] some studies suggest nicotine and alcohol in breast milk may affect milk volume,[34] infant behavior, and sleeping patterns, which could inhibit a willing mother's ability to breastfeed early on, thereby motivating earlier cessation.[35] Mothers who abstained from smoking up to 6 months displayed similar breastfeeding patterns to

TABLE 3 Crude and Mutually Adjusted Cox Proportional Hazard Ratios for Study Effect (2000–2001 UBCS vs 2012–2013 SPATZ) on Noninitiation and Cessation of Breastfeeding Stratified by Maternal Education

Breastfeeding Behavior and Outcome	Hazard Ratio (95% Confidence Interval)			
	Less Education (<12 Years)		More Education (≥12 Years)	
	Crude	Mutually Adjusted[a]	Crude	Mutually Adjusted[a]
Predominant				
Noninitiation	1.40 (1.02–1.92)	1.09 (0.78–1.54)	0.80 (0.52–1.24)	0.86 (0.55–1.34)
Cessation at 6 wk	1.02 (0.79–1.30)	0.81 (0.62–1.06)	0.73 (0.52–1.02)	0.80 (0.56–1.14)
Cessation at 4 mo	1.09 (0.87–1.35)	0.92 (0.73–1.15)	0.72 (0.54–0.95)	0.76 (0.56–1.01)
Any				
Noninitiation	0.91 (0.59–1.42)	0.72 (0.45–1.17)	0.68 (0.33–1.41)	0.77 (0.36–1.63)
Cessation at 6 wk	0.88 (0.66–1.18)	0.70 (0.51–0.95)	0.67 (0.44–1.04)	0.73 (0.47–1.14)
Cessation at 3 mo	0.92 (0.71–1.20)	0.73 (0.55–0.96)	0.74 (0.51–1.07)	0.81 (0.56–1.19)
Cessation at 6 mo	0.98 (0.81–1.20)	0.81 (0.66–1.00)	0.66 (0.51–0.85)	0.64 (0.49–0.83)
Cessation at 9 mo	0.93 (0.79–1.11)	0.82 (0.68–0.98)	0.79 (0.65–0.96)	0.76 (0.62–0.93)

[a] Mutually adjusted for maternal smoking, BMI, delivery mode, age, nationality, and first parity.

TABLE 4 Mutually Adjusted Cox Proportional Hazard Ratios for Noninitiation and Cessation of Breastfeeding in the 2012–2013-SPATZ Cohort

Risk Factor	Hazard Ratio (95% Confidence Interval)					
	Predominant Breastfeeding			Any Breastfeeding		
	Noninitiation	Cessation at 6 Weeks	Cessation at 4 Months	Noninitiation	Cessation at 6 Weeks	Cessation at 6 Months
Education						
≥12 y	ref	ref	ref	ref	ref	ref
<12 y	1.18 (0.75–1.87)	1.44 (1.00–2.09)	1.50 (1.10–2.05)	1.74 (0.83; 3.66)	1.87 (1.18–2.97)	1.66 (1.25–2.21)
Alcohol status						
Never drinker	Reference	Reference	Reference	Reference	Reference	Reference
Abstinent drinker	0.42 (0.19–0.94)	0.44 (0.23–0.84)	0.46 (0.27–0.78)	0.35 (0.07–1.74)	0.35 (0.13–0.96)	0.36 (0.21–0.63)
Resumed at 6 wk to 6 mo	0.76 (0.39–1.52)	0.96 (0.56–1.66)	1.14 (0.73–1.77)	0.77 (0.25–2.40)	0.86 (0.40–1.86)	1.63 (1.10–2.40)
Resumed by 6 wk	1.02 (0.58–1.78)	1.61 (1.00–2.57)	1.52 (1.01–2.30)	1.62 (0.68–3.87)	3.08 (1.71–5.55)	2.13 (1.46–3.12)
Undetermined	0.56 (0.28–1.13)	0.81 (0.43–1.50)	0.88 (0.51–1.52)	0.55 (0.17–1.74)	1.18 (0.55–2.54)	1.08 (0.65–1.80)
Smoking status						
Never smoker	Reference	Reference	Reference	Reference	Reference	Reference
Abstinent smoker	1.41 (0.74–2.67)	1.05 (0.63–1.77)	1.11 (0.71–1.73)	2.26 (0.90–5.68)	1.41 (0.76–2.60)	1.22 (0.82–1.80)
Resumed smoking	1.48 (0.57–3.87)	1.18 (0.53–2.62)	2.11 (1.20–3.70)	0.67 (0.09–5.35)	1.13 (0.43–2.95)	2.03 (1.21–3.38)
Continuous smoker	2.23 (1.18–4.19)	1.69 (0.99–2.88)	1.78 (1.12–2.82)	1.14 (0.41–3.21)	1.02 (0.51–2.04)	1.54 (0.99–2.39)
Undetermined	2.25 (1.10–4.58)	1.63 (0.89–2.98)	1.28 (0.75–2.18)	1.04 (0.34–3.25)	1.08 (0.54–2.16)	1.11 (0.67–1.84)
Prepregnancy BMI						
Normal (≤18.5 to <25)	Reference	Reference	Reference	Reference	Reference	Reference
Underweight (<18.5)	4.22 (1.85–9.61)	3.35 (1.60–7.01)	2.64 (1.30–5.37)	4.92 (1.59–15.23)	3.93 (1.59–9.72)	2.60 (1.25–5.43)
Overweight (≤25 to <30)	2.30 (1.43–3.71)	1.87 (1.28–2.73)	1.51 (1.09–2.09)	1.65 (0.76–3.61)	1.67 (1.04–2.67)	1.34 (0.99–1.81)
Obese (BMI ≥30)	2.85 (1.68–4.85)	2.37 (1.54–3.64)	1.98 (1.37–2.87)	2.05 (0.87–4.85)	2.09 (1.23–3.57)	1.76 (1.25–2.47)
Delivery mode						
Vaginal spontaneous	Reference	Reference	Reference	Reference	Reference	Reference
Elective cesarean	1.73 (1.08–2.77)	1.81 (1.21–2.72)	1.60 (1.11–2.31)	2.29 (1.11–4.73)	1.68 (1.02–2.77)	1.90 (1.36–2.66)
Emergency cesarean	1.55 (0.91–2.65)	1.87 (1.21–2.89)	1.96 (1.35–2.85)	1.83 (0.77–4.36)	1.54 (0.88–2.68)	1.66 (1.16–2.37)
Vaginal assisted	0.70 (0.24–1.97)	1.10 (0.55–2.17)	1.08 (0.62–1.88)	0.51 (0.07–3.96)	0.79 (0.31–2.05)	1.16 (0.72–1.88)
Returned to work after delivery						
Did not work	Reference	Reference	Reference	Reference	Reference	Reference
Month 1–3	0.92 (0.33–2.57)	0.54 (0.20–1.49)	0.72 (0.35–1.49)	1.58 (0.45–5.59)	0.93 (0.33–2.60)	1.24 (0.73–2.10)
Month 4–6	0.80 (0.28–2.29)	0.78 (0.33–1.82)	0.87 (0.42–1.81)	1.51 (0.41–5.51)	1.19 (0.50–2.84)	1.36 (0.80–2.30)
Month 7–12	0.46 (0.14–1.48)	0.72 (0.35–1.51)	0.83 (0.46–1.47)	NA	1.08 (0.46–2.57)	1.12 (0.67–1.87)
Undetermined	1.88 (1.03–3.43)	1.59 (0.94–2.70)	1.98 (1.23–3.18)	3.16 (1.24–8.01)	2.43 (1.28–4.61)	2.57 (1.64–4.04)

NA signifies not applicable (eg, no participants in the numerator).

nonsmokers, and, surprisingly, those who abstained from drinking alcohol were at significantly lower risk for early breastfeeding cessation even when compared with mothers who reported no history of drinking. Given the importance of the postpartum period for motivating long-term changes in health behavior, this finding supports need for stage-matched interventions including promoting continued smoking cessation before and after breastfeeding cessation.[36,37]

CONCLUSIONS

In our cohorts, longer duration of predominant and any breastfeeding observed over time were likely due to upstream events resulting in increased prevalence of higher general education among women and subsequent lower rates of individual risk factors including smoking and obesity. Among lower educated women, <50% met minimum predominant breastfeeding guidelines, whereas <30% met minimum guidelines for overall breastfeeding duration, rates far lower than those observed among higher educated mothers. These results suggest widening socioeconomic and subsequent health-related disparities, which may require specific interventions aimed at improving breastfeeding patterns in Germany and elsewhere. Although programs focusing on obesity, smoking, and cesarean delivery would benefit all mothers, programs tailored specifically toward less educated mothers are necessary.

ACKNOWLEDGMENTS

We thank the midwives, nurses, and obstetricians of the Department of Gynecology and Obstetrics, University Medical Center Ulm, for their study support. We also thank Gisela Breitinger and Christa Johanna Knauß for providing excellent technical assistance.

ABBREVIATIONS

HR: hazard ratio
UBCS: Ulm Birth Cohort Study
SPATZ: Ulm SPATZ Health Study

PEDIATRICS (ISSN Numbers: Print, 0031-4005; Online, 1098-4275).

FINANCIAL DISCLOSURE: The authors have indicated they have no financial relationships relevant to this article to disclose.

FUNDING: The Ulm Birth Cohort Study was supported by grants of the German Research Council (BR 1704/3-1, BR 1704/3-2, BR 1704/3-3). The Ulm SPATZ Health Study was funded through an unrestricted grant by the Medical Faculty of Ulm University. These funders had no role in the study design; in the collection, analysis, and interpretation of data; in the writing of the report; or in the decision to submit the article for publication. The contributing researchers are independent of the funders.

POTENTIAL CONFLICT OF INTEREST: The authors have indicated they have no potential conflicts of interest to disclose.

REFERENCES

1. World Health Organization. UNICEF. *Global Strategy for Infant and Young Child Feeding*. Geneva, Switzerland: World Health Organization; 2003. Available at: http://www.who.int/nutrition/publications/infantfeeding/9241562218/en. Accessed September 1, 2015

2. Hoddinott P, Tappin D, Wright C. Breast feeding. *BMJ*. 2008;336(7649):881–887 10.1136/bmj.39521.566296.BE

3. Horta BL, Bahl R, Martines JC, Victora CG; World Health Organization. *Evidence on the Long-Term Effects of Breastfeeding: Systematic Review and Meta-Analyses*. 2007. Available at: http://www.who.int/iris/handle/10665/43623. Accessed August 10, 2015

4. Lange C, Schenk L, Bergmann R. Distribution, duration and temporal trend of breastfeeding in Germany. Results of the German Health Interview and Examination Survey for Children and Adolescents (KiGGS) [in German]. *Bundesgesundheitsblatt Gesundheitsforschung Gesundheitsschutz*. 2007;50(5-6):624–633 10.1007/s00103-007-0223-9

5. Bundesinstitut für Risikobewertung. Empfehlung der Nationalen Stillkommission am BfR vom 1. March 2004. Available at: http://www.bfr.bund.de/cm/343/stilldauer.pdf. Accessed September 1, 2015

6. Kohlhuber M, Rebhan B, Schwegler U, Koletzko B, Fromme H. Breastfeeding rates and duration in Germany: a Bavarian cohort study. *Br J Nutr*. 2008;99(5):1127–1132 10.1017/S0007114508864835

7. Bertini G, Perugi S, Dani C, Pezzati M, Tronchin M, Rubaltelli FF. Maternal education and the incidence and duration of breast feeding: a prospective study. *J Pediatr Gastroenterol Nutr*. 2003;37(4):447–452

8. Horta BL, Kramer MS, Platt RW. Maternal smoking and the risk of early weaning: a meta-analysis. *Am J Public Health*. 2001;91(2):304–307

9. Prior E, Santhakumaran S, Gale C, Philipps LH, Modi N, Hyde MJ. Breastfeeding after cesarean delivery: a systematic review and meta-analysis of world literature. *Am J Clin Nutr*. 2012;95(5):1113–1135 10.3945/ajcn.111.030254

10. Taveras EM, Capra AM, Braveman PA, Jensvold NG, Escobar GJ, Lieu TA. Clinician support and psychosocial risk factors associated with breastfeeding discontinuation. *Pediatrics*. 2003;112(1 pt 1):108–115

11. Weyermann M, Rothenbacher D, Brenner H. Duration of breastfeeding and risk of overweight in childhood: a prospective birth cohort study from Germany. *Int J Obes 2005*. 2006;30(8):1281–1287. doi:10.1038/sj.ijo.0803260

12. Braig S, Grabher F, Ntomchukwu C, et al. Determinants of maternal hair cortisol concentrations at delivery reflecting the last trimester of pregnancy. *Psychoneuroendocrinology*. 2015;52:289–296 10.1016/j.psyneuen.2014.12.006

13. World Health Organization Dept of Child and Adolescent Health and Development. Indicators for assessing infant and young child feeding practices: part 1. Definitions: conclusions of a consensus meeting held 6 November 8, 2007 in Washington DC, USA. 2008. Available at: http://apps.who.int//iris/handle/10665/43895. Accessed September 1, 2015

14. VanderWeele TJ. Unmeasured confounding and hazard scales: sensitivity analysis for total, direct, and indirect effects. *Eur J Epidemiol*. 2013;28(2):113–117 10.1007/s10654-013-9770-6

15. Zou G. A modified poisson regression approach to prospective studies with binary data. *Am J Epidemiol*. 2004;159(7):702–706

16. Amir LH, Donath SM. Socioeconomic status and rates of breastfeeding in Australia: evidence from three recent national health surveys. *Med J Aust*. 2008;189(5):254–256

17. Scott JA, Binns CW, Oddy WH, Graham KI. Predictors of breastfeeding duration: evidence from a cohort study. *Pediatrics*. 2006;117(4):e646–e655 10.1542/peds.2005-1991

18. Odom EC, Li R, Scanlon KS, Perrine CG, Grummer-Strawn L. Reasons for earlier than desired cessation of breastfeeding. *Pediatrics*. 2013;131(3):e726–e732 10.1542/peds.2012-1295

19. Schirm E, Schwagermann MP, Tobi H, de Jong-van den Berg LTW. Drug use during breastfeeding. A survey from the Netherlands. *Eur J Clin Nutr*. 2004;58(2):386–390 10.1038/sj.ejcn.1601799

20. Amir LH. Managing common breastfeeding problems in the community. *BMJ*. 2014;348:g2954

21. *Referat 24 Mikrozensus*. Stuttgart, Germany: Statistisches Landesamt Baden-Württemberg; 2014

22. Maziak W, Hense HW, Döring A, Keil U. Ten-year trends in smoking behaviour among adults in southern Germany. *Int J Tuberc Lung Dis.* 2002;6(9):824–830

23. Scott JA, Binns CW, Graham KI, Oddy WH. Temporal changes in the determinants of breastfeeding initiation. *Birth.* 2006;33(1):37–45 10.1111/j.0730-7659.2006.00072.x

24. Yang S, Platt RW, Dahhou M, Kramer MS. Do population-based interventions widen or narrow socioeconomic inequalities? The case of breastfeeding promotion. *Int J Epidemiol.* 2014;43(4):1284–1292 10.1093/ije/dyu051

25. Webb AL, Sellen DW, Ramakrishnan U, Martorell R. Maternal years of schooling but not academic skills is independently associated with infant-feeding practices in a cohort of rural Guatemalan women. *J Hum Lact.* 2009;25(3):297–306 10.1177/0890334408330449

26. Menon ST. Toward a model of psychological health empowerment: implications for health care in multicultural communities. *Nurse Educ Today.* 2002;22(1):28–39, discussion 40–43 10.1054/nedt.2001.0721

27. Verret-Chalifour J, Giguère Y, Forest J-C, Croteau J, Zhang P, Marc I. Breastfeeding initiation: impact of obesity in a large Canadian perinatal cohort study. *PLoS One.* 2015;10(2):e0117512 10.1371/journal.pone.0117512

28. Mäkelä J, Vaarno J, Kaljonen A, Niinikoski H, Lagström H. Maternal overweight impacts infant feeding patterns--the STEPS Study. *Eur J Clin Nutr.* 2014;68(1):43–49 10.1038/ejcn.2013.229

29. Hauff LE, Leonard SA, Rasmussen KM. Associations of maternal obesity and psychosocial factors with breastfeeding intention, initiation, and duration. *Am J Clin Nutr.* 2014;99(3):524–534 10.3945/ajcn.113.071191

30. Rasmussen KM, Kjolhede CL. Prepregnant overweight and obesity diminish the prolactin response to suckling in the first week postpartum. *Pediatrics.* 2004;113(5). Available at: www.pediatrics.org/cgi/content/full/113/5/e465

31. Turcksin R, Bel S, Galjaard S, Devlieger R. Maternal obesity and breastfeeding intention, initiation, intensity and duration: a systematic review. *Matern Child Nutr.* 2014;10(2):166–183 10.1111/j.1740-8709.2012.00439.x

32. Kronborg H, Vaeth M, Rasmussen KM. Obesity and early cessation of breastfeeding in Denmark. *Eur J Public Health.* 2013;23(2):316–322 10.1093/eurpub/cks135

33. Donath SM, Amir LH; ALSPAC Study Team. The relationship between maternal smoking and breastfeeding duration after adjustment for maternal infant feeding intention. *Acta Paediatr.* 2004;93(11):1514–1518 10.1111/j.1651-2227.2004.tb02639.x

34. Vio F, Salazar G, Infante C. Smoking during pregnancy and lactation and its effects on breast-milk volume. *Am J Clin Nutr.* 1991;54(6):1011–1016

35. Haastrup MB, Pottegård A, Damkier P. Alcohol and breastfeeding. *Basic Clin Pharmacol Toxicol.* 2014;114(2):168–173 10.1111/bcpt.12149

36. Prochaska JO, Velicer WF. The transtheoretical model of health behavior change. *Am J Health Promot.* 1997;12(1):38–48 10.4278/0890-1171-12.1.38

37. Su A, Buttenheim AM. Maintenance of smoking cessation in the postpartum period: which interventions work best in the long-term? *Matern Child Health J.* 2014;18(3):714–728 10.1007/s10995-013-1298-6

Supplemental Information

SUPPLEMENTAL TABLE 5 Change in Study Effect Point Estimate (2000–2001 UBCS vs 2012–2013 SPATZ) After Single Adjustment for Demographic and Lifestyle Factors

Breastfeeding Behavior and Outcome	Crude Study Effect, HR (95% CI)	Change in Point Estimate After Adjustment for Single Factor						
		Education	Smoking	BMI	Delivery	Age	Nationality	Parity
Predominant								
Noninitiation	1.01 (0.78–1.30)	+0.14[a]	+0.10[a]	(−0.06)[a]	(−0.08)[a]	+0.02[a]	+0.00[a]	+0.00[a]
Cessation at 6 wk	0.76 (0.63–0.93)	+0.14[a]	+0.06	(−0.03)	(−0.04)	+0.05	+0.01	+0.00
Cessation at 4 mo	0.79 (0.67–0.93)	+0.14[a]	+0.04	(−0.02)	(−0.03)	+0.05	+0.01	+0.00
Any								
Noninitiation	0.68 (0.47–0.99)	+0.16[a]	+0.11[a]	(−0.04)	(−0.05)	+0.02[a]	(−0.01)	+0.00
Cessation at 6 wk	0.66 (0.52–0.84)	+0.15[a]	+0.05	(−0.04)	(−0.03)	+0.05	+0.00	+0.00
Cessation at 3 mo	0.71 (0.58–0.88)	+0.15[a]	+0.04	(−0.04)	(−0.04)	+0.05	+0.00	+0.00
Cessation at 6 mo	0.71 (0.60–0.82)	+0.13	+0.02	(−0.03)	(−0.04)	+0.05	+0.01	(−0.01)
Cessation at 9 mo	0.75 (0.66–0.85)	+0.12	+0.03	(−0.02)	(−0.03)	+0.05	+0.01	+0.00

CI, confidence interval; HR, hazard ratio.
[a] Indicates the study effect was not statistically significant after adjustment (ie, the 95% CI includes 1.00).

SUPPLEMENTAL TABLE 6 Mutually Adjusted Cox Proportional Hazard Ratios for Noninitiation and Cessation of Breastfeeding in the 2000–2001 UBCS Cohort

Risk Factor	Hazard Ratio (95% Confidence Interval)					
	Predominant breastfeeding			Any breastfeeding		
	Noninitiation	Cessation at 6 Weeks	Cessation at 4 Months	Noninitiation	Cessation at 6 Weeks	Cessation at 6 Months
Education						
≥12 y	Reference	Reference	Reference	Reference	Reference	Reference
<12 y	1.13 (0.76–1.69)	1.33 (1.00–1.78)	1.20 (0.94–1.54)	1.73 (0.95–3.14)	1.48 (1.03–2.11)	1.26 (1.01–1.57)
Smoking status						
Never smoker	ref	ref	ref	ref	ref	ref
Abstinent smoker	0.30 (0.11–0.83)	0.49 (0.28–0.85)	0.53 (0.34–0.83)	NA	NA	0.75 (0.53–1.07)
Resumed smoking	NA	0.85 (0.34–2.09)	1.30 (0.68–2.48)	NA	0.23 (0.03–1.67)	1.66 (0.96–2.87)
Continuous smoker	2.84 (1.88–4.29)	3.13 (2.32–4.22)	2.99 (2.28–3.92)	4.42 (2.63–7.43)	4.03 (2.89–5.63)	3.16 (2.46–4.06)
Undetermined	2.00 (1.06–3.76)	3.00 (2.00–4.50)	2.95 (2.02–4.30)	3.07 (1.43–6.59)	3.70 (2.35–5.84)	3.22 (2.23–4.65)
Prepregnancy BMI						
Normal (≤18.5 to <25)	Reference	Reference	Reference	Reference	Reference	Reference
Underweight (<18.5)	1.87 (0.81–4.32)	1.42 (0.77–2.64)	1.29 (0.74–2.22)	1.34 (0.32–5.60)	0.95 (0.39–2.35)	0.89 (0.50–1.60)
Overweight (≤25 to <30)	1.38 (0.90–2.09)	1.29 (0.95–1.76)	1.30 (1.00–1.70)	1.21 (0.68–2.13)	1.17 (0.81–1.70)	1.35 (1.06–1.70)
Obese (BMI ≥30)	1.53 (0.88–2.67)	2.02 (1.38–2.94)	1.90 (1.34–2.68)	2.15 (1.15–4.02)	2.18 (1.44–3.32)	1.87 (1.36–2.59)
Delivery mode						
Vaginal spontaneous	Reference	Reference	Reference	Reference	Reference	Reference
Elective cesarean	1.05 (0.50–2.20)	1.26 (0.76–2.09)	1.30 (0.83–2.03)	0.90 (0.35–2.30)	1.03 (0.56–1.89)	1.41 (0.95–2.09)
Emergency cesarean	1.43 (0.86–2.38)	1.35 (0.95–1.93)	1.22 (0.88–1.68)	1.62 (0.85–3.11)	1.37 (0.90–2.08)	1.20 (0.89–1.62)
Vaginal assisted	1.66 (0.76–3.65)	1.27 (0.68–2.35)	1.05 (0.59–1.84)	1.68 (0.51–5.54)	1.30 (0.60–2.81)	1.20 (0.74–1.95)

NA, not applicable (eg, no participants in the numerator).

Impact of Prolonged Breastfeeding on Dental Caries: A Population-Based Birth Cohort Study

Karen Glazer Peres, BDS, PhD,[a] Gustavo G. Nascimento, BDS, PhD,[b,c] Marco Aurelio Peres, BDS, PhD,[a] Murthy N. Mittinty, PhD,[d] Flavio Fernando Demarco, BDS, PhD,[e] Ina Silva Santos, MD, PhD,[e] Alicia Matijasevich, MD, PhD,[f] Aluisio J D Barros, MD, PhD[e]

BACKGROUND: Few studies have assessed the effect of breastfeeding, bottle feeding, and sugar consumption on children's dental caries. We investigated whether the duration of breastfeeding is a risk factor for dental caries in the primary dentition, independently of sugar consumption.

METHODS: An oral health study (*n* = 1303) nested in a birth cohort study was carried out in southern Brazil. The average number of decayed, missing, and filled primary tooth surfaces (dmfs) and severe early childhood caries (S-ECC: dmfs $\geq$6) were investigated at age 5 years. Breastfeeding was the main exposure collected at birth and at 3, 12, and 24 months of age. Data on sugar consumption were collected at 24, 48, and 60 months of age. Marginal structural modeling was used to estimate the controlled direct effect of breastfeeding (0–12, 13–23, and $\geq$24 months) on dmfs and on S-ECC.

RESULTS: The prevalence of S-ECC was 23.9%. The mean number of dmfs was 4.05. Children who were breastfed for $\geq$24 months had a higher number of dmfs (mean ratio: 1.9; 95% confidence interval: 1.5–2.4) and a 2.4 times higher risk of having S-ECC (risk ratio: 2.4; 95% confidence interval: 1.7–3.3) than those who were breastfed up to 12 months of age. Breastfeeding between 13 and 23 months had no effect on dental caries.

CONCLUSIONS: Prolonged breastfeeding increases the risk of having dental caries. Preventive interventions for dental caries should be established as early as possible because breastfeeding is beneficial for children's health. Mechanisms underlying this process should be investigated more deeply.

[a]*Australian Research Centre for Population Oral Health, Adelaide Dental School, and [d]Discipline of Public Health, School of Public Health, University of Adelaide, Adelaide, South Australia, Australia; [b]Graduate Program in Dentistry, School of Dentistry, and [e]Postgraduate Program in Epidemiology, Federal University of Pelotas, Pelotas, Brazil; [f]Department of Preventive Medicine, School of Medicine, University of São Paulo, São Paulo, Brazil; and [c]Section of Periodontology, Department of Dentistry and Oral Health, Aarhus University, Aarhus, Denmark*

Dr K.G. Peres coordinated the oral health data collection, conceptualized the study, and drafted the initial manuscript; Drs Nascimento and Mittinty carried out all statistical analyses and reviewed and revised the manuscript; Dr M.A. Peres trained field workers, supervised data collection, and critically reviewed the manuscript; Dr Demarco coordinated the oral health data collection, trained field workers, supervised data collection, and critically reviewed the manuscript; Dr de Barros, Dr Santos and Dr Matijasevich coordinated all stages of the birth cohort study and critically reviewed the manuscript; and all authors approved the final version of the manuscript and agree to be accountable for all aspects of the work.

DOI: https://doi.org/10.1542/peds.2016-2943

Accepted for publication Apr 7, 2017

WHAT'S KNOWN ON THIS SUBJECT: Despite some evidence on the increased risk of dental caries in children breastfed beyond 12 months of age, these findings are derived from highly heterogeneous studies and lack controlling for key confounders.

WHAT THIS STUDY ADDS: Breastfeeding up to 24 months of age or beyond has a controlled direct effect on the severity of primary dental caries. This risk is noteworthy independent of lifetime sugar consumption.

To cite: Peres KG, Nascimento GG, Peres MA, et al. Impact of Prolonged Breastfeeding on Dental Caries: A Population-Based Birth Cohort Study. *Pediatrics.* 2017; 140(1):e20162943

Untreated dental caries in the primary dentition affects 9% of the world's population.[1] This condition, together with untreated dental caries in permanent teeth, ranked 80th in detailed causes of years lived with disability among 291 investigated health conditions.[1] Untreated dental caries may cause pain and suffering, affecting children's and families' day-to-day life.[2,3] A contemporary publication reinforces dental caries as a sugar-dependent disease.[4]

The American Academy of Pediatrics recommends breastfeeding for at least 12 months, continued subsequently as long as mutually desired by the mother and child, whereas the World Health Organization recommends breastfeeding for ≥ 24 months.[5] There are well-known benefits of breastfeeding for children's health, such as the reduction of infant mortality[6] and several general health infant diseases[5,7,8] and malocclusions.[9] A previous study, however, has suggested that lactation beyond a certain period of time can increase the risk of dental caries,[10] whereas another study was not able to confirm this association.[11] Results often vary depending on the definition of the duration of breastfeeding, the sample used, and whether the investigators adjusted for potential confounders. A systematic review and meta-analysis showed a reduced risk of dental caries in children breastfed up to 12 months, but the reliability of the studies was considered weak.[12] Nevertheless, children breastfed for >12 months had more dental caries when compared with children breastfed for <12 months. This review pointed out the lack of studies that assessed the role played by breastfeeding, bottle feeding, and sugar consumption on children >12 months of age.[12]

One of the most challenging aspects of the reviewed literature is the extent to which children are selected into breastfeeding based on several socioeconomic and demographic components that are concurrently associated with infant feeding practices and long-term child outcomes. Fluoride exposure, certain dietary habits, and oral hygiene practices may influence the effect of breastfeeding on dental caries, particularly considering their long-term effects.[13,14,]

Some methodological aspects may improve the quality of research seeking causal inference, such as a prospective design and the use of analytical tools where potential confounders are considered. For example, by using marginal structural modeling (MSM), it is possible to estimate the controlled direct effect (CDE) of an exposure on an outcome. The CDE quantifies the effect of a given exposure under intervention (eg, prolonged breastfeeding) that sets the mediator (eg, sugar consumption) to a specific value for all individuals in the population creating unobserved (counterfactual) quantities. The CDE can be theorized as a hypothetical experiment using observational data, which allow us to reproduce a randomized controlled trial.[15] Given the aforementioned existing gaps in the literature, this study aimed to address the following research question: Is there a CDE of prolonged breastfeeding (PB) on dental caries at age 5 years?

METHODS

Data Setting and Sample Selection

A population-based birth cohort of 4231 live births in Pelotas, Brazil started in 2004. Infants were examined within 24 hours of birth (99%), and follow-up occurred at 3 months (96%), at 12 months (94.2%), and 4 years of age (93.5%).[16] During these follow-ups, mothers were interviewed face to face, and anthropometric measures were collected from mothers and children.

All children who were born between September and December 2004 and who had participated in the 4-year-old follow-up (n = 1303) were eligible to participate in the 2009 oral health assessment. Pelotas has had a public fluoridated water supply since 1962. At age 5 years, 37.0% of the children had visited a dentist, and 45.7% still received assistance when toothbrushing.[17] This sample size was sufficient to estimate the effect of PB on the presence of severe early childhood caries (S-ECC) with a statistical power of at least 80% (β = 20%). The prevalence of S-ECC in the nonexposed group (breastfeeding <24 months) was equal to 17%, a relative risk of ≥ 1.5 (α = 5%). Household interviews and dental examinations were scheduled by phone using contact details from previous cohort waves. When this approach failed, a household visit was the option.

Outcome

Dental caries was investigated by using the decayed, missing, or filled primary tooth surfaces (dmfs) index according to World Health Organization[18] criteria. Children were examined while seated in an ordinary chair under artificial illumination (head lamp). Two different outcomes were assessed in this study: (1) the average number of dmfs; and (2) the presence of S-ECC (number of dmfs ≥ 6). Eight dentists were trained and calibrated to perform dental examinations, which involved 100 preschool children excluded from the sample. The minimum intraclass correlation coefficient for dmfs values was 0.92.

Main Explanatory Variable

PB was the main explanatory variable, and information was collected immediately after the participant's birth and at 3, 12, and 24 months and 4 years of age by using the following questions: "Is your child being breastfed? If 'No,' when did she/he stop being breastfed?" "Based on the literature,[12] 1 variable with 3 categories was created as follows: (1) Breastfeeding up to and including 12 months; (2) breastfeeding for 13 to 23 months; and (3) breastfeeding ≥24 months.

Covariates

A directed acyclic graph was drawn to depict the proposed conceptual framework and to identify possible causal pathways (Fig 1). The baseline confounders in the causal relationship between PB and dental caries included socioeconomic conditions and maternal age at child's birth. Information on family income was collected in Brazilian reals (1 US dollar = 3.15 Brazilian reals during the data gathering) and then categorized into quintiles. Maternal level of education was categorized into 4 groups (≤4, ≥5–8, 9–11, and ≥12 full years of schooling), and maternal age was collected in years and analyzed in 4 groups (<20, 20–29, 30–39, ≥40 years of age).

Information on sugar consumption was obtained at 24 and 48 months and at 5 years of age. Food consumption at 24 and 48 months was assessed by using a list of food items or food groups consumed in the 24 hours before the interview. The mother was asked whether each food item in a list had been consumed in each of 7 meals or periods of the day: on waking, morning, lunch, afternoon, dinner, evening, and night.[19] The list was as follows: breast milk, cow's milk, milk powder, coffee, water or tea, juice, bread/cookies, yogurt, fruits, eggs, rice, beans, vegetables/legumes, pasta, potato or cassava, meat, and powdered chocolate milk drinks. Soft drinks were added to the food list for children aged 48 months. The frequency of habitual consumption of chocolate, powdered chocolate milk drinks, candies, lollipops, soft drinks, and chewing gums was compiled in a single sugar group and was categorized by time of day at 24 months of age as follows: "low sugar consumption" (0 or <2 times per day) and "high sugar consumption" (≥2 times per

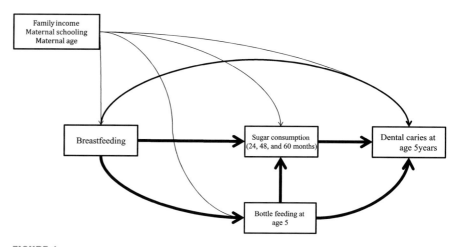

FIGURE 1
Directed acyclic graph to depict the relationship between PB and dental caries at age 5 years. The 2004 Pelotas Birth Cohort, 2004 to 2009, Pelotas, Brazil.

day). Information at 48 months was categorized as "low sugar consumption" (≤2 times per day) and "high sugar consumption" (>2 times per day). Finally, dietary information at age 5 years was collected by using the question "How many times a day does <child> eat sweet foods between meals (eg, cookies, candies, lollipops, chewing gum, chocolate)?" and was categorized as "low sugar consumption" (≤2 times per day) and "high sugar consumption" (>2 times per day). Because not only the frequency of sugar exposure[20] but also the pattern of sugar consumption over time[4] may be important for the progress of dental caries, a categorical variable was created as follows: (1) low (low sugar consumption during the 3 analyzed periods); (2) infrequently (high sugar consumption only at 48 months and/or at 60 months); (3) infrequently but including a critical period (high sugar consumption only at 24 months, or at 24 and 48 or 60 months); (4) high (high sugar consumption in 3 analyzed periods). The critical period (24 months of age) was considered when the teeth are most susceptible to dental caries soon after they erupt.

Sugar consumption was considered a later exposure to dental caries because it is chronologically placed between the main exposure and

the outcome. Information on the use of bottle feeding at night was collected at 5 years of age (never/yes, but stopped versus yes, still in use). This variable was considered a sugar consumption–dental caries confounder (Fig 1).

Oral behavior variables (frequency of tooth brushing and dental visits) were not included in the analyses because there is no direct path from oral behaviors to dental caries. Additionally, the only possible backdoor path between oral behaviors and breastfeeding was blocked after controlling for the sociodemographic variables (Supplemental Fig 2).

Data Quality Control

A total of 15% of the interviews were repeated by telephone to assess data quality. The questionnaire was pretested, including questions regarding the pattern of dental attendance during the child's life, age at the first dental visit, and the reason for the first dental visit.

Statistical Analyses

Descriptive analysis included absolute and relative frequencies and outcome prevalence estimates according to independent variables. Both multiplicative and additive interaction between PB and sugar consumption were tested, including the cross-product term in the analytical model (Supplemental Tables 3 and 4). Because an interaction was not detected, the cross-product term was not included in the analysis.[21] Since the use of the conventional regression approach provides biased estimates when conditioning on later exposure of the effect between the exposure and the outcome (collider bias),[22] we used MSM to estimate the CDE of PB on dental caries taking into account the pattern of sugar consumption throughout the life course.[23] Detailed information of how MSM was applied to estimate the CDE can be found in the MSM section of the Supplemental Material.

Ethical Considerations

The Ethics Committee of the Federal University of Pulutuo approved the project (number 100/2009). All examinations and interviews were carried out after authorization by the parent or the legal guardian of the participant through a consent letter.

RESULTS

Out of the 1303 eligible children, 86.6% (1129) had complete data on dental caries and had responded to the questionnaire at age 5 years. The prevalence of S-ECC was 23.9% (Table 1); 542 (48%) children had at least 1 surface affected by dental caries (mean number of dmfs: 4.05; SD: 7.38; median: 0; range: 0–69). Among those who had experienced dental caries, the mean number of dmfs was 8.40 (SD: 8.75), whereas the median number of dmfs was 5 (range: 1–69). Approximately half of the children's mothers were between 20 and 29 years of age and had between 5 and 8 years of schooling. Nearly one-quarter of the sample was breastfed for ≥24 months. About 7% of the children had never consumed sugar, whereas 11% consumed sugar at 24, 48, and 60 months of age. Almost half of the sample was still bottle fed at age 5 years.

Unadjusted analyses revealed that the lower the family income and the less maternal schooling, the greater the level of dental caries and risk of having S-ECC. PB was associated with both outcomes, and high sugar consumption was only associated with a greater risk of having S-ECC when compared with those who consumed little sugar (Table 1).

Table 2 shows the CDE of PB on the outcomes. Those children who were breastfed for ≥24 months presented higher levels of dental caries than those who were breastfed for <12 months (mean ratio: 1.9; 95% confidence interval [CI]: 1.5–2.4). Moreover, children breastfed for ≥24 months had a 2.4 times higher risk of S-ECC than those breastfed for <12 months (risk ratio: 2.4; 95% CI: 1.7–3.3).

Supplemental Table 5 presents the results of the sensitivity analysis for unmeasured confounders (U). This table presents hypothetical scenarios where the presence of U would eliminate the CDE of PB on dental caries. For example, to eliminate the CDE of PB on S-ECC, a U not included in the analysis should increase the risk of dental caries by at least 3.0 times (γ in column 6, line 6) and should be 9.0 times more prevalent among those exposed (P1) than those unexposed (P2). In this case, the probability of the presence of U should be equal to 80% (P1 − P2).

DISCUSSION

Being breastfed for ≥24 months increased the risk of having dental caries at 5 years of age. Likewise, those children were more likely to develop S-ECC. These effects were not mediated by sugar consumption during the life course. Our finding corroborates studies conducted in another Brazilian city[10,14,] as well as in high-income countries.[24,25,] However, these studies investigated different cut-off points for breastfeeding. For example, any type of breastfeeding for ≥20 months was significantly associated with

dental caries in Southern Italy,[24] whereas breastfeeding for >12 months increased the risk of S-ECC in Germany.[25]

Some mechanisms have been proposed to explain such a relationship. First, PB may be associated with a higher frequency of breastfeeding[10] and nocturnal breastfeeding on demand,[26,27,] when cleaning teeth is difficult. A meta-analysis with 5 studies, including only 1 cohort study, reported an ~7 times greater risk of having dental caries among children who were exposed to longer nocturnal breastfeeding versus shorter periods of nocturnal breastfeeding.[12] Second, some authors highlighted the concept that genes and environmental components can modify the susceptibility to caries in children, even within the same dentition[28]; however, the role of breastfeeding in this relationship has not been investigated. A recent study[29] suggested that the genetic diversity of *Streptococcus mutans*, the most common bacterium associated with the development of dental caries, may be associated with caries susceptibility in those children who present such bacteria. Nevertheless, the presence of PB remained associated with S-ECC despite the presence of *S mutans* in this study.[29] PB may contribute to S-ECC because it facilitates the colonization of *S mutans*.[30] Another potential explanation is related to the composition of human milk and its potential cariogenicity, because dental caries is a sugar-dependent disease. Human milk produces more caries than cows' milk on smooth surfaces, but exhibits lower cariogenicity than infant formula or sucrose. The high concentration of lactose found in human milk has the potential to reduce the pH of dental plaque, leading to dental caries.[31]

The major strengths of this study are the population-based study design, the high response in all cohort waves, the high level of diagnostic

TABLE 1 Sample Description According to Independent Variables and Outcomes

Variables	Sample n (%)	Mean dmfs	95% CI	Crude Rate Ratio[a]	95% CI	S-ECC	95% CI	Crude Risk Ratio[b]	95% CI
Maternal age, y (n = 1121)									
<20	214 (18.9)	5.1	4.1 to 6.0	1.0	—	32.9	26.5 to 39.2	1.0	—
20–29	544 (48.2)	4.1	3.5 to 4.8	0.8	0.6 to 1.1	23.4	19.8 to 26.9	0.6	0.4 to 0.9
30–39	340 (30.1)	3.2	2.5 to 3.9	0.6	0.4 to 0.9	18.6	14.4 to 22.7	0.5	0.3 to 0.7
≥40	30 (2.7)	5.3	2.1 to 8.4	1.0	0.5 to 2.3	30.0	12.6 to 47.4	0.9	0.4 to 2.0
Family income quintiles (Brazilian real)[c] (n = 1129)									
5 (highest)	225 (19.9)	2.2	1.6 to 2.9	1.0	—	15.2	10.4 to 19.9	1.0	—
4	187 (16.6)	3.1	2.2 to 4.0	1.37	0.9 to 2.0	19.9	14.1 to 25.7	1.4	0.8 to 2.3
3	265 (23.5)	4.0	3.2 to 4.8	1.8	1.2 to 2.6	23.9	18.8 to 29.1	1.8	1.1 to 2.8
2	190 (16.8)	4.3	3.4 to 5.3	1.9	1.3 to 2.9	27.0	20.6 to 33.4	2.1	1.3 to 3.3
1 (lowest)	262 (23.2)	6.1	4.9 to 7.3	2.7	1.9 to 3.9	31.9	21.2 to 37.6	2.6	1.7 to 4.1
Maternal level of education, y (n = 1106)									
≥12	123 (11.2)	1.8	0.9 to 2.8	1.0	—	10.5	5.0 to 16.1	1.0	—
9–11	394 (35.7)	3.2	2.6 to 3.8	1.7	1.1 to 2.6	20.7	16.7 to 24.7	2.2	1.2 to 4.1
5–8	445 (40.2)	4.6	4.0 to 5.3	2.5	1.6 to 3.8	28.1	23.9 to 32.3	3.3	1.8 to 6.1
≤4	144 (13.0)	6.9	5.1 to 8.6	3.7	2.2 to 6.1	32.6	24.9 to 40.4	4.1	2.1 to 8.0
Breastfeeding (n = 1128)									
0–12	741 (65.7)	3.4	2.9 to 3.9	1.0	—	19.8	16.9 to 22.7	1.0	—
13–23	129 (11.4)	3.1	2.2 to 4.0	0.9	0.6 to 1.3	20.1	13.1 to 27.2	1.0	0.6 to 1.6
≥24	258 (22.9)	6.4	5.3 to 7.5	1.9	1.4 to 2.5	37.5	31.5 to 43.5	2.4	1.8 to 3.3
Sugar consumption during lifetime (n = 1065)									
Low[d]	74 (6.9)	2.8	1.5 to 4.1	1.0	—	18.9	9.8 to 28.1	1.0	—
Infrequently[e]	531 (49.9)	3.8	3.2 to 4.4	1.3	0.8 to 2.3	22.2	18.7 to 25.8	1.2	0.7 to 2.2
Infrequently with critical period[f]	346 (32.5)	4.1	3.3 to 4.9	1.4	0.8 to 2.5	23.1	18.6 to 27.6	1.3	0.7 to 2.4
High[g]	114 (10.7)	4.9	3.7 to 6.1	1.8	0.9 to 3.2	35.1	26.2 to 44.0	2.3	1.1 to 4.6
Bottle feeding at night – 5 y (n = 1126)									
Never/yes, but stopped	565 (50.2)	4.4	3.8 to 5.0	1.0	—	26.5	22.8 to 30.1	1.0	—
Yes, still use	561 (49.8)	3.7	3.1 to 4.3	0.9	0.7 to 1.1	21.1	17.6 to 24.4	0.8	0.6 to 1.1
S-ECC (n = 1122)									
dmfs <6	854 (76.1)	0.9	0.7 to 1.0	—	—	—	—	—	—
dmfs ≥6	268 (23.9)	14.2	13.1 to 15.3	—	—	—	—	—	—

—, reference category.
[a] Mean ratio estimated by negative binomial regression for level of dmfs as the outcome.
[b] Risk ratio estimated by log-linear regression for S-ECC as the outcome.
[c] 1 US dollar = 3.15 Brazilian reals (January 6, 2004).
[d] Low, low sugar consumption (0 or <2 times per day) at 12 and 24 months and 5 years of age.
[e] Infrequently, high sugar consumption (>2 times per day) only at 48 months and/or at 5 years of age.
[f] Infrequently with critical period, high sugar consumption (>2 times per day) only at 24 months, or at 24 and 48 months of age, or at 24 and 48 months of age.
[g] High, high sugar consumption (>2 times per day) at 12 and 24 months and 5 years of age.

TABLE 2 CDE of Breastfeeding on Dental Caries From MSM

	Dental Caries	Severe Dental Caries
	MSM: Mean Ratio[a] (95% CI)	MSM: Relative Risk[a] (95% CI)
Breastfeeding		
Up to 12 mo	1.0	1.0
13–23 mo	0.9 (0.6 to 1.3)	1.0 (0.6 to 1.6)
≥24 mo or beyond	1.9 (1.5 to 2.4)	2.4 (1.7 to 3.3)
Sugar exposure		
Low	1.0	1.0
Infrequently	1.4 (0.8 to 2.4)	1.3 (0.7 to 2.6)
Infrequently including critical period	1.6 (0.9 to 2.7)	1.5 (0.7 to 2.9)
High	1.8 (1.0 to 3.1)	2.3 (1.1 to 4.9)

2004 Pelotas Birth Cohort, Pelotas, Brazil, 2004 to 2009.
[a] Adjusted for family income, maternal schooling, maternal age, sugar consumption, and bottle feeding at age 5 years.

reliability, and the methodological and analytical approach employed. The sample distribution of our study was similar to that of the general cohort study,[16] suggesting no selection bias. Recall bias was unlikely, because the information used was collected during or shortly after exposure, leading to short recall periods. Observation bias is also unlikely to have occurred, because observers, when performing oral examinations, were unaware of the duration of breastfeeding for the children. MSM provided estimates that allowed a causal interpretation between PB and dental caries at age 5 years. The strength of our findings is ensured by the fulfillment of conditions required by MSM, such as positivity and correct model specification. The sensitivity analysis for unmeasured confounding ensured the robustness of our findings. To eliminate the CDE of PB on dental caries, the difference in the prevalence of U and the effect of U on the outcome showed rates that are unlikely to be observed in the real world. However, a certain degree of unmeasured confounding can always exist in observational studies.

This study helps to close existing gaps in the literature by including information on the use of bottle feeding and dietary habits suggested in a recent systematic review.[12] Moreover, it included some key confounders, such as socioeconomic conditions, and, therefore, a range of food/drink consumption over the studied period, information that is absent

from many earlier studies. However, the generalizability of our findings is uncertain and may only be warranted for populations with similar patterns of breastfeeding and fluoride exposure.

Our study has limitations; for example, we did not collect information on other potentially cariogenic sources and the frequency of nocturnal breastfeeding, which may have led to residual confounding. The absence of information on dental caries experience before the age of 5 years did not permit a better understanding of the long-term effect of breastfeeding on dental caries experience in the earlier stages. Furthermore, the presence of only cavitated smooth surfaces was not considered S-ECC,[32] which may have underestimated the prevalence of S-ECC. Nevertheless, children with severe caries are still the focus of our research. Finally, another limitation is related to the period when information regarding sugar consumption was collected. Patterns of sugar consumption are established in early childhood[33] and may be associated with S-ECC.[34]

We distinguish between different effects of PB; first, the average number of teeth with dental caries, and second, the severity of dental caries. Breastfeeding exclusively for 6 months and breastfeeding until 12 months of age protect against malocclusion[9] and dental caries,[12] respectively, and these practices should be encouraged in public

policies, meeting the rationale of the common risk factor approach.[35] From the health practitioner's perspective, a positive and informative relationship with mothers may include emphasizing the importance of breastfeeding for oral health and allows tooth brushing recommendations to be provided. Mothers may be encouraged to clean their children's teeth before going to bed and to use fluoride toothpaste in adequate amounts, avoiding demineralization of teeth.[36] Fluoride toothpaste can reduce tooth demineralization, but this depends on sugar consumption. However, the effect of PB on S-ECC was not mediated by dietary factors.

S-ECC is a public health issue because it is a major but preventable condition that leads to pain and suffering that may affect children's quality of life.[37] S-ECC impacts on the wider society; it is the most common reason for hospitalization and the use of general anesthesia among children in some countries, particularly for those from disadvantaged socioeconomic groups.[38] This intervention is resource-intensive, costly, and not without risk for individuals and society.[39]

CONCLUSIONS

Breastfeeding for ≥24 months increases the risk of having S-ECC. We suggest adopting measures to prevent dental caries in childhood as early as possible, because breastfeeding is beneficial for children's health.

ABBREVIATIONS

CDE: controlled direct effect
CI: confidence interval
dmfs: decayed, missing, and filled primary tooth surface
MSM: marginal structural model
PB: prolonged breastfeeding
S-ECC: severe early childhood caries
U: unmeasured confounder

Address correspondence to Karen Glazer Peres, BDS, PhD, Australian Research Centre for Population Oral Health, Adelaide Dental School, University of Adelaide, 122, Frome St, Adelaide, Australia 5000. E-mail: karen.peres@adelaide.edu.au

PEDIATRICS (ISSN Numbers: Print, 0031-4005; Online, 1098-4275).

FINANCIAL DISCLOSURE: The authors have indicated they have no financial relationships relevant to this article to disclose.

FUNDING: The Wellcome Trust supported the 2004 birth cohort study. The World Health Organization, National Support Program for Centers of Excellence (PRONEX), Brazilian National Research Council (CNPq), Brazilian Ministry of Health, and Children's Pastorate supported previous phases of the study. Drs Matijasevich, Santos, de Barros, and Demarco are supported by the CNPq. The oral health study was supported by CNPq (process 402372/2008-5, to Dr K.G. Peres).

POTENTIAL CONFLICT OF INTEREST: The authors have indicated they have no potential conflicts of interest to disclose.

REFERENCES

1. Marcenes W, Kassebaum NJ, Bernabé E, et al. Global burden of oral conditions in 1990-2010: a systematic analysis. *J Dent Res.* 2013;92(7):592–597

2. Peres KG, Peres MA, Araujo CL, Menezes AM, Hallal PC. Social and dental status along the life course and oral health impacts in adolescents: a population-based birth cohort. *Health Qual Life Outcomes.* 2009;7:95

3. Kramer PF, Feldens CA, Ferreira SH, Bervian J, Rodrigues PH, Peres MA. Exploring the impact of oral diseases and disorders on quality of life of preschool children. *Community Dent Oral Epidemiol.* 2013;41(4):327–335

4. Moynihan PJ, Kelly SA. Effect on caries of restricting sugars intake: systematic review to inform WHO guidelines. *J Dent Res.* 2014;93(1):8–18

5. Kramer MS, Kakuma R. Optimal duration of exclusive breastfeeding. *Cochrane Database Syst Rev.* 2012;(8):CD003517

6. Sankar MJ, Sinha B, Chowdhury R, et al. Optimal breastfeeding practices and infant and child mortality: a systematic review and meta-analysis. *Acta Paediatr.* 2015;104(467):3–13

7. Horta BL, Loret de Mola C, Victora CG. Breastfeeding and intelligence: a systematic review and meta-analysis. *Acta Paediatr.* 2015;104(467):14–19

8. Horta BL, Loret de Mola C, Victora CG. Long-term consequences of breastfeeding on cholesterol, obesity, systolic blood pressure and type 2 diabetes: a systematic review and meta-analysis. *Acta Paediatr.* 2015;104(467):30–37

9. Peres KG, Cascaes AM, Nascimento GG, Victora CG. Effect of breastfeeding on malocclusions: a systematic review and meta-analysis. *Acta Paediatr.* 2015;104(467):54–61

10. Chaffee BW, Feldens CA, Vítolo MR. Association of long-duration breastfeeding and dental caries estimated with marginal structural models. *Ann Epidemiol.* 2014;24(6):448–454

11. Nunes AM, Alves CM, Borba de Araújo F, et al. Association between prolonged breast-feeding and early childhood caries: a hierarchical approach. *Community Dent Oral Epidemiol.* 2012;40(6):542–549

12. Tham R, Bowatte G, Dharmage SC, et al. Breastfeeding and the risk of dental caries: a systematic review and meta-analysis. *Acta Paediatr.* 2015;104(467):62–84

13. Thitasomakul S, Piwat S, Thearmontree A, Chankanka O, Pithpornchaiyakul W, Madyusoh S. Risks for early childhood caries analyzed by negative binomial models. *J Dent Res.* 2009;88(2):137–141

14. Feldens CA, Giugliani ER, Vigo Á, Vítolo MR. Early feeding practices and severe early childhood caries in four-year-old children from southern Brazil: a birth cohort study. *Caries Res.* 2010;44(5):445–452

15. VanderWeele TJ. Bias formulas for sensitivity analysis for direct and indirect effects. *Epidemiology.* 2010;21(4):540–551

16. Santos IS, Barros AJ, Matijasevich A, Domingues MR, Barros FC, Victora CG. Cohort profile: the 2004 Pelotas (Brazil) birth cohort study. *Int J Epidemiol.* 2011;40(6):1461–1468

17. Camargo MBJ, Barros AJD, Frazão P, et al. Predictors of dental visits for routine check-ups and for the resolution of problems among preschool children. *Rev Saude Publica.* 2012;46(1):87–97

18. World Health Organization. *Oral Health Survey: Basic Methods. Report of a WHO Consultation.* 4th ed. Geneva, Switzerland: World Health Organization; 1997

19. Gatica G, Barros AJ, Madruga S, Matijasevich A, Santos IS. Food intake profiles of children aged 12, 24 and 48 months from the 2004 Pelotas (Brazil) birth cohort: an exploratory analysis using principal components. *Int J Behav Nutr Phys Act.* 2012;9:43

20. Anderson CA, Curzon ME, Van Loveren C, Tatsi C, Duggal MS. Sucrose and dental caries: a review of the evidence. *Obes Rev.* 2009;10(suppl 1):41–54

21. Vansteelandt S. Estimation of direct and indirect effects. In: Berzuini C, Dawid P, Bernardinell L, eds. *Causality: Statistical Perspectives and Applications.* Hoboken, NJ: Wiley & Sons; 2012

22. Robins JM, Greenland S. Identifiability and exchangeability for direct and indirect effects. *Epidemiology.* 1992;3(2):143–155

23. Lange T, Rasmussen M, Thygesen LC. Assessing natural direct and indirect effects through multiple pathways. *Am J Epidemiol.* 2014;179(4):513–518

24. Nobile CG, Fortunato L, Bianco A, Pileggi C, Pavia M. Pattern and severity of early childhood caries in Southern Italy: a preschool-based cross-sectional study. *BMC Public Health.* 2014;14:206

25. Bissar A, Schiller P, Wolff A, Niekusch U, Schulte AG. Factors contributing to severe early childhood caries in south-west Germany. *Clin Oral Investig.* 2014;18(5):1411–1418

26. al-Dashti AA, Williams SA, Curzon ME. Breast feeding, bottle feeding and dental caries in Kuwait, a country with low-fluoride levels in the water supply. *Community Dent Health*. 1995;12(1):42–47

27. van Palenstein Helderman WH, Soe W, van 't Hof MA. Risk factors of early childhood caries in a Southeast Asian population. *J Dent Res*. 2006;85(1):85–88

28. Wang X, Willing MC, Marazita ML, et al. Genetic and environmental factors associated with dental caries in children: the Iowa Fluoride Study. *Caries Res*. 2012;46(3):177–184

29. Yu LX, Tao Y, Qiu RM, Zhou Y, Zhi QH, Lin HC. Genetic polymorphisms of the sortase A gene and social-behavioural factors associated with caries in children: a case-control study. *BMC Oral Health*. 2015;15:54

30. Vachirarojpisan T, Shinada K, Kawaguchi Y, Laungwechakan P, Somkote T, Detsomboonrat P. Early childhood caries in children aged 6-19 months. *Community Dent Oral Epidemiol*. 2004;32(2):133–142

31. Prabhakar AR, Kurthukoti AJ, Gupta P. Cariogenicity and acidogenicity of human milk, plain and sweetened bovine milk: an in vitro study. *J Clin Pediatr Dent*. 2010;34(3):239–247

32. Drury TF, Horowitz AM, Ismail AI, Maertens MP, Rozier RG, Selwitz RH. Diagnosing and reporting early childhood caries for research purposes. A report of a workshop sponsored by the National Institute of Dental and Craniofacial Research, the Health Resources and Services Administration, and the Health Care Financing Administration. *J Public Health Dent*. 1999;59(3):192–197

33. Rossow I, Kjaernes U, Holst D. Patterns of sugar consumption in early childhood. *Community Dent Oral Epidemiol*. 1990;18(1):12–16

34. Chaffee BW, Feldens CA, Rodrigues PH, Vítolo MR. Feeding practices in infancy associated with caries incidence in early childhood. *Community Dent Oral Epidemiol*. 2015;43(4):338–348

35. Sheiham A, Watt RG. The common risk factor approach: a rational basis for promoting oral health. *Community Dent Oral Epidemiol*. 2000;28(6):399–406

36. Duggal MS, Toumba KJ, Amaechi BT, Kowash MB, Higham SM. Enamel demineralization in situ with various frequencies of carbohydrate consumption with and without fluoride toothpaste. *J Dent Res*. 2001;80(8):1721–1724

37. Gomes MC, Pinto-Sarmento TC, Costa EM, Martins CC, Granville-Garcia AF, Paiva SM. Impact of oral health conditions on the quality of life of preschool children and their families: a cross-sectional study. *Health Qual Life Outcomes*. 2014;12:55

38. Australian Institute of Health and Welfare. *Australia's Health 2012*. Canberra, Australia: Australian Institute of Health and Welfare; 2012

39. Cartwright DP. Death in the dental chair. *Anaesthesia*. 1999;54(2):105–107

Supplemental Information

MSMS

MSMs are a new class of causal models that distinguishes between confounder and mediators in the analysis, reducing the gap left by conventional regression methods to assess mediation.[40] Furthermore, by dealing with potential confounding by measured covariates through weighting rather than conditioning on covariates, MSMs allow for the identification of direct effects even in settings in which conventional approaches are biased.[22]

This technique is also considerably relevant for observational studies when exposures cannot be randomly allocated, such as breastfeeding, because it simulates a randomized controlled trial scenario. Moreover, in the absence of unmeasured confounding and measurement error, the results from an observational inverse probability treatment weight analysis may have causal interpretation and can overcome the issue of selection bias.[41] Thus, a MSM was used to estimate the CDE of PB on severe dental caries considering the sugar consumption pattern, whereas the CDE is defined as the effect of breastfeeding on dental caries at age 5 years regardless of sugar consumption during the life course. In the absence of interaction between breastfeeding and sugar consumption, the CDE may be interpreted as the total natural direct effect.[42] Stabilized weights are more efficient than inverse-probability-to-treatment weights, because stabilized weight precludes extreme differences in weights for the exposed and unexposed groups. Moreover, it maintains the original sample size in the weighted data set and provides a robust CI.[43] Stabilized weights (SW) were calculated for breastfeeding (1) and sugar consumption (2) separately according to the following formulas:

$$SW_i^{breastfeeding} = \frac{f(BF)}{f(BF|C)} \; ; \; (1)$$

$$SW_i^{sugar} = \frac{f(sugar|BF)}{f(sugar|BF,L,C)}, \; (2)$$

where BF is PB; sugar is sugar consumption; C represents baseline confounders; and L represents the sugar consumption-dental caries confounder. Also, in the formula, f(BF) is the function of breastfeeding (BF), and f(BF|C) is the function of breastfeeding (BF) conditional on baseline confounders (C); whereas f(sugar|BF) is the function of sugar consumption (sugar) conditional on breastfeeding (BF), and f(sugar|BF, L,C) is the function of sugar consumption (sugar) conditional on breastfeeding (BF), baseline (C), and sugar consumption-dental caries (L) confounders.

The final stabilized weight was computed as:

$$SW = SW_i^{breastfeeding} \times SW_i^{sugar}.$$

The distribution of stabilized weights was: stabilized weight for BF: mean = 1.00; range = 0.59 to 1.76; interquartile range = 0.93 to 1.05; stabilized weight for sugar consumption: mean = 1.00; range = 0.57 to 2.46; interquartile range = 0.93 to 1.06; and final stabilized weight: mean = 1.00; range = 0.48 to 2.66; interquartile range = 0.87 to 1.09. All analyses were conducted by using Stata version 13.0 (Stata Corp, College Station, TX).

SENSITIVITY ANALYSES FOR U

MSMs rely on the assumption that there is no unmeasured confounding between the mediator and outcome, exposure and mediator, and exposure and outcome. Although these assumptions may not be analytically verified, some alternatives have been suggested for conducting sensitivity analysis for unmeasured confounding (U).[15] For conducting this analysis, following VanderWeele,[15] we needed to assume 2 aspects, (1) the prevalence of U and (2) the effect of U on the outcome. We also assumed there was no relative excess risk due to interaction between exposure and U. The parameters of U, such as γ (conditional increase in the risk of dental caries), P1 [P(U = 1|BF, sugar, C)], and P2 [P(U = 1|BF*, sugar, C)] were specified from systematic reviews. We used the following model given by VanderWeele[15] to calculate the bias introduced by U that could invalidate the CDE:

$$Bias \; CD \; E_{BF, BF*|C}^{RR}(sugar) =$$

$$\frac{1 + (\gamma - 1)P1(U = 1|BF, sugar, C)}{1 + (\gamma - 1)P2(U = 1|BF*, sugar, C)}$$

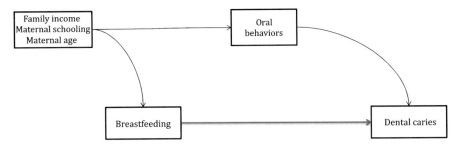

SUPPLEMENTAL FIGURE 2
Directed acyclic graph displays the backdoor path of oral behaviors blocked by socioeconomic variables.

SUPPLEMENTAL TABLE 3 Multiplicative Interaction Between Breastfeeding and Sugar Consumption

Parameter	Estimate	95% CI	SE	P
S-ECC				
Sugar#BF	−0.14	−0.32 to 0.07	0.11	.192
Intercept	−1.91	−260 to −1.21	0.35	<.001
Dental caries				
Sugar#BF	−0.07	−0.21 to 0.08	0.09	.403
Intercept	0.78	0.22 to 1.35	0.29	<.001

signifies interaction between conditions.

SUPPLEMENTAL TABLE 4 Relative Excess Risk Due to Interaction Between Breastfeeding and Sugar Consumption

Parameter	Estimate	95% CI	SE	P
S-ECC				
RERI	−0.37	−5.02 to 4.27	2.37	.875
BF (0 and 2)				
Sugar (0 and 3)				
RERI	−0.07	−0.49 to 0.35	0.21	.732
BF (1 and 2)				
Sugar (2 and 3)				
RERI	−0.27	−2.76 to 2.23	1.27	.833
BF (0 and 2)				
Sugar (1 and 3)				
Dental caries				
RERI	1.19	−2.39 to 4.47	1.82	.515
BF (0 and 2)				
Sugar (0 and 3)				
RERI	0.12	−0.35 to 0.59	0.24	.625
BF (1 and 2)				
Sugar (0 and 3)				
RERI	0.68	−1.59 to 2.95	1.16	.557
BF (0 and 2)				
Sugar (1 and 3)				

Numbers in parentheses in column 1 indicate the levels of each variable considered in the RERI analysis. BF, breastfeeding; RERI, relative excess risk due to interaction.

SUPPLEMENTAL TABLE 5 Sensitivity Analysis for U Considering the Estimates of PB on Severe Dental Carries

γ	P1	P2	P1 – P2	RR	γ	P1	P2	P1 – P2	RR	γ	P1	P2	P1-P2	RR
2	40	10	30	1.27	3	40	10	30	1.50	4	40	10	30	1.70
2	50	10	40	1.32	3	50	10	40	1.67	4[a]	50[a]	10[a]	40[a]	1.92[a,b]
2	60	10	50	1.45	3	60	10	50	1.83	4[a]	60[a]	10[a]	50[a]	2.15[a,b]
2	70	10	60	1.54	3[a]	70[a]	10[a]	60[a]	2.00[a,b]	4[a]	70[a]	10[a]	60[a]	2.38[a,c]
2	80	10	70	1.63	3[a]	80[a]	10[a]	70[a]	2.16[a,b]	4	80	10	70	2.60[a,c]
2	90	10	80	1.72	3[a]	90[a]	10[a]	80[a]	2.33[a,c]	4	90	10	80	2.80[a,c]
2	40	20	20	1.16	3	40	20	20	1.28	4	40	20	20	1.37
2	50	20	30	1.25	3	50	20	30	1.42	4	50	20	30	1.56
2	60	20	40	1.33	3	60	20	40	1.57	4	60	20	40	1.75
2	70	20	50	1.42	3	70	20	50	1.70	4[a]	70[a]	20[a]	50[a]	1.93[a,b]
2	80	20	60	1.50	3	80	20	60	1.85	4[a]	80[a]	20[a]	60[a]	2.10[a,b]
2	90	20	70	1.60	3[a]	90[a]	20[a]	70[a]	2.00[a,b]	4[a]	90[a]	20[a]	70[a]	2.30[a,b]
2	40	30	10	1.07	3	40	30	10	1.12	4	40	30	10	1.15
2	50	30	20	1.15	3	50	30	20	1.25	4	50	30	20	1.31
2	60	30	30	1.23	3	60	30	30	1.38	4	60	30	30	1.47
2	70	30	40	1.31	3	70	30	40	1.50	4	70	30	40	1.63
2	80	30	50	1.36	3	80	30	50	1.62	4	80	30	50	1.78
2	90	30	60	1.46	3	90	30	60	1.75	4[a]	90[a]	30[a]	60[a]	1.94[a,b]
2	50	40	10	1.07	3	50	40	10	1.10	4	50	40	10	1.13
2	60	40	20	1.14	3	60	40	20	1.20	4	60	40	20	1.27
2	70	40	30	1.21	3	70	40	30	1.30	4	70	40	30	1.41
2	80	40	40	1.28	3	80	40	40	1.44	4	80	40	40	1.54
2	90	40	50	1.36	3	90	40	50	1.55	4	90	40	50	1.68
2	60	50	10	1.06	3	60	50	10	1.10	4	60	50	10	1.12
2	70	50	20	1.13	3	70	50	20	1.20	4	70	50	20	1.24
2	80	50	30	1.20	3	80	50	30	1.30	4	80	50	30	1.36
2	90	50	40	1.27	3	90	50	40	1.40	4	90	50	40	1.48

It is noteworthy that U must be strongly associated with dental caries (γ should be at least 3) and unequally distributed among the exposed (P1) and nonexposed (P2) groups. This seems unlikely to be observed in the real world, because no condition related to breastfeeding and dental caries satisfy these parameters. Thus, it ensures the robustness of the observed findings. γ, conditional increase in the risk for dental caries; P1, prevalence in exposed group (breastfed for ≥24 months); P2, prevalence in nonexposed group (breastfed for ≤12 mo); P1 – P2, calculated differences in the probability of U; RR, relative risk.
[a] Indicates scenario where U would nullify the CDE of PB on dental caries.
[b] Results would eliminate the CDE of 24 months of breastfeeding on dental caries.
[c] Results would eliminate the CDE of 24 months of breastfeeding on S-ECC.

SUPPLEMENTAL REFERENCES

40. Robins JM, Hernán MA, Brumback B. Marginal structural models and causal inference in epidemiology. *Epidemiology*. 2000;11(5):550–560

41. Evans RJ, Didelez V. Recovering from selection bias using marginal structure in discrete models. In: Advances in Causal Inference Workshop; *July 16, 2015*; Amsterdam, Netherlands

42. De Stavola BL, Daniel RM. Marginal structural models: the way forward for life-course epidemiology? *Epidemiology*. 2012;23(2):233–237

43. Xu S, Ross C, Raebel MA, Shetterly S, Blanchette C, Smith D. Use of stabilized inverse propensity scores as weights to directly estimate relative risk and its confidence intervals. *Value Health*. 2010;13(2):273–277

Breastfeeding and Improved Cognitive/Noncognitive Development: Does the Effect Last Post Infancy and Toddlerhood?

Dr Lewis First, MD, MA, Editor in Chief, *Pediatrics*

There are many great reasons to recommend breastfeeding as the preferred feeding method to new mothers, one of which has been the data from studies suggesting improved cognitive and noncognitive development in babies who breastfeed. But how valid and reliable is that evidence especially when you look up the road at the developmental trajectories of children who did and did not breastfeed? Girard et al. (10.1542/peds.2016-1848) investigated this question in approximately 8000 families in Ireland. Children in this cohort were randomly selected to participate by sharing parent and teacher reports and combining these with developmental assessments on these children at 3 and 5 years looking at who did and did not breastfeed (based on maternal report of breastfeeding with propensity score matching). While breastfeeding at first glance showed better developmental outcomes in cognitive and noncognitive development, once propensity matching occurred, only 1 of 13 developmental outcomes remained as being statistically significant—i.e. the level of hyperactivity being less for those children who breastfed for at least 6 months and even this disappeared by age 5. Does this mean that breastfeeding not be recommended due to the lack of differences in development when compared to those who did not breastfeed for at least a half a year? No—of course not, given the many other reasons why breastfeeding is best for a baby. To further help explain the unexpected findings in this study and to note some limitations of the data findings as presented, Dr. Lydia Furman, an expert on lactation issues, provides an important commentary (10.1542/peds.2017-0150) to better frame this study in a larger context. Dr. Furman's commentary adds a nice perspective that may enable you to appreciate the negative findings in this study but await confirmation in future studies before you can generalize the findings. In the meantime, hopefully this study will not by itself stop you from continuing to advocate as strongly as ever for mothers of new babies to breastfeed for at least six months if not the first year of life.

Breastfeeding: What Do We Know, and Where Do We Go From Here?

Lydia Furman, MD

Exclusive breastfeeding through age 6 months with continued breastfeeding to 12 months and beyond is the optimal infant feeding method because of its lifesaving benefits for children and mothers worldwide.[1,2] Breastfeeding reduces all-cause and infection-related child mortality, sudden infant death syndrome–related mortality, and maternal breast cancer and cardiovascular risk; the effect of breast milk is dose-dependent, with exclusivity and longer duration increasing benefits.[3–5] With this background, Dr Lisa-Christine Girard and colleagues have conducted a unique and thoughtful study to examine the impact of breastfeeding on language, problem behaviors, and cognition in Irish children at ages 3 and 5 years.[6]

In their sample of >8000 children, the breastfed and not-breastfed groups were clinically and statistically different. This difference is especially important because there may be differences between mothers who do and do not breastfeed that are not known to the researchers (or anyone else) that either directly affect the outcome being studied or affect the outcome indirectly via another social or environmental factor (ie, as a mediator). Even randomization does not ensure perfect distribution of unknown variables between study groups, but it is the optimal study design. Indeed, the main challenge facing researchers who seek to examine the impact of breastfeeding on child outcomes is an inability to randomly assign individual mothers to breastfeed or not. Dr Girard and colleagues tackled this problem in 2 ways. Without the ability to randomly assign mothers to feeding choice, the authors chose to use propensity score matching to approximate randomization by matching for suspected confounders, and they used structural equation modeling to use their full data set and examine for mediator and moderator effects. One challenge of propensity score matching is that it causes data loss because not everyone can be matched; structural equation modeling thus served as a strong complementary analytical method.

The data set of Dr Girard et al has some limitations that should be acknowledged. Although most infants in the breastfeeding cohort were exclusively breastfed at ≤31 days, <5% were fully breastfed at >180 days, which limits the ability to examine optimal breastfeeding. Duration of breastfeeding was captured in broad time bands (≤31 days, 32–180 days, >180 days), which combines infants with very different feeding experiences and may dilute the impact of longer durations of breast milk receipt, depending on when exclusivity ends. Both exclusivity and duration are important, because dose response is well established for breast milk benefits.[3–5] Maternal IQ was not measured, as the authors appropriately note; ideally we need this information to consider child cognitive ability. Understanding these study limitations still does not diminish the value of the study, which is a thoughtful contribution to the breastfeeding literature.

Department of Pediatrics, University Hospitals Rainbow Babies and Children's Hospital and Case Western Reserve University School of Medicine, Cleveland, Ohio

Opinions expressed in these commentaries are those of the author and not necessarily those of the American Academy of Pediatrics or its Committees.

DOI: 10.1542/peds.2017-0150

Accepted for publication Jan 17, 2017

Address correspondence to Lydia Furman, MD, Division of General Pediatrics and Adolescent Medicine, Room 784, MS 6019, Department of Pediatrics, Rainbow Babies and Children's Hospital, 11100 Euclid Ave, Cleveland, OH 44016. E-mail: lydia.furman@uhhospitals.org

PEDIATRICS (ISSN Numbers: Print, 0031-4005; Online, 1098-4275).

FINANCIAL DISCLOSURE: The author has indicated she has no financial relationships relevant to this article to disclose.

FUNDING: No external funding.

POTENTIAL CONFLICT OF INTEREST: The author has indicated she has no potential conflicts of interest to disclose.

COMPANION PAPER: A companion to this article can be found online at www.pediatrics.org/cgi/doi/10.1542/peds.2016-1848.

To cite: Furman L. Breastfeeding: What Do We Know, and Where Do We Go From Here?. *Pediatrics.* 2017;139(4):e20170150

COMMENTARY

We can place the study of Girard et al in context by examining childhood outcomes from the PROBIT study, in which 31 Belarus hospitals were prospectively cluster randomized to a breastfeeding intervention based on the World Health Organization Baby-Friendly Hospital Initiative versus regular care, with significantly increased exclusive breastfeeding at 3 and 6 months and beyond among intervention hospital infants.[7] This large trial examined similar behavioral outcomes and is in agreement with Girard and colleagues; among the 13 889 children (81.5%) followed up at age 6.5 years, there was no effect of duration or exclusivity of breastfeeding on several validated measures of child behavior or on maternal relationship measures.[8] Finally, although Girard et al found no effect of breastfeeding on cognitive ability, the PROBIT study reported a mean IQ increase of 7.5 points (95% confidence interval, 0.8–14.3) at age 6.5 years in children from intervention hospitals.[9] Although the topic is controversial, and a recent systematic review identified heterogeneity between studies, among the 4 studies with the least bias (each >500 subjects, controlled for maternal IQ, breastfeeding recall duration <3 years) breastfeeding improved performance on IQ testing by 1.76 points (95% confidence interval, 0.25–3.26), suggesting a small but durable impact of breastfeeding on intelligence.[10]

But on what breastfeeding outcomes should we now focus? At this point, we know well that breastfeeding has an array of life-saving maternal, child, and societal benefits, even if childhood behavioral outcomes are not affected. The many known benefits of breastfeeding are neither fully realized nor equitably distributed, however, at least in part because not all women and their partners receive the preconception, prenatal, and postnatal education and support needed to initiate and continue breastfeeding as recommended.[11-14] Younger, unmarried, poor, and less educated women of racial and ethnic minorities are less likely to breastfeed, as we witness in the study of Girard et al (Table 1) and in national and international data alike.[6,14,15] How can we change the landscape so that all mothers can have opportunity and resources to have the chance to choose to breastfeed and to succeed if they so choose? This is the much-needed breastfeeding research that we hope to read about before the next breastfeeding commentary is published in *Pediatrics*.

REFERENCES

1. American Academy of Pediatrics, Section on Breastfeeding. Breastfeeding and the use of human milk. *Pediatrics*. 2012;129(3). Available at: www.pediatrics.org/cgi/content/full/129/3/e827

2. World Health Organization. Infant and young child nutrition: global strategy for infant and young child feeding. April 16, 2002. Geneva, Switzerland: World Health Organization. Available at: http://apps.who.int/gb/archive/pdf_files/WHA55/ea5515.pdf?ua=1. Accessed November 11, 2015

3. Sankar MJ, Sinha B, Chowdhury R, et al. Optimal breastfeeding practices and infant and child mortality: a systematic review and meta-analysis. *Acta Paediatr*. 2015;104(467):3–13

4. Hauck FR, Thompson JM, Tanabe KO, Moon RY, Vennemann MM. Breastfeeding and reduced risk of sudden infant death syndrome: a meta-analysis. *Pediatrics*. 2011;128(1):103–110

5. Chowdhury R, Sinha B, Sankar MJ, et al. Breastfeeding and maternal health outcomes: a systematic review and meta-analysis. *Acta Paediatr*. 2015;104(467):96–113

6. Girard LC, Doyle O, Tremblay RE. Breastfeeding, cognitive and noncognitive development in early childhood: a population study. *Pediatrics*. 2017;139(4):e20161848

7. Kramer MS, Chalmers B, Hodnett ED, et al; PROBIT Study Group (Promotion of Breastfeeding Intervention Trial). Promotion of Breastfeeding Intervention Trial (PROBIT): a randomized trial in the Republic of Belarus. *JAMA*. 2001;285(4):413–420

8. Kramer MS, Fombonne E, Igumnov S, et al; Promotion of Breastfeeding Intervention Trial (PROBIT) Study Group. Effects of prolonged and exclusive breastfeeding on child behavior and maternal adjustment: evidence from a large, randomized trial. *Pediatrics*. 2008;121(3). Available at: www.pediatrics.org/cgi/content/full/121/3/e435

9. Kramer MS, Aboud F, Mironova E, et al; Promotion of Breastfeeding Intervention Trial (PROBIT) Study Group. Breastfeeding and child cognitive development: new evidence from a large randomized trial. *Arch Gen Psychiatry*. 2008;65(5):578–584

10. Horta BL, Loret de Mola C, Victora CG. Breastfeeding and intelligence: a systematic review and meta-analysis. *Acta Paediatr*. 2015;104(467):14–19

11. Bartick MC, Stuebe AM, Schwarz EB, Luongo C, Reinhold AG, Foster EM. Cost analysis of maternal disease associated with suboptimal breastfeeding. *Obstet Gynecol*. 2013;122(1):111–119

12. McKinney CO, Hahn-Holbrook J, Chase-Lansdale PL, et al; Community Child Health Research Network. Racial and ethnic differences in breastfeeding. *Pediatrics*. 2016;138(2):e20152388

13. Logan C, Zittel T, Striebel S, et al. Changing societal and lifestyle factors and breastfeeding patterns over time. *Pediatrics*. 2016;137(5):e20154473

14. Roberts TJ, Carnahan E, Gakidou E. Can breastfeeding promote child health equity? A comprehensive analysis of breastfeeding patterns across the developing world and what we can learn from them. *BMC Med*. 2013;11:254

15. Centers for Disease Control and Prevention. Breastfeeding among US children born 2001–2013, CDC National Immunization Survey. Available at: https://www.cdc.gov/breastfeeding/data/nis_data/rates-any-exclusive-bf-socio-dem-2013.htm. Accessed January 4, 2017

Breastfeeding, Cognitive and Noncognitive Development in Early Childhood: A Population Study

Lisa-Christine Girard, PhD,[a,b] Orla Doyle, PhD,[b,c] Richard E. Tremblay, PhD[a,b,d,e,f]

abstract

BACKGROUND AND OBJECTIVES: There is mixed evidence from correlational studies that breastfeeding impacts children's development. Propensity score matching with large samples can be an effective tool to remove potential bias from observed confounders in correlational studies. The aim of this study was to investigate the impact of breastfeeding on children's cognitive and noncognitive development at 3 and 5 years of age.

METHODS: Participants included ~8000 families from the Growing Up in Ireland longitudinal infant cohort, who were identified from the Child Benefit Register and randomly selected to participate. Parent and teacher reports and standardized assessments were used to collect information on children's problem behaviors, expressive vocabulary, and cognitive abilities at age 3 and 5 years. Breastfeeding information was collected via maternal report. Propensity score matching was used to compare the average treatment effects on those who were breastfed.

RESULTS: Before matching, breastfeeding was associated with better development on almost every outcome. After matching and adjustment for multiple testing, only 1 of the 13 outcomes remained statistically significant: children's hyperactivity (difference score, −0.84; 95% confidence interval, −1.33 to −0.35) at age 3 years for children who were breastfed for at least 6 months. No statistically significant differences were observed postmatching on any outcome at age 5 years.

CONCLUSIONS: Although 1 positive benefit of breastfeeding was found by using propensity score matching, the effect size was modest in practical terms. No support was found for statistically significant gains at age 5 years, suggesting that the earlier observed benefit from breastfeeding may not be maintained once children enter school.

WHAT'S KNOWN ON THIS SUBJECT: The medical benefits of breastfeeding for mother and child are considered numerous, yet the effect of breastfeeding on cognitive abilities remains largely debated given selection into breastfeeding. The effect on behavior is even less well understood.

WHAT THIS STUDY ADDS: In applying quasi-experimental techniques which mimic random assignment, this study supports limited positive impacts of breastfeeding for children's cognitive and noncognitive development. Although significant, the effect of breastfeeding on noncognitive development is small in practical terms.

To cite: Girard L, Doyle O, Tremblay RE. Breastfeeding, Cognitive and Noncognitive Development in Early Childhood: A Population Study. *Pediatrics.* 2017;139(4):e20161848

[a]School of Public Health, Physiotherapy, and Sports Science, [b]Geary Institute for Public Policy, and [c]UCD School of Economics, University College Dublin, Dublin, Ireland; and [d]Research Unit on Children's Psychosocial Maladjustment (GRIP), Departments of [e]Pediatrics, and [f]Psychology, Université de Montreal, Montreal, Canada

Dr Girard conceptualized the study, carried out the initial analyses, interpreted the data, and drafted the initial manuscript; Drs Doyle and Tremblay conceptualized the study and critically reviewed and revised the manuscript; and all authors approved the final manuscript as submitted and agree to be accountable for all aspects of the work.

An earlier partial version of this work (age 3 data only) was presented as an oral presentation at the Growing Up in Ireland annual research conference; December 2015; Dublin, Ireland; and at 2 university seminar series; Life Course Centre, University of Queensland, Brisbane, Queensland, Australia and Melbourne Institute of Applied Economic and Social Research, Melbourne, Victoria, Australia; February 2016.

DOI: 10.1542/peds.2016-1848

Accepted for publication Jan 17, 2017

ARTICLE

The medical benefits of breastfeeding for both mother and child are considered numerous and well documented.[1-5] Yet the effect of breastfeeding on general cognitive abilities has been a topic of debate for nearly a century.[6] The mechanism argued to be responsible for these effects is the nutrients found in breast milk.[7,8] Two specific types of long-chain polyunsaturated fatty acids, namely docosahexaenoic (DHA) and arachidonic acid, have been implicated in both visual and neural development and functioning through neural maturation, which is important for cognitive abilities, such as problem solving.[9-11]

The link with nutrients may also impact specific cognitive abilities like language development. For example, language abilities, such as vocabulary, are highly dependent on working and long-term memory given the consolidation and retrieval processes needed during acquisition.[12,13] In rats, deficiency of fatty acids, such as DHA, during lactation resulted in poor memory retention during learning tasks, whereas supplementation of DHA had reversal effects.[14] If the hypothesized "causal" mechanism of superior nutrition in breast milk is true, coupled with the specific impact of DHA on memory, breastfeeding should also impact language abilities. To date, ~20 studies have investigated this association and all but 1[15] examined a combined measure of language (receptive and expressive) or receptive language only. There remains debate as to whether expressive and receptive language in early childhood form distinct modalities of language,[16,17] raising the question of whether breastfeeding would be equally beneficial to each modality in the case of a 2-factor language model.

Less studied is the impact of breastfeeding on behavior. Breastfeeding may lead to reduced behavioral problems as a result of early skin-to-skin contact, which helps form a secure mother-infant bond.[18] Any effects of breastfeeding on cognitive and language development could also prevent the development of behavior problems. The absence of early behavior problems has social, economic, and medical value to society through reduced prevalence of delinquency, incarceration rates, and substance abuse,[19-21] making this an important area of research. With few exceptions, there remains a dearth of high-quality studies examining behavior,[22-25] and among them, consensus is not evident.

Without randomization of mothers to breastfeeding and formula conditions, it is challenging to confirm the causal impact of these hypotheses. One study randomized the provision of a breastfeeding intervention, modeled on the Baby-Friendly Hospital Initiative, and found that the children of mothers in the intervention group had higher intelligence scores compared with controls at age 6 years.[26] The strongest effects were for verbal intelligence. This study offers the best support to date for a causal link between breastfeeding and cognitive development. However, it is the only cluster randomized trial on human lactation.

The majority of studies in this field are observational, thus the causal implications of breastfeeding are questionable given the inherent difficulty in controlling for selection into breastfeeding. For example, initial associations with cognitive development are often reduced after adjustments for confounders, such as parental education/IQ (ie, from an average 5-point to 3-point difference[27]), and, in some cases, the associations are no longer statistically significant.[28] A variety of observational studies now apply quasi-experimental methods to better address the issue of selection bias, making inroads toward a better understanding of potential causal paths. The techniques used include propensity score matching (PSM), instrument variables, and sibling pair models. This study uses PSM because the sibling pair model limits the available pool of participants and instrument variables are extremely sensitive to the validity of the chosen instrumentation, which should be associated with the exposure but not with the outcome except for via the exposure.

Using a large longitudinal population sample, we applied PSM, which mimics random assignment, in an effort to investigate the potential impacts of breastfeeding on children's cognitive ability, expressive vocabulary, and behavior problems. Both breastfeeding duration and intensity were examined. Significant advantages for children who were breastfed, after matching, were expected for all outcomes. Grounded in the recommendations of the World Health Organization,[29] it was expected that larger effect sizes would be observed for children who were fully breastfed and for longer durations.

METHODS

Participants

Participants included families enrolled in the Growing Up in Ireland infant cohort. Families with infants born between December 2007 and May 2008 were identified from the Child Benefit Register and randomly selected to participate. The overall recruitment response rate was 65% ($N = 11 134$). A detailed description of the study design can be found elsewhere.[30] We used data collected at 9 months and 3 and 5 years of age. Only families with complete data for all confounders when children were 9 months and children who were born full term were included ($N = 9854$; 88.5% of the initial sample). Boys represented 50.6% ($N = 4991$)

TABLE 1 Family, Maternal, Infant, and Medical Characteristics: Infant Cohort at 9 Months

	Ever Breastfed (N = 5940)	Never Breastfed (N = 3914)	P
	n (%)	n (%)	
Resident spouse/partner (yes)	5469 (92.1)	3213 (82.1)	≤.001
Social class			≤.001
Professional/managerial	3486 (58.7)	1449 (37.0)	
Nonmanual/skilled manual	1533 (25.8)	1419 (36.3)	
Semiskilled/unskilled	505 (8.5)	397 (10.1)	
Unknown/never worked	416 (7.0)	649 (16.6)	
Medical card status (yes)	1336 (22.8)	1433 (36.6)	≤.001
Maternal education			≤.001
Primary level/no education	65 (1.1)	152 (3.9)	
Second level	1782 (30.0)	2269 (58.0)	
Third level	4093 (68.9)	1493 (38.1)	
Maternal working status (yes)	4828 (81.3)	2865 (73.2)	≤.001
Maternal age, y			≤.001
≤ 24	456 (7.7)	653 (16.7)	
25–29	1178 (19.8)	883 (22.6)	
30–34 y	2202 (37.1)	1240 (31.7)	
≥35 y	2104 (35.4)	1138 (29.1)	
Maternal ethnicity (Irish)	4209 (70.9)	3725 (95.2)	≤.001
Maternal depression (yes)	222 (3.7)	201 (5.3)	.001
Smoking in dwelling during pregnancy (yes)	1535 (25.8)	1646 (42.1)	≤.001
Delivery mode (cesarean)	1348 (22.7)	1063 (27.2)	≤.001
Birth weight (≥2500 g; yes)	5842 (98.4)	3810 (97.3)	<.001
Visit to the NICU (yes)	575 (9.7)	420 (10.7)	.090
Infant sex (boy)	2944 (49.6)	2047 (52.3)	.008
Siblings living in dwelling (yes)	3248 (54.7)	2614 (66.8)	≤.001

Medical card coverage is a means-tested card issued by health services on the basis of financial need. There are 2 tiers of medical card coverage: "full coverage," which includes visits to general practitioners plus prescriptions and "general practitioner only coverage," which excludes prescriptions. Regarding the maternal education variable, primary level/no formal education is approximately equivalent to having an elementary to middle school education in the US system; second level is approximately equivalent to a high school diploma or technical trade/vocational diploma in the US system; and third level is equivalent to a college or bachelor's degree, graduate degree, or doctorate. Maternal working status refers to employment before pregnancy. Categorization of maternal depression refers to a score of ≥11 on the Center for Epidemiologic Studies Depression Scale.

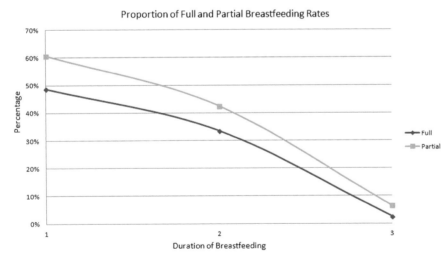

Proportion of Full and Partial Breastfeeding Rates

FIGURE 1
The category "1" on the x-axis represents breastfeeding up to 31 days; "2" represents between 32 and 180 days; and "3" represents ≥181 days.

5 years resulted in 7478 children being included in these analyses. Demographic characteristics of the families and rates of breastfeeding engagement can be found in Table 1 and Fig 1. Ethics approval was obtained from the Research Ethics Committee, Department of Children and Youth Affairs Ireland, and written consent was collected from parents/guardians before data collection.

Measures

Children's cognitive abilities and expressive vocabulary were measured by using 2 scales from the British Abilities Scale[31]. The pictures similarities scale assessed problem-solving skills and the naming vocabulary scale assessed expressive vocabulary. The construct validity of each scale was derived by using the Wechsler Preschool and Primary Scale of Intelligence-Revised

of the sample. Attrition across waves reduced the sample size to 8715 children at 3 years and 8032 at 5 years. Some children had missing data on the cognitive and vocabulary scales, resulting in 8535 and 8241 children respectively at age 3 and 7972 and 7942 children respectively at age 5. Additionally, missing teacher reports for behavior at age

TABLE 2 Bivariate Correlations Between Parent and Teacher SDQ Scores and Means (SDs) of Children's Outcomes at 3 and 5 Years of Age

	Conduct Problems, 5 y (Teacher)	Hyperactivity, 5 y (Teacher)	Difficulties, 5 y (Teacher)	Means (SD)	Minimum–Maximum
Conduct problems, 5 y (parent)	$r = 0.23^{***}$	$r = 0.21^{***}$	$r = 0.22^{***}$	1.44 (1.46)	0–10
Hyperactivity, 5 y (parent)	$r = 0.22^{***}$	$r = 0.35^{***}$	$r = 0.32^{***}$	3.23 (2.40)	0–10
Difficulties, 5 y (parent)	$r = 0.22^{***}$	$r = 0.29^{***}$	$r = 0.32^{***}$	7.10 (4.71)	0–32
Conduct problems, 5 y (teacher)	—	—	—	0.73 (1.33)	0–10
Hyperactivity, 5 y (teacher)	$r = 0.51^{***}$	—	—	2.96 (2.81)	0–10
Difficulties, 5 y (teacher)	$r = 0.70^{***}$	$r = 0.82^{***}$	—	5.92 (5.25)	0–32
Conduct problems, 3 y (parent)	—	—	—	2.15 (1.80)	0–10
Hyperactivity, 3 y (parent)	—	—	—	3.10 (2.14)	0–10
Difficulties, 3 y (parent)	—	—	—	7.71 (4.53)	0–32
Nonverbal reasoning, 5 y	—	—	—	58.89 (10.61)	20–80
Nonverbal reasoning, 3 y	—	—	—	53.30 (10.77)	20–80
Expressive vocabulary, 5 y	—	—	—	55.27 (12.22)	20–80
Expressive vocabulary, 3 y	—	—	—	51.16 (12.75)	20–80

$^{***} P \leq .001.$

($r = 0.74$ and 0.83, respectively).[31] Standardized scores that adjusted for performance as compared with other children of the same age, with a mean of 50 and a SD of 10, were used. Age was adjusted in 3-month age bands.

The Strengths and Difficulties Questionnaire (SDQ[32]) was used to assess children's problem behaviors. The parent version was used at age 3 years and both the parent and teacher versions were used at age 5 years. The SDQ is comprised of 5 scales (emotional symptoms, conduct problems, hyperactivity/inattention, peer relationship problems, and prosocial behavior) with ratings of applicability of behaviors on a 3-point scale. A total difficulties scale is included, combining the 4 problem scales, to yield an overall difficulties score. We used the conduct problems, hyperactivity/inattention, and difficulties scales given our focus on externalizing problems. Validation of the SDQ has been extensively documented.[33] Table 2 reports the correlations between parent and teacher SDQ reports and the means and SDs for all child outcomes.

Breastfeeding information was collected retrospectively when infants were 9 months old via maternal report. Support for the reliability of recall in previous breastfeeding studies has been established.[34] However, given the lower reliability regarding the timing of the introduction of additional fluids/solids, Labbok and Krasovec's definition of full (ie, exclusive or almost exclusive) and partial breastfeeding are used.[35] Two breastfeeding variables were created to assess whether the infant was fully or partially breastfed and the duration of each. Mothers were asked 4 questions: "Was <baby> ever breastfed," "How old was <baby> when he/she completely stopped being breastfed," "Was <baby> ever exclusively breastfed," and "How old was <baby> when he/she completely stopped being exclusively breastfed?" First, infants were grouped by breastfeeding status, both full and partial (5940) and never breastfed (3914). Of those who had ever been breastfed, 4795 had full breastfeeding at some point. Next, breastfeeding duration was grouped into 3 intervals; breastfed up to 31 days, 32 to 180 days, and ≥181 days. Each category of duration was treated as mutually exclusive, dummy coded, and compared against infants who had never been breastfed for the purpose of matching.

Confounders have been suggested in part to account for the associations found between breastfeeding and child outcomes. We matched groups (breastfed, never breastfed) on 14 of the most pertinent factors. At the child level, factors included sex (boy/girl), birth weight (≥2500 g), and having neonatal intensive care (yes/no). At the maternal level, factors included age (≤24 years, 25–29 years, 30–34 years, or ≥35 years), highest level of education (primary level/no education, second level, or third level), working status before pregnancy (yes/no), ethnicity (Irish, any other white background, African or any other black background, Asian background, or other, including mixed background), depression (a score of ≥11 on the Center for Epidemiologic Studies Depression Scale), and type of delivery (vaginal or caesarean). Family-level factors included having a partner in the residence (yes/no), social class (professional/managerial, other nonmanual/skilled manual, or semiskilled/unskilled), medical card status (free medical care, free general practitioner care, or no free medical care), total number of household members who smoked during the pregnancy (none, or ≥1), and whether the cohort infant had siblings living in the household.

Statistical Analysis

PSM reduces selection bias by matching children who were breastfed to children who were not, but who had a similar probability of being breastfed based on their measured characteristics. We used PSM logit models with nearest neighbor 1:1 matching techniques. In nearest neighbor matching, the sample is randomly ordered with matching occurring sequentially between the treatment (breastfed) and control (not breastfed) group based on participants' propensity scores. Typically, the pair is then removed from the list and the next match is created. To ensure optimal matches, we imposed a caliper so that pairs could only be matched if the propensity score was within a tenth of a SD of the other. We also allowed matching with replacement given the low rates of longer durations and full breastfeeding in this cohort. Although matching with replacement has been argued to increase variance in the data, it also arguably reduces bias in the sample by ensuring better quality of matches.[36] Balance checks in all models revealed substantial reductions of bias between matched groups on all individual confounders (ie, 0%–13.9% remaining bias in partial breastfeeding models, 0%–18.1% remaining bias in full models; data available on request). The remaining overall mean bias across models ranged from 3.2% to 8.5%. The ≤20% remaining bias has been suggested as the acceptable cutoff after matching.[37] Thus, we concluded that the analytic matching technique resulted in good matches between conditions. Matching resulted in all participants falling within the area of common support. The average treatment effect on those who were treated (ie, children who were breastfed) is reported. Adjustments were made for multiple hypothesis testing by using the Holmes-Bonferroni method. All statistical analyses for PSM were conducted by using Stata version 13 software (Stata Corp, College Station, TX).

To note, although PSM is advantageous in mimicking random assignment, a drawback is the challenge in evaluating a linear dose-response association, which has previously been found. Structural equation modeling (SEM) offers an alternative approach to examining this dose-response association.

Additionally, SEM uses the full sample and has greater power. Thus, the data were also modeled by using SEM, where confounders were treated as correlated exogenous variables, the duration of breastfeeding was treated as a continuous mediating variable, and child outcomes were treated as correlated, which could be influenced by both breastfeeding and confounders. These results can be found in the Supplemental Material.

RESULTS

Postmatching results for children fully breastfed up to 31 days revealed no statistically significant differences between groups on any outcome at age 3 or 5 years (Table 3). Similarly, for children who were fully breastfed between 33 and 100 days, no statistically significant differences were found for any outcomes at either age postmatching (Table 4). Finally, for children who were fully breastfed for ≥6, statistically significant differences were found postmatching for only 2 outcomes, problem solving and hyperactivity at age 3 years. Children who were fully breastfed scored 2.95 (SE = 1.39, P = .048) points higher on the problem-solving scale compared with children who were never breastfed and –0.84 (SE = 0.25, $P \leq$ .001) points lower on the hyperactivity scale. After adjustment for multiple testing, cognition was no longer statistically significant. However, children who were fully breastfed had slightly lower parent-rated hyperactivity compared with controls, and this remained statistically significant after adjustment (Table 5). Of note, results of the partial breastfeeding models were similar to the full models, however, after adjustment for multiple testing, neither cognitive ability nor hyperactivity at age 3 years remained statistically significant. These results can be found in the Supplemental Material.

DISCUSSION

Without randomized controlled trials, the issue of causality will necessarily remain open, however the present results contribute important insights to the long-standing debate of potential "causal effects" versus artifacts of confounding that are not properly accounted for. This study also provides new perspectives on breastfeeding and children's externalizing behavior. To the best of our knowledge, this is among the first studies to examine expressive vocabulary as an individual outcome and to consider externalizing behavior. It should be noted that our results apply only to infants born full term.

After adjustment for multiple testing, the initial support found for breastfeeding and better problem solving at age 3 years if the child was breastfed for a minimum of 6 months was no longer statistically significant. In addition, no statistically significant effects were found for cognitive ability at age 5 years. These results are in contrast to some studies that have used PSM techniques to examine the effects of breastfeeding and general cognitive abilities.[38–40] However, differences in both analytical choices of the PSM approach used (eg, replacement, calipers) and differing selection of covariates may help to explain these differences across studies. Nonetheless, our findings were surprising in the context of the nutrients in breast milk being responsible for increased cognitive development. Regarding expressive vocabulary, no statistically significant advantages were observed for children who were breastfed at either age 3 or age 5.

The limited research on breastfeeding and behavior problems is inconsistent, despite the relatively consistent reliance on the SDQ. Of interest, studies that have dichotomized the SDQ scales into abnormal scores (ie, at the 85th or 90th percentile) have not found

TABLE 3 Full Breastfeeding up to 31 Days and Child Outcomes at 3 and 5 Years of Age: Pre- and Postmatching

	Prematching				Postmatching			
	T	C	Difference	SE	T	C	Difference	SE
Problem solving, 3 y	53.75	52.52	1.23***	0.35	53.75	53.05	0.70	0.79
Problem solving, 5 y	59.30	58.06	1.24***	0.35	59.30	58.03	1.26	0.83
Vocabulary, 3 y	52.22	50.34	1.88***	0.40	52.22	50.91	1.30	0.95
Vocabulary, 5 y	56.09	55.40	0.69†	0.39	56.09	56.51	−0.41	0.89
Conduct, 3 y	2.11	2.31	−0.20***	0.05	2.11	2.14	−0.03	0.14
Conduct, 5 y	1.43	1.56	−0.13**	0.05	1.43	1.39	0.04	0.11
Hyperactivity, 3 y	3.07	3.27	−0.19**	0.07	3.07	3.04	0.03	0.16
Hyperactivity, 5 y	3.31	3.43	−0.11	0.08	3.31	3.01	0.29	0.18
Difficulties, 3 y	7.63	8.11	−0.47**	0.14	7.63	7.50	0.13	0.35
Difficulties, 5 y	7.15	7.49	−0.33*	0.16	7.15	6.54	0.60	0.36
Conduct, 5 y (teacher)	0.73	0.74	−0.01	0.04	0.73	0.67	0.06	0.10
Hyperactivity, 5 y (teacher)	2.95	3.12	−0.16†	0.09	2.95	3.03	−0.07	0.21
Difficulties, 5 y (teacher)	5.77	6.21	−0.44*	0.18	5.77	5.94	−0.16	0.40

Postmatching results have been adjusted for multiple hypothesis testing. Ns at age 3 years for the treatment group varied between 1262 and 1337 and between 3335 and 3419 for the control group. Ns at age 5 for the treatment group varied between 1229 and 1243 (teacher outcomes, 1154) and between 3078 and 3105 (teacher outcomes 2887) for the control group. C, control (not breastfed); Diff, difference in scores between groups; T, treatment (breastfed).
*** $P \le .001$.
** $P \le .01$.
* $P \le .05$.
† $P \le .10$.

TABLE 4 Full Breastfeeding 32 to 180 Days and Child Outcomes at 3 and 5 Years of Age: Results Pre- and Postmatching

	Prematching				Postmatching			
	T	C	Difference	SE	T	C	Difference	SE
Problem solving, 3 y	54.26	52.52	1.73***	0.27	54.26	52.91	1.34	1.02
Problem solving, 5 y	59.72	58.06	1.66***	0.28	59.72	58.81	0.91	1.03
Vocabulary, 3 y	52.17	50.34	1.83***	0.33	52.17	50.72	1.44	1.24
Vocabulary, 5 y	55.34	55.40	−0.05	0.32	55.34	56.41	−1.06	1.11
Conduct, 3 y	2.02	2.31	−0.29***	0.04	2.02	2.09	−0.06	0.16
Conduct, 5 y	1.32	1.56	−0.24***	0.03	1.32	1.35	−0.02	0.13
Hyperactivity, 3 y	2.92	3.27	−0.34***	0.05	2.92	3.17	−0.24	0.19
Hyperactivity, 5 y	2.94	3.43	−0.48***	0.06	2.94	2.93	0.01	0.22
Difficulties, 3 y	7.30	8.11	−0.81***	0.11	7.30	7.37	−0.07	0.41
Difficulties, 5 y	6.56	7.49	−0.93***	0.12	6.56	6.47	0.08	0.45
Conduct, 5 y (teacher)	0.68	0.74	−0.06†	0.03	0.68	0.69	−0.01	0.12
Hyperactivity, 5 y (teacher)	2.75	3.12	−0.36***	0.07	2.75	3.01	−0.26	0.27
Difficulties 5 y, teacher	5.56	6.21	−0.65***	0.14	5.56	6.06	−0.49	0.52

Postmatching results have been adjusted for multiple hypothesis testing. Ns at age 3 years for the treatment group varied between 2524 and 2742 and between 3335 and 3419 for the control group. Ns at age 5 years for the treatment group varied between 2514 and 2548 (teacher outcomes, 2402) between 3077 and 3105 for the control group (teacher outcomes 2877). C, control (not breastfed); Diff, difference in scores between groups; T, treatment (breastfed).
*** $P \le .001$.
† $P \le .10$.

statistically significant differences,[23–25] suggesting that breastfeeding is not likely to be a contributor to behavioral problems at clinical levels. When the SDQ scales are treated as continuous, small effects under certain conditions have been found.[22] In this study, we treated all 3 scales as continuous and found that children who were fully breastfed for ≥6 months had lower parent-rated scores on the hyperactivity scale at age 3 years only. This result remained statistically significant after adjustment for multiple testing. Our results suggest that longer durations of breastfeeding might help to reduce hyperactive behaviors for children who display mild to moderate levels in the short term, but that these benefits are not maintained even in the medium term.

This result would seemingly support the recommendation of the World Health Organization, suggesting that breastfeeding for at least 6 months is necessary for early gains to be observed.

The inherent strengths of this study include the use of a particularly large longitudinal developmental dataset, the use of a quasi-experimental

TABLE 5 Full Breastfeeding ≥181 Days and Child Outcomes at 3 and 5 Years of Age: Results Pre- and Postmatching

	Prematching				Postmatching			
	T	C	Difference	SE	T	C	Difference	SE
Problem solving, 3 y	54.43	52.52	1.90*	0.77	54.43	51.48	2.95	1.39
Problem solving, 5 y	59.54	58.06	1.47†	0.79	59.54	58.30	1.24	1.48
Vocabulary, 3 y	50.85	50.34	0.51	0.90	50.85	49.42	1.42	1.80
Vocabulary, 5 y	53.29	55.40	−2.10**	0.85	53.29	52.14	1.15	1.80
Conduct, 3 y	1.88	2.31	−0.42***	0.12	1.88	1.95	−0.06	0.22
Conduct, 5 y	1.20	1.56	−0.35**	0.11	1.20	1.43	−0.22	0.16
Hyperactivity, 3 y	2.52	3.27	−0.74***	0.15	2.52	3.37	−0.84***	0.25
Hyperactivity, 5 y	2.69	3.43	−0.74***	0.17	2.69	2.87	−0.18	0.27
Difficulties, 3 y	6.73	8.11	−1.37***	0.32	6.73	7.67	−0.93	0.57
Difficulties, 5 y	6.07	7.49	−1.42***	0.36	6.07	6.41	−0.34	0.56
Conduct, 5 y (teacher)	0.64	0.74	−0.09	0.10	0.64	0.52	0.11	0.15
Hyperactivity, 5 y (teacher)	2.61	3.12	−0.50*	0.21	2.61	2.82	−0.21	0.36
Difficulties, 5 y (teacher)	5.39	6.21	−0.82*	0.40	5.39	5.56	−0.16	0.66

Postmatching results have been adjusted for multiple hypothesis testing. Ns at age 3 years for the treatment group varied between 195 and 220 and between 3335 and 3419 for the control group. Ns at age 5 years for the treatment group varied between 211 and 213 (teacher outcomes, 185) and between 3306 and 3337 (teacher outcomes 2877) for the control group. C, control (not breastfed); Diff, difference in scores between groups; T, treatment (breastfed).

*** $P ≤ .001.$
** $P ≤ .01.$
* $P ≤ .05.$
† $P ≤ .10.$

statistical approach, the use of a repeated measures design, the use of multiple informants and simultaneous standardized assessments thereby limiting potential shared method variance, the comparatively large number of confounders controlled (ie, 14) in contrast to previous studies (ie, an average of 7.7 ± 3.4 in higher-quality studies[28];), and assessments in both cognitive and noncognitive domains of child development. Despite these strengths, some limitations must be noted. First, information on breastfeeding was collected retrospectively. Although the reliability of recall has been established,[34] it must be acknowledged that recall bias may nevertheless be present, particularly regarding the duration of full breastfeeding. Second, only parent-reported SDQs were collected when children were 3 years of age. Studies have found that parents typically rate their children as having higher levels of problem behaviors as compared with teacher reports, with weak associations between these 2 types of informants,[24] as was found in the current study for behavior ratings at age 5 years between parents and teachers. Having access to child care staff reports at age 3 years would have increased

the reliability of the maternal-rated hyperactivity finding. Third, no information pertaining to direct breastfeeding versus expressed breast milk feeding was collected. Thus, it is not possible to investigate whether the association with reduced hyperactivity at age 3 years was the result of skin-to-skin contact or due to the nutrients in breast milk. This is an important direction for future studies examining behavioral outcomes. Fourth, although maternal education was included as a confounder, maternal IQ was not collected in this cohort. In the few studies that controlled for maternal IQ, the findings suggested that it accounted for a large part of the association between breastfeeding and cognitive outcomes.[39,41] Thus, the inclusion of maternal IQ in future studies that employ PSM is warranted. Finally, PSM does not address selection on unobservables. Causal estimates may only be estimated by using PSM if selection is on observable characteristics or, in cases where unobservable factors influence selection into breastfeeding, the balancing on observables also balances on these unobservables. Despite these limitations, the results of this study add to the growing literature by showing

that some statistically significant positive noncognitive benefits may result from longer durations of breastfeeding. Yet, beyond the statistical implications, the practical implications appear minimal and short lived. It is important to note, however, that these findings do not contradict the many medical benefits afforded to both mother and child as a result of breastfeeding.

ACKNOWLEDGMENTS

We thank the Irish Social Science Data Archive for permission to use the infant cohort data from the Growing Up in Ireland study. We also thank the participants and their families for their long-term commitment to this study.

ABBREVIATIONS

DHA: docosahexaenoic
PSM: propensity score matching
SDQ: strengths and difficulties questionnaire
SEM: structural equation modeling

Address correspondence to Lisa-Christine Girard, PhD, School of Public Health, Physiotherapy, and Sports Science, University College Dublin, Geary Institute for Public Policy, Room B205, Belfield, Dublin 4, Ireland. E-mail: lisa.girard@ucd.ie

PEDIATRICS (ISSN Numbers: Print, 0031-4005; Online, 1098-4275).

FINANCIAL DISCLOSURE: The authors have indicated they have no financial relationships relevant to this article to disclose.

FUNDING: Dr Girard is supported by a Marie Curie International Incoming Fellowship. The research that led to these results was funded by the People Programme (Marie Curie Actions) of the European Union's Seventh Framework Programme FP7/2007-2013/ under the Research Executive Agency grant agreement 625014.

POTENTIAL CONFLICT OF INTEREST: The authors have indicated they have no potential conflicts of interest to disclose.

COMPANION PAPER: A companion to this article can be found online at www.pediatrics.org/cgi/doi/10.1542/peds.2017-0150.

REFERENCES

1. Ip S, Chung M, Raman G, Trikalinos TA, Lau J. A summary of the Agency for Healthcare Research and Quality's evidence report on breastfeeding in developed countries. *Breastfeed Med.* 2009;4(suppl 1):S17–S30

2. Narod SA. Modifiers of risk of hereditary breast cancer. *Oncogene.* 2006;25(43):5832–5836

3. Taylor JS, Kacmar JE, Nothnagle M, Lawrence RA. A systematic review of the literature associating breastfeeding with type 2 diabetes and gestational diabetes. *J Am Coll Nutr.* 2005;24(5):320–326

4. Horta BL, Loret de Mola C, Victora CG. Long-term consequences of breastfeeding on cholesterol, obesity, systolic blood pressure and type 2 diabetes: a systematic review and meta-analysis. *Acta Paediatr.* 2015;104(S467):30–37

5. Victora CG, Bahl R, Barros AJ, et al; Lancet Breastfeeding Series Group. Breastfeeding in the 21st century: epidemiology, mechanisms, and lifelong effect. *Lancet.* 2016;387(10017):475–490

6. Hoefer C, Hardy MC. Later development of breastfed and artificially fed infants: Comparison of physical and mental growth. *J Am Med Assoc.* 1929;92(8):615–619

7. Auestad N, Scott DT, Janowsky JS, et al. Visual, cognitive, and language assessments at 39 months: a follow-up study of children fed formulas containing long-chain polyunsaturated fatty acids to 1 year of age. *Pediatrics.* 2003;112(3 pt 1). Available at: www.pediatrics.org/cgi/content/full/112/3/e177

8. Horwood LJ, Fergusson DM. Breastfeeding and later cognitive and academic outcomes. *Pediatrics.* 1998;101(1). Available at: www.pediatrics.org/cgi/content/full/101/1/e9

9. Brenna JT, Varamini B, Jensen RG, Diersen-Schade DA, Boettcher JA, Arterburn LM. Docosahexaenoic and arachidonic acid concentrations in human breast milk worldwide. *Am J Clin Nutr.* 2007;85(6):1457–1464

10. Das UN, Fams. Long-chain polyunsaturated fatty acids in the growth and development of the brain and memory. *Nutrition.* 2003;19(1):62–65

11. McCann JC, Ames BN. Is docosahexaenoic acid, an n-3 long-chain polyunsaturated fatty acid, required for development of normal brain function? An overview of evidence from cognitive and behavioral tests in humans and animals. *Am J Clin Nutr.* 2005;82(2):281–295

12. Baddeley A. Working memory and language: an overview. *J Commun Disord.* 2003;36(3):189–208

13. Baddeley A. Working memory. *Science.* 1992;255(5044):556–559

14. García-Calatayud S, Redondo C, Martín E, Ruiz JI, García-Fuentes M, Sanjurjo P. Brain docosahexaenoic acid status and learning in young rats submitted to dietary long-chain polyunsaturated fatty acid deficiency and supplementation limited to lactation. *Pediatr Res.* 2005;57(5 pt 1):719–723

15. Silva PA, Buckfield P, Spears GF. Some maternal and child developmental characteristics associated with breast feeding: a report from the Dunedin Multidisciplinary Child Development Study. *Aust Paediatr J.* 1978;14(4):265–268

16. Fenson L, Dale PS, Reznick JS, Bates E, Thal DJ, Pethick SJ. Variability in early communicative development. *Monogr Soc Res Child Dev.* 1994;59(5):1–173; discussion 174–185

17. Tomblin JB, Zhang X. The dimensionality of language ability in school-age children. *J Speech Lang Hear Res.* 2006;49(6):1193–1208

18. Britton JR, Britton HL, Gronwaldt V. Breastfeeding, sensitivity, and attachment. *Pediatrics.* 2006;118(5). Available at www.pediatrics.org/cgi/content/full/118/5/e1436

19. Copeland WE, Miller-Johnson S, Keeler G, Angold A, Costello EJ. Childhood psychiatric disorders and young adult crime: a prospective, population-based study. *Am J Psychiatry.* 2007;164(11):1668–1675

20. Pingault JB, Côté SM, Galéra C, et al. Childhood trajectories of inattention, hyperactivity and oppositional behaviors and prediction of substance abuse/dependence: a 15-year longitudinal population-based study. *Mol Psychiatry.* 2013;18(7):806–812

21. Schultz TW. Investment in human capital. *Am Econ Rev.* 1961;51(1):1–17

22. Borra C, Iacovou M, Sevilla A. The effect of breastfeeding on children's cognitive and noncognitive development. *Labour Econ.* 2012;19(4):496–515

23. Heikkilä K, Sacker A, Kelly Y, Renfrew MJ, Quigley MA. Breastfeeding and child behaviour in the Millennium Cohort Study. *Arch Dis Child*. 2011;96(7)635–642

24. Kramer MS, Fombonne E, Igumnov S, et al; Promotion of Breastfeeding Intervention Trial (PROBIT) Study Group. Effects of prolonged and exclusive breastfeeding on child behavior and maternal adjustment: evidence from a large, randomized trial. *Pediatrics*. 2008;121(3). Available at: www.pediatrics.org/cgi/content/full/121/3/e435

25. Lind JN, Li R, Perrine CG, Schieve LA. Breastfeeding and later psychosocial development of children at 6 years of age. *Pediatrics*. 2014;134(suppl 1):S36–S41

26. Kramer MS, Aboud F, Mironova E, et al; Promotion of Breastfeeding Intervention Trial (PROBIT) Study Group. Breastfeeding and child cognitive development: new evidence from a large randomized trial. *Arch Gen Psychiatry*. 2008;65(5):578–584

27. Anderson JW, Johnstone BM, Remley DT. Breast-feeding and cognitive development: a meta-analysis. *Am J Clin Nutr*. 1999;70(4):525–535

28. Walfisch A, Sermer C, Cressman A, Koren G. Breast milk and cognitive development--the role of confounders: a systematic review. *BMJ Open*. 2013;3(8):e003259

29. World Health Organization. *UNICEF. Global Strategy for Infant and Young Child Feeding*. Geneva, Switzerland: WHO Press; 2003

30. Williams J, Greene S, McNally S, Murray A, Quail A. *Growing up in Ireland; National Longitudinal Study of Children: The Infants and Their Families*. Dublin, Ireland: The Stationery Office; 2010

31. Elliott CD, Smith P, McCullock K. *British Abilities Scale (BAS II) Technical Manual*. Windsor, United Kingdom: nferNelson; 1997

32. Goodman R. The Strengths and Difficulties Questionnaire: a research note. *J Child Psychol Psychiatry*. 1997;38(5):581–586

33. Theunissen MH, Vogels AG, de Wolff MS, Reijneveld SA. Characteristics of the strengths and difficulties questionnaire in preschool children. *Pediatrics*. 2013;131(2). Available at: www.pediatrics.org/cgi/content/full/131/2/e446

34. Li R, Scanlon KS, Serdula MK. The validity and reliability of maternal recall of breastfeeding practice. *Nutr Rev*. 2005;63(4):103–110

35. Labbok M, Krasovec K. Toward consistency in breastfeeding definitions. *Stud Fam Plann*. 1990;21(4):226–230

36. Caliendo M, Kopeinig S. Some practical guidance for the implementation of propensity score matching. *J Econ Surv*. 2008;22(1):31–72

37. Rosenbaum PR, Rubin DB. The bias due to incomplete matching. *Biometrics*. 1985;41(1):103–116

38. Boutwell BB, Beaver KM, Barnes JC. Role of breastfeeding in childhood cognitive development: a propensity score matching analysis. *J Paediatr Child Health*. 2012;48(9):840–845

39. Jiang M, Foster EM, Gibson-Davis CM. Breastfeeding and the child cognitive outcomes: a propensity score matching approach. *Matern Child Health J*. 2011;15(8):1296–1307

40. Smithers LG, Brazionis L, Golley RK, et al. Associations between dietary patterns at 6 and 15 months of age and sociodemographic factors. *Eur J Clin Nutr*. 2012;66(6):658–666

41. Der G, Batty GD, Deary IJ. Effect of breast feeding on intelligence in children: prospective study, sibling pairs analysis, and meta-analysis. *BMJ*. 2006;333(7575):945

Supplemental Information

SUPPLEMENTAL TABLE 6 Partial Breastfeeding ≤31 Days and Child Outcomes at 3 and 5 Years of Age: Results Pre- and Postmatching

	Prematching				Postmatching			
	T	C	Difference	SE	T	C	Difference	SE
Problem solving, 3 y	53.51	52.53	0.97**	0.33	53.51	53.71	−0.20	0.76
Problem solving, 5 y	59.19	58.07	1.11***	0.33	59.19	58.41	0.77	0.77
Vocabulary, 3 y	52.07	50.35	1.72***	0.38	52.07	50.83	1.23	0.92
Vocabulary, 5 y	55.67	55.40	0.26	0.37	55.67	56.12	−0.45	0.84
Conduct, 3 y	2.11	2.31	−0.20***	0.05	2.11	2.15	−0.03	0.12
Conduct, 5 y	1.44	1.55	−0.11*	0.04	1.44	1.35	0.08	0.10
Hyperactivity, 3 y	3.13	3.26	−0.12*	0.06	3.13	3.14	−0.00	0.14
Hyperactivity, 5 y	3.36	3.42	−0.05	0.07	3.36	3.01	0.35	0.17
Difficulties, 3 y	7.78	8.11	−0.32*	0.14	7.78	7.66	0.11	0.32
Difficulties, 5 y	7.27	7.48	−0.21	0.15	7.27	6.72	0.54	0.35
Conduct, 5 y (teacher)	0.75	0.074	0.01	0.04	0.75	0.74	0.01	0.09
Hyperactivity, 5 y (teacher)	3.01	3.11	−0.09	0.09	3.01	3.08	−0.06	0.20
Difficulties, 5 y (teacher)	5.93	6.20	−0.27	0.17	5.93	5.98	−0.05	0.37

Postmatching results have been adjusted for multiple hypothesis testing. *N*s at age 3 years for the treatment group varied between 1503 and 1598 and between 3337 and 3422 for the control group. *N*s at age 5 years for the treatment group varied between 1481 and 1500 (teacher outcomes, 1392) and between 3080 and 3108 (teacher outcomes 2880) for the control group. C, control (not breastfed); Diff, difference in scores between groups; T, treatment (breastfed).
*** $P \le .001$.
** $P \le .01$.
* $P \le .05$.

SUPPLEMENTAL TABLE 7 Partial Breastfeeding 32 to 180 Days and Child Outcomes at 3 and 5 Years of Age: Results Pre- and Postmatching

	Prematching				Postmatching			
	T	C	Difference	SE	T	C	Difference	SE
Problem solving, 3 y	53.55	52.53	1.01**	0.31	53.55	53.28	0.26	0.93
Problem solving, 5 y	59.10	58.07	1.02**	0.32	59.10	58.72	0.37	0.95
Vocabulary, 3 y	52.16	50.35	1.81***	0.37	52.16	50.66	1.49	1.10
Vocabulary, 5 y	55.65	55.40	0.24	0.35	55.65	56.36	−0.71	1.00
Conduct, 3 y	2.03	2.31	−0.27***	0.05	2.03	2.20	−0.16	0.15
Conduct, 5 y	1.37	1.55	−0.18***	0.04	1.37	1.35	0.01	0.12
Hyperactivity, 3 y	3.02	3.26	−0.24***	0.06	3.02	3.10	−0.08	0.18
Hyperactivity, 5 y	3.07	3.42	−0.34***	0.07	3.07	2.83	0.23	0.20
Difficulties, 3 y	7.38	8.11	−0.72***	0.13	7.38	7.44	−0.05	0.39
Difficulties, 5 y	6.82	7.48	−0.65***	0.14	6.82	6.27	0.55	0.40
Conduct, 5 y (teacher)	0.72	0.74	−0.01	0.04	0.72	0.68	0.04	0.11
Hyperactivity, 5 y (teacher)	2.86	3.11	−0.24**	0.08	2.86	2.94	−0.07	0.25
Difficulties, 5 y (teacher)	5.74	6.20	−0.46**	0.16	5.74	6.01	−0.27	0.47

Postmatching results have been adjusted for multiple hypothesis testing. *N*s at age 3 years for the treatment group varied between 1696 and 1812 and between 3337 and 3422 for the control group. *N*s at age 5 years for the treatment group varied between 1673 and 1689 (teacher outcomes, 1594) and between 3080 and 3108 (teacher outcomes 2880) for the control group. C, control (not breastfed); Diff, difference in scores between groups; T, treatment (breastfed).
*** $P \le .001$.
** $P \le .01$.

SUPPLEMENTAL TABLE 8 Partial Breastfeeding ≥181 Days and Child Outcomes at 3 and 5 Years of Age: Results Pre- and Postmatching

	Prematching				Postmatching			
	T	C	Difference	SE	T	C	Difference	SE
Problem solving, 3 y	54.28	52.53	1.75***	0.31	54.28	52.24	2.04	1.06
Problem solving, 5 y	59.86	58.07	1.78***	0.32	59.86	58.13	1.72	1.14
Vocabulary, 3 y	50.91	50.35	0.56	0.37	50.91	49.25	1.66	1.27
Vocabulary, 5 y	54.30	55.40	−1.09**	0.36	54.30	54.47	−0.16	1.22
Conduct 3, y	1.99	2.31	−0.32***	0.05	1.99	2.16	−0.16	0.17
Conduct 5, y	1.29	1.55	−0.26***	0.04	1.29	1.42	−0.13	0.13
Hyperactivity, 3 y	2.84	3.26	−0.42***	0.06	2.84	3.34	−0.50	0.20
Hyperactivity, 5 y	2.90	3.42	−0.52***	0.07	2.90	2.97	−0.07	0.24
Difficulties, 3 y	7.24	8.11	−0.86***	0.13	7.24	7.57	−0.32	0.42
Difficulties, 5 y	6.54	7.48	−0.93***	0.14	6.54	6.64	−0.10	0.48
Conduct, 5 y (teacher)	0.66	0.74	−0.07†	0.04	0.66	0.65	0.01	0.13
Hyperactivity, 5 y (teacher)	2.74	3.11	−0.37***	0.08	2.74	2.91	−0.17	0.27
Difficulties, 5 y (teacher)	5.56	6.20	−0.64***	0.16	5.56	5.78	−0.22	0.51

Postmatching results have been adjusted for multiple hypothesis testing. Ns at age 3 years for the treatment group varied between 1691 and 1869 and between 3337 and 3422 for the control group. Ns at age 5 years for the treatment group varied between 1694 and 1721 (teacher outcomes, 1599) and between 3080 and 3108 (teacher outcomes 2880) for the control group. C, control (not breastfed); Diff, difference in scores between groups; T, treatment (breastfed).

*** $P \leq .001$.

** $P \leq .01$.

† $P \leq .10$.

SUPPLEMENTAL TABLE 9 Breastfeeding and Child Outcomes at 3 and 5 Years of Age Using a SEM Approach

	Age 3				Age 5			
	B (SE)	95% CI	P	β	B (SE)	95% CI	P	β
Cognition								
Direct effects of								
Full breastfeeding	0.007 (0.002)	0.003–0.011	<.001	0.040	0.005 (0.002)	0.001–0.009	.010	0.030
Partner in residence	0.772 (0.508)	−0.224 to 1.768	.129	0.023	0.607 (0.510)	−0.393 to 1.606	.234	0.018
Maternal age	−0.219 (0.142)	−0.498 to 0.060	.124	−0.020	−0.095 (0.145)	−0.380 to 0.190	.514	−0.009
Maternal education	1.392 (0.259)	0.885–1.900	<.001	0.070	1.189 (0.262)	0.676–1.703	<.001	0.061
Social class	−0.132 (0.088)	−0.304 to 0.040	.133	−0.026	−0.161 (0.086)	−0.329 to 0.007	.060	−0.032
Medical card status	0.370 (0.177)	0.024–0.717	.036	0.030	0.303 (0.186)	−0.060 to 0.667	.102	0.025
Maternal working status	0.347 (0.321)	−0.281 to 0.976	.279	0.013	0.763 (0.328)	0.120–1.406	.020	0.030
Maternal ethnicity	−0.504 (0.113)	−0.725 to −0.283	<.001	−0.056	0.081 (0.111)	−0.136 to 0.299	.463	0.009
Maternal depression	−0.052 (0.574)	−1.177 to 1.073	.928	−0.001	−0.851 (0.563)	−1.955 to 0.252	.131	−0.016
Smoking during pregnancy	−0.398 (0.266)	−0.918 to 0.123	.134	−0.017	−0.103 (0.268)	−0.629 to 0.423	.701	−0.005
Sibling status	−0.844 (0.262)	−1.358 to −0.330	.001	−0.038	−0.826 (0.272)	−1.360 to −0.293	.002	−0.038
Visit to the NICU	−0.363 (0.359)	−1.068 to 0.341	.312	−0.011	−0.546 (0.359)	−1.249 to 0.158	.128	−0.016
Birth weight	1.545 (0.898)	−0.214 to 3.304	.085	0.020	0.972 (0.855)	−0.704 to 2.647	.256	0.013
Child sex	2.363 (0.229)	1.913–2.812	<.001	0.110	1.326 (0.235)	0.865–1.787	<.001	0.062
Type of delivery	−0.056 (0.079)	−0.211 to 0.099	.479	−0.008	−0.076 (0.081)	−0.234 to 0.082	.346	−0.011
Indirect effects of breastfeeding								
Partner in residence	0.042 (0.018)	0.007–0.077	.020	0.001	0.031 (0.016)	0.000–0.063	.050	0.001
Maternal age	0.043 (0.013)	0.018–0.069	.001	0.004	0.032 (0.013)	0.007–0.058	.012	0.003
Maternal education	0.137 (0.039)	0.060–0.214	.001	0.007	0.102 (0.04)	0.023–0.181	.011	0.005
Social class	−0.008 (0.003)	−0.015 to −0.002	.016	−0.002	−0.006 (0.003)	−0.012 to 0.000	.040	−0.001
Medical card status	−0.001 (0.006)	−0.013 to 0.010	.798	0.000	−0.001 (0.004)	−0.010 to 0.007	.799	0.000
Maternal working status	−0.032 (0.014)	−0.060 to −0.004	.027	−0.001	−0.024 (0.012)	−0.048 to 0.000	.055	−0.001
Maternal ethnicity	0.073 (0.021)	0.032–0.115	<.001	0.008	0.055 (0.021)	0.013–0.097	.010	0.006
Maternal depression	−0.024 (0.018)	−0.060 to 0.012	.195	0.000	−0.018 (0.015)	−0.046 to 0.011	.222	0.000
Smoking during pregnancy	−0.055 (0.018)	−0.090 to −0.021	.002	−0.002	−0.041 (0.017)	−0.075 to −0.007	.017	−0.002
Sibling status	−0.040 (0.015)	−0.070 to −0.011	.007	−0.002	−0.030 (0.014)	−0.057 to −0.003	.027	−0.001
Visit to the NICU	−0.015 (0.013)	−0.041 to 0.011	.270	0.000	−0.011 (0.01)	−0.031 to 0.010	.294	0.000
Birth weight	0.084 (0.036)	0.014–0.154	.018	0.001	0.063 (0.032)	0.001–0.124	.047	0.001
Child sex	0.032 (0.012)	0.009–0.055	.007	0.001	0.024 (0.011)	0.002–0.045	.030	0.001
Type of delivery	−0.025 (0.007)	−0.040 to −0.010	.001	−0.003	−0.019 (0.007)	−0.033 to −0.004	.013	−0.003
Vocabulary								
Direct effects of								
Full breastfeeding	0.003 (0.002)	−0.001 to 0.008	.151	0.017	−0.004 (0.002)	−0.008 to 0.001	.117	−0.018
Partner in residence	−0.010 (0.579)	−1.146 to 1.125	.986	0.000	−2.058 (0.590)	−3.215 to −0.901	<.001	−0.054
Maternal age	0.478 (0.168)	0.148–0.807	.004	0.037	0.955 (0.164)	0.633–1.277	<.001	0.077
Maternal education	1.769 (0.299)	1.184–2.355	<.001	0.074	1.823 (0.294)	1.247–2.399	<.001	0.080
Social class	−0.342 (0.100)	−0.539 to −0.146	.001	−0.057	−0.409 (0.102)	−0.609 to −0.209	<.001	−0.071
Medical card status	0.874 (0.216)	0.451–1.297	<.001	0.059	1.080 (0.213)	0.663–1.496	<.001	0.077
Maternal working status	0.774 (0.379)	0.031–1.517	.041	0.025	0.038 (0.372)	−0.691 to 0.768	.918	0.001
Maternal ethnicity	−2.375 (0.148)	−2.665 to −2.085	<.001	−0.221	−2.545 (0.148)	−2.835 to −2.254	<.001	−0.247
Maternal depression	−0.022 (0.645)	−1.286 to 1.243	.973	0.000	0.877 (0.653)	−0.404 to 2.158	.179	0.014
Smoking during pregnancy	−0.737 (0.308)	−1.340 to −0.134	.017	−0.027	−0.31 (0.299)	−0.895 to 0.275	.299	−0.012
Sibling status	−1.796 (0.313)	−2.409 to −1.184	<.001	−0.069	−1.137 (0.300)	−1.725 to −0.549	<.001	−0.045

TABLE 9 Continued

	Age 3				Age 5			
	B (SE)	95% CI	P	β	B (SE)	95% CI	P	β
Visit to the NICU	−0.672 (0.426)	−1.507 to 0.163	.115	−0.01	−0.867 (0.403)	−1.656 to −0.078	.031	−0.022
Birth weight	1.242 (0.931)	−0.582 to 3.066	.182	0.01	0.917 (0.957)	−0.960 to 2.793	.338	0.011
Child sex	3.599 (0.266)	3.078–4.121	<.001	0.14	1.306 (0.260)	0.796–1.817	<.001	0.053
Type of delivery	−0.167 (0.092)	−0.346 to 0.013	.069	−0.01	−0.022 (0.091)	−0.201 to 0.157	.807	−0.003
Indirect effects of breastfeeding								
Partner in residence	0.021 (0.016)	−0.011 to 0.052	.196	0.00	−0.022 (0.016)	−0.052 to 0.009	.161	−0.001
Maternal age	0.021 (0.015)	−0.008 to 0.051	.156	0.00	−0.022 (0.014)	−0.051 to 0.006	.120	−0.002
Maternal education	0.067 (0.047)	−0.025 to 0.159	.153	0.00	−0.071 (0.045)	−0.160 to 0.018	.119	−0.003
Social class	−0.004 (0.003)	−0.010 to 0.002	.187	−0.00	0.004 (0.003)	−0.002 to 0.010	.161	0.001
Medical card status	−0.001 (0.003)	−0.006 to 0.005	.801	0.00	0.001 (0.003)	−0.005 to 0.007	.801	0.000
Maternal working status	−0.016 (0.012)	−0.039 to 0.008	.201	−0.00	0.016 (0.012)	−0.007 to 0.040	.171	0.001
Maternal ethnicity	0.036 (0.025)	−0.013 to 0.086	.151	0.00	−0.038 (0.024)	−0.086 to 0.010	.118	−0.004
Maternal depression	−0.012 (0.012)	−0.035 to 0.011	.318	0.00	0.012 (0.012)	−0.011 to 0.036	.300	0.000
Smoking during pregnancy	−0.027 (0.019)	−0.065 to 0.009	.159	−0.001	0.029 (0.019)	−0.008 to 0.066	.128	0.001
Sibling status	−0.020 (0.015)	−0.049 to 0.009	.176	−0.001	0.021 (0.014)	−0.007 to 0.049	.140	0.001
Visit to the NICU	−0.007 (0.008)	−0.023 to 0.009	.370	0.000	0.008 (0.008)	−0.008 to 0.023	.346	0.000
Birth weight	0.041 (0.032)	−0.021 to 0.103	.192	0.000	−0.043 (0.031)	−0.103 to 0.016	.155	−0.001
Child sex	0.016 (0.011)	−0.007 to 0.038	.175	0.001	−0.016 (0.011)	−0.039 to 0.006	.149	−0.001
Type of delivery	−0.012 (0.009)	−0.029 to 0.005	.157	−0.001	0.013 (0.008)	−0.003 to 0.029	.123	0.002
Conduct problems								
Direct effects of								
Full breastfeeding	−0.001 (0.000)	−0.001 to 0.000	.037	−0.022	−0.001 (0.000)	−0.001 to 0.000	.018	−0.026
Partner in residence	−0.129 (0.091)	−0.307 to 0.049	.156	−0.023	−0.158 (0.080)	−0.315 to −0.001	.049	−0.035
Maternal age	−0.150 (0.024)	−0.196 to −0.103	<.001	−0.082	−0.075 (0.021)	−0.115 to −0.035	<.001	−0.051
Maternal education	−0.099 (0.042)	−0.182 to −0.016	.019	−0.030	−0.078 (0.036)	−0.150 to −0.007	.031	−0.029
Social class	0.024 (0.015)	−0.006 to 0.053	.115	0.028	0.018 (0.013)	−0.008 to 0.045	.175	0.027
Medical card status	−0.058 (0.030)	−0.117 to 0.000	.050	−0.028	−0.072 (0.026)	−0.123 to −0.022	.005	−0.043
Maternal working status	0.042 (0.054)	−0.064 to 0.147	.442	0.010	0.041 (0.046)	−0.050 to 0.132	.373	0.012
Maternal ethnicity	0.012 (0.017)	−0.021 to 0.045	.464	0.008	−0.023 (0.015)	−0.052 to 0.006	.122	−0.019
Maternal depression	0.440 (0.113)	0.218–0.661	<.001	0.050	0.422 (0.092)	0.241–0.602	<.001	0.058
Smoking during pregnancy	0.213 (0.044)	0.126–0.300	<.001	0.055	0.164 (0.037)	0.091–0.238	<.001	0.053
Sibling status	0.147 (0.044)	0.060–0.233	.001	0.040	0.115 (0.037)	0.042–0.188	.002	0.039
Visit to the NICU	−0.021 (0.058)	−0.135 to 0.093	.715	−0.004	−0.025 (0.050)	−0.122 to 0.072	.613	−0.005
Birth weight	−0.088 (0.145)	−0.372 to 0.195	.541	−0.007	−0.080 (0.128)	−0.331 to 0.171	.532	−0.008
Child sex	−0.154 (0.038)	−0.228 to −0.079	<.001	−0.043	−0.204 (0.032)	−0.266 to −0.141	<.001	−0.070
Type of delivery	−0.018 (0.013)	−0.043 to 0.008	.178	−0.015	−0.018 (0.011)	−0.040 to 0.004	.106	−0.018
Indirect effects of breastfeeding:								
Partner in residence	−0.004 (0.002)	−0.008 to 0.001	.086	−0.001	−0.004 (0.002)	−0.008 to 0.000	.062	−0.001
Maternal age	−0.004 (0.002)	−0.008 to 0.000	.041	−0.002	−0.004 (0.002)	−0.007 to −0.001	.021	−0.003
Maternal education	−0.013 (0.006)	−0.025 to −0.001	.039	−0.004	−0.012 (0.005)	−0.022 to −0.002	.019	−0.004
Social class	0.001 (0.000)	0.000–0.002	.078	0.001	0.001 (0.000)	0.000–0.001	.054	0.001
Medical card status	0.000 (0.001)	−0.001 to 0.001	.799	0.000	0.000 (0.001)	−0.001 to 0.001	.799	0.000
Maternal working status	0.003 (0.002)	−0.001 to 0.006	.096	0.001	0.003 (0.002)	0.000–0.006	.070	0.001
Maternal ethnicity	−0.007 (0.003)	−0.013 to 0.000	.038	−0.005	−0.007 (0.003)	−0.012 to −0.001	.018	−0.005
Maternal depression	0.002 (0.002)	−0.002 to 0.006	.249	0.000	0.002 (0.002)	−0.001 to 0.006	.235	0.000

TABLE 9 Continued

	Age 3				Age 5			
	B (SE)	95% CI	P	β	B (SE)	95% CI	P	β
Smoking during pregnancy	0.005 (0.003)	0.000–0.010	.049	0.001	0.005 (0.002)	0.001–0.009	.027	0.002
Sibling status	0.004 (0.002)	0.000–0.008	.062	0.001	0.004 (0.002)	0.000–0.007	.037	0.001
Visit to the NICU	0.001 (0.001)	−0.001 to 0.004	.312	0.000	0.001 (0.001)	−0.001 to 0.004	.298	0.000
Birth weight	−0.008 (0.004)	−0.017 to 0.001	.080	−0.001	−0.007 (0.004)	−0.015 to 0.000	.061	−0.001
Child sex	−0.003 (0.002)	−0.006 to 0.000	.067	−0.001	−0.003 (0.001)	−0.006 to 0.000	.044	−0.001
Type of delivery	0.002 (0.001)	0.000–0.005	.042	0.002	0.002 (0.001)	0.000–0.004	.021	0.002
Hyperactivity								
Direct effects of								
Full breastfeeding	−0.001 (0.000)	−0.002 to −0.001	<.001	−0.044	−0.002 (0.000)	−0.002 to −0.001	<.001	−0.043
Partner in residence	−0.183 (0.102)	−0.382 to 0.016	.071	−0.028	−0.369 (0.118)	−0.601 to −0.137	.002	−0.050
Maternal age	−0.193 (0.028)	−0.248 to −0.138	<.001	−0.089	−0.186 (0.033)	−0.251 to −0.121	<.001	−0.077
Maternal education	−0.336 (0.049)	−0.432 to −0.239	<.001	−0.085	−0.311 (0.057)	−0.423 to −0.199	<.001	−0.070
Social class	0.041 (0.017)	0.008–0.073	.015	0.040	0.026 (0.019)	−0.012 to 0.064	.179	0.023
Medical card status	−0.062 (0.034)	−0.129 to 0.005	.069	−0.025	−0.096 (0.040)	−0.174 to −0.018	.016	−0.035
Maternal working status	0.022 (0.062)	−0.100 to 0.143	.728	0.004	0.079 (0.073)	−0.065 to 0.222	.283	0.014
Maternal ethnicity	0.100 (0.020)	0.060–0.140	<.001	0.056	0.018 (0.023)	−0.028 to 0.063	.445	0.009
Maternal depression	0.395 (0.127)	0.146–0.645	.002	0.037	0.470 (0.148)	0.179–0.760	.002	0.040
Smoking during pregnancy	0.131 (0.051)	0.030–0.231	.011	0.029	0.214 (0.060)	0.096–0.331	<.001	0.042
Sibling status	−0.224 (0.053)	−0.327 to −0.121	<.001	−0.051	−0.282 (0.060)	−0.400 to −0.165	<.001	−0.058
Visit to the NICU	0.110 (0.078)	−0.043 to 0.262	.158	0.016	0.187 (0.083)	0.024–0.349	.024	0.024
Birth weight	−0.166 (0.163)	−0.485 to 0.153	.308	−0.011	−0.431 (0.203)	−0.828 to −0.033	.034	−0.025
Child sex	−0.460 (0.044)	−0.547 to −0.373	<.001	−0.107	−0.677 (0.052)	−0.778 to −0.576	<.001	−0.141
Type of delivery	−0.006 (0.015)	−0.037 to 0.024	.675	−0.005	−0.006 (0.018)	−0.041 to 0.029	.734	−0.004
Indirect effects via breastfeeding								
Partner in residence	−0.009 (0.004)	−0.016 to −0.002	.014	−0.001	−0.010 (0.004)	−0.018 to −0.002	.015	−0.001
Maternal age	−0.009 (0.002)	−0.014 to −0.005	<.001	−0.004	−0.010 (0.003)	−0.016 to −0.005	<.001	−0.004
Maternal education	−0.030 (0.007)	−0.044 to −0.015	<.001	−0.007	−0.033 (0.008)	−0.049 to −0.016	<.001	−0.007
Social class	0.002 (0.001)	0.000–0.003	.010	0.002	0.002 (0.001)	0.000–0.003	.011	0.002
Medical card status	0.000 (0.001)	−0.002 to 0.003	.798	0.000	0.000 (0.001)	−0.002 to 0.003	.798	0.000
Maternal working status	0.007 (0.003)	0.001 to 0.013	.019	0.001	0.008 (0.003)	0.001–0.014	.021	0.001
Maternal ethnicity	−0.016 (0.004)	−0.024 to −0.008	<.001	−0.009	−0.018 (0.004)	−0.026 to −0.009	<.001	−0.009
Maternal depression	0.005 (0.004)	−0.003 to 0.013	.187	0.000	0.006 (0.004)	−0.003 to 0.014	.194	0.000
Smoking during pregnancy	0.012 (0.003)	0.005–0.019	<.001	0.003	0.013 (0.004)	0.006–0.021	.001	0.003
Sibling status	0.009 (0.003)	0.003–0.014	.003	0.002	0.010 (0.003)	0.003–0.016	.003	0.002
Visit to the NICU	0.003 (0.003)	−0.002 to 0.009	.268	0.000	0.004 (0.003)	−0.003 to 0.010	.265	0.000
Birth weight	−0.018 (0.007)	−0.032 to −0.004	.012	−0.001	−0.02 (0.008)	−0.036 to −0.004	.013	−0.001
Child sex	−0.007 (0.002)	−0.012 to −0.002	.004	−0.002	−0.008 (0.003)	−0.013 to −0.002	.005	−0.002
Type of delivery	0.005 (0.001)	0.003–0.008	<.001	0.004	0.006 (0.002)	0.003–0.009	<.001	0.004
Total difficulties								
Direct effects of								
Full breastfeeding	−0.002 (0.001)	−0.004 to −0.001	.001	−0.033	−0.003 (0.001)	−0.005 to −0.001	<.001	−0.039
Partner in residence	−0.422 (0.221)	−0.854 to 0.011	.056	−0.030	−0.890 (0.250)	−1.379 to −0.400	<.001	−0.061
Maternal age	−0.459 (0.059)	−0.576 to −0.343	<.001	−0.100	−0.351 (0.065)	−0.479 to −0.223	<.001	−0.074
Maternal education	−0.688 (0.103)	−0.890 to −0.486	<.001	−0.082	−0.623 (0.114)	−0.845 to −0.400	<.001	−0.071
Social class	0.085 (0.037)	0.013–0.158	.021	0.040	0.058 (0.041)	−0.023 to 0.139	.163	0.026

TABLE 9 Continued

	Age 3				Age 5			
	B (SE)	95% CI	P	β	B (SE)	95% CI	P	β
Medical card status	−0.246 (0.073)	−0.390 to −0.103	.001	−0.04	−0.305 (0.081)	−0.464 to −0.145	<.001	−0.056
Maternal working status	0.101 (0.132)	−0.158 to 0.360	.446	0.00	0.134 (0.147)	−0.154 to 0.423	.360	0.012
Maternal ethnicity	0.244 (0.045)	0.157–0.332	<.001	0.06	0.083 (0.049)	−0.012 to 0.178	.088	0.021
Maternal depression	1.525 (0.270)	0.995–2.055	<.001	0.06	1.851 (0.311)	1.242–2.459	<.001	0.079
Smoking during pregnancy	0.477 (0.109)	0.263–0.691	<.001	0.04	0.466 (0.118)	0.235–0.697	<.001	0.046
Sibling status	−0.436 (0.111)	−0.653 to −0.219	<.001	−0.04	−0.614 (0.116)	−0.843 to −0.386	<.001	−0.064
Visit to the NICU	0.252 (0.156)	−0.054–0.559	.106	0.01	0.316 (0.162)	−0.002 to 0.633	.052	0.021
Birth weight	−0.417 (0.320)	−1.045 to 0.211	.193	−0.01	−0.727 (0.413)	−1.536 to 0.082	.078	−0.022
Child sex	−0.766 (0.093)	−0.948 to −0.583	<.001	−0.08	−0.913 (0.101)	−1.111 to −0.714	<.001	−0.097
Type of delivery	−0.027 (0.033)	−0.091 to 0.037	.402	−0.00	−0.032 (0.035)	−0.101 to 0.037	.367	−0.010
Indirect effects of breastfeeding								
Partner in residence	−0.015 (0.007)	−0.028 to −0.002	.027	−0.00	−0.018 (0.008)	−0.033 to −0.003	.018	−0.001
Maternal age	−0.015 (0.005)	−0.025 to −0.005	.002	−0.00	−0.019 (0.005)	−0.029 to −0.008	.001	−0.004
Maternal education	−0.048 (0.015)	−0.078 to −0.018	.002	−0.00	−0.059 (0.017)	−0.091 to −0.027	<.001	−0.007
Social class	0.003 (0.001)	0.000–0.005	.021	0.00	0.004 (0.001)	0.001–0.006	.015	0.002
Medical card status	0.001 (0.002)	−0.003 to 0.005	.798	0.00	0.001 (0.003)	−0.004 to 0.006	.798	0.000
Maternal working status	0.011 (0.005)	0.001 to 0.021	.033	0.001	0.014 (0.006)	0.002 to 0.026	.025	0.001
Maternal ethnicity	−0.026 (0.008)	−0.042 to −0.010	.001	−0.007	−0.032 (0.009)	−0.049 to −0.014	<.001	−0.008
Maternal depression	0.008 (0.007)	−0.004 to 0.021	.202	0.000	0.010 (0.008)	−0.005 to 0.026	.198	0.000
Smoking during pregnancy	0.019 (0.007)	0.006–0.033	.004	0.002	0.024 (0.008)	0.009–0.039	.002	0.002
Sibling status	0.014 (0.005)	0.003–0.025	.010	0.002	0.017 (0.006)	0.005–0.030	.005	0.002
Visit to the NICU	0.005 (0.005)	−0.004 to 0.014	.280	0.000	0.006 (0.006)	−0.005 to 0.018	.268	0.000
Birth weight	−0.029 (0.013)	−0.055 to −0.004	.024	−0.001	−0.036 (0.015)	−0.066 to −0.006	.018	−0.001
Child sex	−0.011 (0.004)	−0.020 to −0.002	.013	−0.001	−0.014 (0.005)	−0.024 to −0.004	.008	−0.001
Type of delivery	0.009 (0.003)	0.003–0.014	.002	0.003	0.011 (0.003)	0.005–0.017	.001	0.003

Modeling breastfeeding and child outcomes by using a SEM approach, which does not attempt to identify causality, revealed differing patterns of associations whereby linear dose-response associations were statistically significant for cognitive outcomes at age 3 and 5 years (for both partial and full breastfeeding), conduct problems at 3 (full breastfeeding) and 5 years (both partial and full breastfeeding), hyperactivity at 3 and 5 years (full breastfeeding), and total difficulties at 3 and 5 years (full breastfeeding). Data for partial breastfeeding models available on request.

AAP News

Study: Breastfeeding for at Least 2 Months Decreases Risk of SIDS

Melissa Jenco, News Content Editor

Breastfeeding for at least two months could cut the risk of sudden infant death syndrome (SIDS) nearly in half, according to a new study.

"Even if mothers are unable to exclusively breastfeed, they can feel reassured that any breastfeeding provides protection against SIDS to their infants," authors wrote in the study "Duration of Breastfeeding and Risk of SIDS: An Individual Participant Data (IPD) Meta-analysis" (Thompson JMD, et al. *Pediatrics*. Oct. 30, 2017, https://doi.org/10.1542/peds.2017-1324).

AAP policies note that breastfeeding has been linked to lower rates of SIDS. The Academy recommends exclusive breastfeeding for six months and continuation until the child is at least 1 year.

Rachel Y. Moon, M.D., FAAP, lead author of the AAP SIDS policy, was among the researchers involved in this new study that set out to look at how long a mother needs to breastfeed to protect her baby and the impact of breastfeeding exclusively. The team looked at eight studies from around the world involving 2,267 SIDS cases and 6,837 control infants.

Univariate analysis found breastfeeding had a protective effect against SIDS even for small amounts of time, but the multivariable analysis showed the effect began at two months and increased over time. Adjusted odds ratios were 0.91 for those breastfed less than two months, 0.6 for those breastfed two to four months, 0.4 for four to six months and 0.36 for over six months.

"It is thus important that public health messages about SIDS risk reduction emphasize that breastfeeding, if it is to be protective, must continue for at least 2 months," authors wrote.

Breastfeeding exclusively did not provide more protection than partial breastfeeding, despite the team's previous research to the contrary.

Authors said it was unclear why breastfeeding protected infants from SIDS but discussed several possibilities, including better arousal from sleep in breastfed babies. Breast milk also boosts infants' immune systems and supports their brain development.

Data from 2007 showed roughly 89% of infants in the European Union, 85% in New Zealand, 77% in the United Kingdom, 75% in the U.S. and 42% in Ireland had ever been breastfed. The World Health Organization has set a target of half of infants being exclusively breastfed for at least six months by 2025.

"Further increases in breastfeeding rates will result in lower infant mortality as a whole," authors wrote, "and decreases in SIDS rates, specifically."

Duration of Breastfeeding and Risk of SIDS: An Individual Participant Data Meta-analysis

John M.D. Thompson, PhD,[a] Kawai Tanabe, MPH,[b] Rachel Y. Moon, MD,[c] Edwin A. Mitchell, FRSNZ, FRACP, FRCPCH, DSc (Med),[a] Cliona McGarvey, PhD,[d] David Tappin, MBBS, MD, MSc,[e] Peter S. Blair, PhD,[f] Fern R. Hauck, MD, MS[b]

abstract

CONTEXT: Sudden infant death syndrome (SIDS) is a leading cause of postneonatal infant mortality. Our previous meta-analyses showed that any breastfeeding is protective against SIDS with exclusive breastfeeding conferring a stronger effect. The duration of breastfeeding required to confer a protective effect is unknown.

OBJECTIVE: To assess the associations between breastfeeding duration and SIDS.

DATA SOURCES: Individual-level data from 8 case-control studies.

STUDY SELECTION: Case-control SIDS studies with breastfeeding data.

DATA EXTRACTION: Breastfeeding variables, demographic factors, and other potential confounders were identified. Individual study and pooled analyses were performed.

RESULTS: A total of 2267 SIDS cases and 6837 control infants were included. In multivariable pooled analysis, breastfeeding for <2 months was not protective (adjusted odds ratio [aOR]: 0.91, 95% confidence interval [CI]: 0.68–1.22). Any breastfeeding ≥2 months was protective, with greater protection seen with increased duration (2–4 months: aOR: 0.60, 95% CI: 0.44–0.82; 4–6 months: aOR: 0.40, 95% CI: 0.26–0.63; and >6 months: aOR: 0.36, 95% CI: 0.22–0.61). Although exclusive breastfeeding for <2 months was not protective (aOR: 0.82, 95% CI: 0.59–1.14), longer periods were protective (2–4 months: aOR: 0.61, 95% CI: 0.42–0.87; 4–6 months: aOR: 0.46, 95% CI: 0.29–0.74).

LIMITATIONS: The variables collected in each study varied slightly, limiting our ability to include all studies in the analysis and control for all confounders.

CONCLUSIONS: Breastfeeding duration of at least 2 months was associated with half the risk of SIDS. Breastfeeding does not need to be exclusive to confer this protection.

[a]Department of Paediatrics: Child and Youth Health and Obstetrics and Gynaecology, University of Auckland, Auckland, New Zealand; Departments of [b]Family Medicine and [c]Pediatrics, University of Virginia, Charlottesville, Virginia; [d]National Paediatric Mortality Register, Temple Street Children's University Hospital, Dublin, Ireland; [e]Department of Child Health, School of Medicine, University of Glasgow, Glasgow, United Kingdom; and [f]School of Social and Community Medicine, University of Bristol, Bristol, United Kingdom

Dr Thompson conceptualized and designed the study, conducted the analyses, and drafted the initial manuscript; Ms Tanabe and Drs Moon and Hauck conceptualized and designed the study, participated in the interpretation of the data, and critically reviewed and revised the manuscript; Drs Mitchell, McGarvey, Tappin, and Blair provided data for the study and reviewed and revised the manuscript; and all authors approved the final manuscript as submitted.

DOI: https://doi.org/10.1542/peds.2017-1324

Accepted for publication Aug 7, 2017

Address correspondence to John M.D. Thompson, PhD, Department of Paediatrics: Child and Youth Health, University of Auckland, Private Bag 92019, Auckland 1142, New Zealand. E-mail: j.thompson@auckland.ac.nz

To cite: Thompson J.M.D., Tanabe K, Moon RY, et al. Duration of Breastfeeding and Risk of SIDS: An Individual Participant Data Meta-analysis. *Pediatrics.* 2017;140(5):e20171324

REVIEW ARTICLE

Breastfeeding has been shown in several studies to be associated with a decreased risk of sudden infant death syndrome (SIDS).[1–3] In a previous meta-analysis, we have shown that breastfeeding is protective against SIDS (adjusted odds ratio [aOR]: 0.55, 95% confidence interval [CI]: 0.44–0.69 for any breastfeeding) and that this protective effect is stronger with exclusive breastfeeding (odds ratio [OR]: 0.27, 95% CI: 0.24–0.31).[3]

However, it has been difficult to determine what duration of breastfeeding is required to confer a protective effect against SIDS. This may partly be because the incidence of breastfeeding across countries and different cultures varies and because the authors of different studies investigating the association with SIDS use different definitions for any breastfeeding, exclusive breastfeeding, and the duration of either practice. Meta-analyses of breastfeeding duration at the study level are difficult to undertake, and, so far, the effect size and the duration of breastfeeding required to confer this protective effect have not been quantified.

We therefore aimed to use individual-level data from international studies and, with cooperation of the individual authors, to assess the associations between duration of any breastfeeding versus exclusive breastfeeding and SIDS.

METHODS

We used the same review protocol as that in our previously reported meta-analysis.[3] We searched the Ovid Medline database (January 1966 through December 2009) to collect data on breastfeeding and its association with SIDS. The search strategy included published articles limited to humans with the medical subject headings terms "sudden infant death" and "breast feeding" and with the key words "sudden infant death syndrome," "SIDS," "cot death," and "breastfeeding." Of the 18 studies included in the meta-analysis, individual level data were provided from 8 large case-control studies of SIDS deaths, which comprise all of the published case-control studies with individual-level data about breastfeeding status. In all studies, there were strict definitions and protocols for determining SIDS cases. The cause of death had to be ascertained by local medical examiners or pediatric or forensic pathologists. No studies without individual-level data were included. All data were obtained via direct contact with the original investigators for each case-control study. Data were checked by the original investigators for completeness and consistency before being released for this analysis. The studies included are detailed below.

The New Zealand Cot Death Study

The New Zealand Cot Death Study (NZCDS) was a national case-control study of all SIDS deaths that took place from November 1987 through October 1990. The authors of the study successfully recruited and obtained data from 393 case patients and 1592 controls, who were randomly selected from all birth cohorts, but with an age distribution to match the age of patients from cases from 1979 to 1984.[4] Data were obtained by an interviewer-administered questionnaire and from hospital obstetric records, which included data about the type of feeding at the time of hospital discharge. Parents were asked whether the infant received any breast milk at any stage of life, in the first 4 weeks, and in the last 2 days. In addition, parents of infants who received any breast milk were asked at what stage breastfeeding stopped (age in weeks). Coding was available for never started and still breastfeeding.

The Chicago Infant Mortality Study

The authors of the Chicago Infant Mortality Study (CIMS) studied all SIDS deaths in Chicago, Illinois, between November 1993 and April 1996, and they included 260 case patients and 260 controls, who were matched by maternal ethnicity, age at death, and birth weight.[5] Data on breastfeeding were collected by a standardized interviewer-administered questionnaire. Parents were asked if the child had ever been breastfed, if the child was still being breastfed, and how old the child was when breastfeeding stopped. In addition, data on other methods of feeding and when they were started were collected so that duration of exclusive breastfeeding could be calculated.

The German SIDS Study

The German SIDS Study (GeSID) was conducted in 11 of 18 states in the former Federal Republic of Germany between November 1998 and October 2001. The study included 333 SIDS case patients and 998 controls, who were matched by geographic region, age, sex, and reference sleep (ie, time of sleep was matched to the time of death for the respective case).[6] Data on breastfeeding were collected by a standardized, interviewer-administered questionnaire. Questions were asked about breastfeeding at 2 weeks of age and at each month of age through 12 months (when applicable) and about whether this breastfeeding was exclusive.

The Scottish Cot Death Trust Study

The Scottish Cot Death Trust study took place between January 1996 and May 2000. Data were collected on 131 SIDS case patients and 278 control infants, who were matched by age, season, and obstetric unit.[7] Data on breastfeeding were collected by a standardized, interviewer-administered questionnaire.

Questions were asked about which types of feeding the infant had and, if not breastfed currently, whether they had ever breastfed and when they stopped.

European Concerted Action on SIDS

The European Concerted Action on SIDS (ECAS) comprised case-control studies in 20 regions in Europe between September 1992 and April 1996.[8] Data for the current analyses were restricted to those centers for which we had not obtained data from elsewhere (Sweden, Norway, Denmark, Netherlands, Austria, Hungary, Ukraine, Spain, Italy, Russia, Slovenia, France, Belgium, Poland, and the United Kingdom [Cambridge]). Data were collected for 382 SIDS case patients and 1159 controls. Data on breastfeeding exclusivity and duration were collected by interviewer-administered questionnaires. Questions were asked about how the infant was being fed at the time of death or interview.

Irish Study of Infant Death

The Irish study was part of an ongoing case-control study of infant death in the Republic of Ireland that began collecting data in 1994 and continued until 2010.[9,10] Controls were matched by date of birth and geographical location. The data included in this analysis comprise 363 case patients and 1163 controls for the period from 1994 to 2003. Data on breastfeeding exclusivity and duration were collected during standardized home interviews.

Confidential Inquiry Into Stillbirth and Deaths in Infancy

The Confidential Inquiry Into Stillbirth and Deaths in Infancy (CESDI) included 5 regions of England between 1993 and 1996.[11] Data were collected for 325 SIDS case patients and 1300 controls, who were matched by age and health visitor. Data were collected for

duration of breastfeeding; however, no information on the duration of exclusive breastfeeding was collected.

South-West England Infant Sleep Study

The South-West England Infant Sleep Study (SWISS) included 2 regions in the South-West of England between 2003 and 2006.[12] Data were collected for 80 SIDS case patients and 87 controls. Data were collected for the duration of breastfeeding; however, no information on the duration of exclusive breastfeeding was collected.

Definitions of Breastfeeding Variables

Duration of any breastfeeding was defined as the length of time that the infant received any human milk, through breastfeeding or expressed breast milk, either exclusively or in combination with other foods (including infant formula). We defined the duration of any breastfeeding as a continuous variable; we created a categorical variable for the duration of any breastfeeding (0–2, 2–4, 4–6, and >6 months).

Duration of exclusive breastfeeding was defined as the length of time that the infant received only human milk, either through breastfeeding or expressed breast milk.[13] We defined the duration of exclusive breastfeeding as a continuous variable; we created a categorical variable for the duration of exclusive breastfeeding (0–2, 2–4, and >4 months). A variable for >6 months was not created because of the small numbers in this group in most of the studies.

Statistical Analysis

Analysis was performed for each study individually, and then data were combined for a pooled analysis. A pooled univariable analysis, using all 8 studies, was conducted,

controlling for study. A multivariable model was then fitted by using 3 of the studies (the NZCDS, CIMS, and GeSID) for which all 19 potential confounders were available (model 1). These confounders had initially been assessed as being available and consistent across these 3 studies at the inception of each study and have been identified as risk or protective factors for SIDS: sleep position at last sleep (supine, side, prone), maternal smoking during pregnancy (yes/no), bed-sharing in the last sleep (infant sleeping with another person on the same surface) (yes/no), room-sharing in the last sleep (infant sleeping in the same room as an adult caregiver but on a separate surface) (yes/no), use of a dummy or pacifier in the last sleep (yes/no), maternal age, prenatal care received (yes/no), marital status (married/not married), parity (primiparous/multiparous), maternal education (university graduate or not), socioeconomic status (SES) (low, middle, high), infant age (<13, 13–19, 20–26, and >26 weeks), infant sex, admission to a special care infant unit (yes/no), season at death, birth weight (<2500 g, 2500–2999 g, 3000–3499 g, and ≥3500 g), gestational age at birth (28–33, 34–37, and 38+ weeks), multiple pregnancy (yes/no), and cesarean delivery (yes/no). Additional models were then fitted to include the other 5 studies, at the expense of reducing the number of confounders but increasing the sample size. These sequential models did not include the following confounders: cesarean delivery (the CESDI and SWISS included in model, model 2), SES and season (the Irish and ECAS studies included, model 3), and, finally, antenatal care and maternal education level (the Scottish study included, model 4).

All analyses were conducted in SAS version 9.4 (SAS Institute, Cary, NC). ORs were estimated by using the proc logistic procedure,

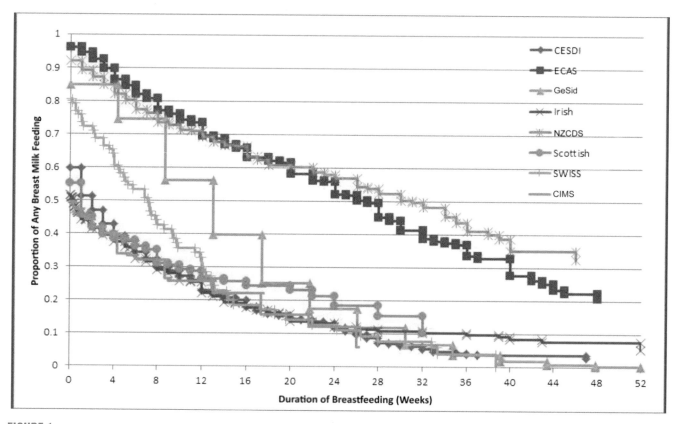

FIGURE 1
Kaplan-Meier survival curves for the proportion of controls still breastfeeding, stratified by study.

with a strata statement for study in pooled analyses. Survival curves were produced for duration of any breastfeeding for control groups by using proc lifetest, with data censored if breastfeeding was still taking place. Statistical significance was defined at the 5% level.

This study was approved by the institutional review board at the University of Virginia. In addition, the individual studies were approved by the institutional ethical review boards and/or ethics committees according to the laws and standards of each country.

RESULTS

There are 8 SIDS case-control studies with individual-level data; all were included (see Supplemental Fig 2 flow diagram). A total of 2267 SIDS case patients and 6837 control infants were included in this analysis.

There was great variability in the rates of any breastfeeding and exclusive breastfeeding in the studies (log rank: 1659.6, $P < .0001$). This is illustrated in Fig 1, which shows survival curves for any breastfeeding for controls from each of the studies. Breastfeeding rates were highest in New Zealand and lowest in the United States, with the European countries having intermediate rates. At 6 months, the rate of any breastfeeding ranged from over 50% in the NZCDS and ECAS to <10% in several of the studies.

Any Breastfeeding

The univariable effects of any breastfeeding stratified by study and the pooled analyses are shown in Table 1. The analysis categorizing duration of any breastfeeding showed that those who breastfed for <2 months incurred a protective effect (OR: 0.61, 95% CI: 0.54–0.69)

and that those breastfeeding for 2 to 4 months had a greater protective effect (OR: 0.26, 95% CI: 0.22–0.30). Breastfeeding duration beyond 4 months provided further small increases in protection (4–6 months: OR: 0.18, 95% CI: 0.14–0.23; 6+ months: OR: 0.13, 95% CI: 0.10–0.18). The multivariable pooled analysis for the 3 studies with all 19 confounders controlled for found ongoing protective effects of any breastfeeding beyond 2 months (2–4 months: aOR: 0.60, 95% CI: 0.44–0.82; 4–6 months: aOR: 0.40, 95% CI: 0.26–0.63; and 6+ months: aOR: 0.36, 95% CI: 0.22–0.61) (Table 2). However, breastfeeding for 0 to 2 months did not have a statistically significant protective effect (aOR: 0.91, 95% CI: 0.68–1.21). The removal of cesarean delivery from the model had little effect on the ORs; however, the removal of SES and season in model 3 saw the protective effects of any breastfeeding become

TABLE 1 Stratified and Pooled Univariable ORs (95% CIs) of SIDS for Duration of Any and Exclusive Breastfeeding

	NZCDS	GeSID	CIMS	Scottish	ECAS	CESDI	SWISS	Irish	Pooled
Any breastfeeding, mo									
Never	1.00	1.00	1.00	1.00	1.00	1.00	1.00	1.00	1.00
>0–2	0.79 (0.55–1.13)	0.70 (0.48–1.02)	0.43 (0.28–0.65)	0.65 (0.41–1.05)	0.56 (0.36–0.88)	0.61 (0.46–0.81)	0.79 (0.37–1.67)	0.68 (0.51–0.92)	0.61 (0.54–0.69)
>2–4	0.49 (0.33–0.71)	0.18 (0.13–0.25)	0.07 (0.03–0.21)	0.16 (0.06–0.47)	0.21 (0.13–0.33)	0.42 (0.28–0.64)	0.42 (0.16–1.12)	0.16 (0.09–0.29)	0.26 (0.22–0.30)
>4–6	0.32 (0.19–0.53)	0.10 (0.06–0.16)	0.06 (0.01–0.51)	0.20 (0.04–0.90)	0.20 (0.12–0.33)	0.39 (0.20–0.78)	0.15 (0.02–1.40)	0.04 (0.01–0.26)	0.18 (0.14–0.23)
>6	0.19 (0.09–0.37)	0.15 (0.10–0.25)	Undefined	Undefined	0.07 (0.03–0.14)	0.25 (0.09–0.70)	0.11 (0.01–0.95)	0.22 (0.07–0.72)	0.13 (0.10–0.18)
Exclusive breastfeeding, mo									
Never	1.00	1.00	1.00	1.00	1.00	Not available	Not available	1.00	1.00
>0–2	0.88 (0.58–1.34)	0.40 (0.28–0.56)	0.46 (0.28–0.76)	0.63 (0.39–1.03)	0.98 (0.73–1.32)			0.40 (0.28–0.58)	0.61 (0.53–0.71)
>2–4	0.41 (0.27–0.64)	0.22 (0.15–0.33)	0.18 (0.02–1.51)	0.21 (0.06–0.73)	0.29 (0.21–0.41)			0.12 (0.05–0.30)	0.25 (0.20–0.30)
4–6	0.32 (0.10–1.03)	0.13 (0.09–0.20)	Undefined	Undefined	0.19 (0.12–0.31)			0.48 (0.16–1.41)	0.16 (0.12–0.21)

stronger. The further removal of maternal education and antenatal care in model 4 had little additional influence on the aOR, but this result reached statistical significance (aOR: 0.83, 95% CI: 0.70–0.99).

Exclusive Breastfeeding

The stratified and pooled analysis for the univariable effects of exclusive breastfeeding is shown in Table 1. The analysis categorizing the duration of exclusive breastfeeding showed that those who exclusively breastfed for <2 months incurred a protective effect (OR: 0.61 95% CI: 0.53–0.71) and that those breastfeeding 2 to 4 months had a greater protective effect (OR: 0.25, 95% CI: 0.20–0.30). Exclusive breastfeeding for >4 months provided a further increase in protection (OR: 0.16, 95% CI: 0.12–0.21). As in the multivariable analysis for any breastfeeding, which controlled for all potential confounders, those who breastfed exclusively for <2 months did not see any statistically significant protective effect (aOR: 0.82, 95% CI: 0.59–1.14), but those who breastfed for longer than 2 months incurred a protective effect (aOR: 0.61, 95% CI: 0.42–0.97) for 2 to 4 months, with increasing protection with longer duration (aOR: 0.46, 95% CI: 0.29–0.74) for those exclusively breastfeeding >4 months. Similarly, the removal of SES and season from the model made the effect sizes slightly stronger (Table 3).

DISCUSSION

We conducted a pooled analysis of individual-level data from 8 major international case-control studies with 2259 case patients and 6894 controls to assess the association between duration of any breastfeeding versus exclusive breastfeeding and SIDS. Although there was some protection seen with breastfeeding for <2 months in univariable analysis, after controlling for potential confounders, we found no statistically significant protection against SIDS until infants had breastfed for at least 2 months. After 2 months, the aOR for any breastfeeding was 0.60 (95% CI: 0.44–0.82), whereas the aOR for exclusive breastfeeding was 0.61 (95% CI: 0.42–0.87). It is thus important that public health messages about SIDS risk reduction emphasize that breastfeeding, if it is to be protective, must continue for at least 2 months. This analysis does not reveal any advantage to exclusive breastfeeding over partial breastfeeding, which may be reassuring to some parents who cannot or do not wish to exclusively breastfeed their infant.

It is yet unclear why breastfeeding offers protective effects against SIDS. The authors of physiologic, neuropathologic, and genetic studies point to dysfunctional arousal responses as a mechanism that creates an intrinsic vulnerability in the infant, which predisposes the infant to SIDS,[14] and breastfed infants are more easily aroused from sleep than are formula-fed infants.[15,16] There are also differences in maternal responses to an infant's behavioral cues, depending on feeding mode, which may impact infant sleep and arousal patterns.[17,18] Additionally, breastfeeding provides immune benefits and is associated with a lower incidence of viral infections, which are associated with an increased risk of SIDS.[19–21] Breast milk contains substances that may contribute to myelin development; Kinney and co-authors found that infants who died of SIDS had delayed myelination of the brain compared with control infants.[22] Breast milk also contains higher levels than formula of docosahexaenoic acid, which is an important structural and functional component of the developing infant brain. One study of autopsied brains of SIDS infants

TABLE 2 Stratified and Pooled Multivariable ORs (95% CIs) of SIDS for Duration of Any Breastfeeding

Duration, mo	NZCDS	GeSID	CIMS	Scottish	ECAS	CESDI	SWISS	Irish	Pooled Model 1a (n = 3386)	Pooled Model 2b (n = 5008)	Pooled Model 3c (n = 6121)	Pooled Model 4d (n = 7842)
Never	1.00	1.00	1.00	1.00	1.00	1.00	1.00	1.00	1.00	1.00	1.00	1.00
>0–2	0.86 (0.53–1.40)	0.89 (0.49–1.63)	0.69 (0.36–1.31)	0.69 (0.31–1.52)	0.79 (0.25–2.51)	0.96 (0.65–1.40)	0.12 (0.01–2.18)	1.13 (0.59–2.17)	0.91 (0.68–1.21)	0.90 (0.72–1.12)	0.83 (0.69–1.01)	0.83 (0.70–0.99)
>2–4	0.67 (0.40–1.11)	0.51 (0.29–0.88)	0.16 (0.04–0.71)	0.38 (0.09–1.54)	0.82 (0.25–2.73)	0.78 (0.45–1.34)	0.02 (<0.001–0.93)	0.19 (0.07–0.51)	0.60 (0.44–0.82)	0.62 (0.48–0.80)	0.52 (0.41–0.65)	0.46 (0.37–0.56)
>4–6	0.39 (0.19–0.80)	0.37 (0.18–0.74)	0.16 (0.01–1.72)	0.20 (0.03–1.57)	0.94 (0.23–3.94)	0.64 (0.24–1.75)	<0.001 (<0.001–3.50)	0.08 (0.01–0.86)	0.40 (0.26–0.63)	0.42 (0.29–0.61)	0.38 (0.27–0.54)	0.40 (0.30–0.53)
>6	0.44 (0.17–1.13)	0.30 (0.15–0.63)	Undefined	Undefined	0.06 (0.00–0.94)	0.26 (0.05–1.25)	0.001 (<0.001–1.71)	0.45 (0.06–3.09)	0.36 (0.22–0.61)	0.34 (0.22–0.54)	0.33 (0.21–0.50)	0.25 (0.17–0.37)

a Model 1 controlled for sleep position at last sleep, maternal smoking during pregnancy, bed-sharing in the last sleep (infant sleeping with another person on the same surface), room-sharing in the last sleep (infant sleeping in the same room as an adult caregiver but on a separate surface), dummy or pacifier in the last sleep, maternal age, prenatal care, marital status, parity, maternal education, SES, infant age, infant sex, admission to a special care infant unit, season at death, birth weight, gestational age, multiple pregnancy, and cesarean delivery.

b Model 2 controlled for variables in model 1, except for cesarean delivery, to include the CESDI and SWISS studies.

c Model 3 controlled for variables in model 2, except season and SES, to include the ECAS and Irish studies.

d Model 4 controlled for variables in model 3, except for antenatal care and maternal education, to include the Scottish study.

TABLE 3 Stratified and Pooled Multivariable ORs (95% CIs) of SIDS for Duration of Exclusive Breastfeeding

Duration mo	NZCDS	GeSID	SIMS	Scottish	ECAS	CESDI	SWISS	Irish	Pooled Model 1a (n = 3397)	Pooled Model 2b	Pooled Model 3c (n = 4319)	Pooled Model 4d (n = 6006)
Never	1.00	1.00	1.00	1.00	1.00	Not available	Not available	1.00	1.00	—	1.00	1.00
>0–2	1.02 (0.56–1.84)	0.70 (0.41–1.19)	0.81 (0.39–1.69)	0.61 (0.26–1.44)	1.27 (0.46–3.48)	Not available	Not available	0.68 (0.33–1.42)	0.82 (0.59–1.14)	—	0.75 (0.58–0.98)	0.82 (0.67–1.01)
>2–4	0.47 (0.27–0.83)	0.51 (0.29–0.90)	0.61 (0.04–8.83)	0.63 (0.12–3.23)	0.48 (0.15–1.53)			0.09 (0.02–0.53)	0.61 (0.42–0.87)	—	0.44 (0.32–0.60)	0.40 (0.31–0.51)
4–6	0.56 (0.15–2.07)	0.31 (0.17–0.58)	Undefined	Undefined	0.60 (0.14–2.54)			3.14 (0.56–17.55)	0.46 (0.29–0.74)	—	0.47 (0.31–0.71)	0.37 (0.26–0.52)

—, Data were not available because these 2 studies had no data on exclusive breastfeeding.

a Model 1 controlled for sleep position at last sleep, maternal smoking during pregnancy, bed-sharing in the last sleep (infant sleeping with another person on the same surface), room-sharing in the last sleep (infant sleeping in the same room as an adult caregiver but on a separate surface), dummy or pacifier in the last sleep, maternal age, prenatal care, marital status, parity, maternal education, SES, infant age, infant sex, admission to a special care infant unit, season at death, birth weight, gestational age, multiple pregnancy, and cesarean delivery.

b Model 2 could not be run because the CESDI and SWISS studies had no data on exclusive breastfeeding.

c Model 3 controlled for variables in model 2, except season and SES, to include the ECAS and Irish studies.

d Model 4 controlled for variables in model 3, except for antenatal care and maternal education, to include the Scottish study.

found that the frontal lobes of the breastfed infants had higher levels of docosahexaenoic acid than those of formula-fed infants; it is unknown if this difference exists in non-SIDS infants.[23] Finally, it is possible that breastfeeding is a distal marker of or proxy for complex protective infant care practices that have not yet been measured, although we would expect that such a marker would be related to sociodemographic variables that have been controlled for in these analyses.

It is unclear why exclusive breastfeeding did not offer any additional protection against SIDS than any, that is, partial, breastfeeding. This is a common challenge in studies in which the differential effects of exclusive and partial breastfeeding have been examined, because of the differing definitions of breastfeeding and confounding factors.[1,24] The analysis accounted for as many demographic and risk factor variables as were possible, but we acknowledge that the effects reported could be caused by residual confounding, although this would be unlikely. It was notable that the inclusion of studies that did not have data on SES increased the protective effect further from the null, thus seemingly showing the importance of SES as a confounder in relation to breastfeeding. Given that lower SES is a risk factor for SIDS, it is possible that the protective effect of SES may in part be explained by increased breastfeeding rates. However, model 3, which did not have data on SES, also did not have data on season. Although SES is associated with breastfeeding, it is unlikely that there is a relationship between season and breastfeeding; thus, we believe that these changes in estimates are likely to be associated with SES.

Other limitations of this study are related to issues with combining data in the individual case-control studies. These case-control studies were all conducted in a rigorous manner and are the basis for most of the current infant safe sleep guidelines in developed countries.[25–27] However, as noted above, the variables collected in the course of each study varied slightly, limiting our ability to include all studies in the analysis and control for all confounders. However, the results of the univariable analysis using only the 3 countries included in the completely controlled multivariable model (model 1) did not differ greatly from the univariable analysis with all 8 studies, so it is unlikely that including the additional studies would have changed the results of the analysis in any meaningful way.

Given these findings, there should be ongoing concerted efforts to increase the rates of breastfeeding initiation and maintenance. Among the control infants in 5 of the 8 countries in this analysis, the proportion of infants who were breastfeeding was <50% at 2 months of age and <30% at 4 months of age. In more recent years, national breastfeeding rates have increased; 2007 Organisation for Economic Co-operation and Development data show that the proportions of infants who were ever breastfed in the countries included in our study were 42% in Ireland, 75% in the United States, 77% in the United Kingdom, 85% in New Zealand, and 89% in the European Union.[28] The World Health Organization's 2025 targets for breastfeeding are to have >50% of infants exclusively breastfeeding for at least 6 months.[13] Further increases in breastfeeding rates will result in lower infant mortality as a whole[24,29] and in decreases in SIDS rates,[3] specifically.

CONCLUSIONS

Breastfeeding duration of a minimum of 2 months appears to be necessary to confer a significant protective effect against SIDS, with an almost halving of the risk. The protective benefits of breastfeeding increase as the duration increases. However, exclusive breastfeeding does not confer additional benefits over partial breastfeeding with regards to SIDS risk reduction. Therefore, mothers should be encouraged to breastfeed for at least 2 months (and preferably longer). Even if mothers are unable to exclusively breastfeed, they can feel reassured that any breastfeeding provides protection against SIDS for their infants. Further study is still needed to better understand the mechanisms by which breastfeeding offers protection.

ACKNOWLEDGMENTS

We acknowledge Drs Robert Carpenter (deceased) and Mechtild Vennemann for their work in data collection and data analysis for this study.

ABBREVIATIONS

aOR: adjusted odds ratio
CESDI: Confifential Inquiry into Stillbirth and Deaths in Infancy
CI: confidence interval
CIMS: Chicago Infant Mortality Study
ECAS: European Concerted Action on SIDS
GeSID: German SIDS Study
NZCDS: New Zealand Cot Death Study
OR: odds ratio
SES: socioeconomic status
SIDS: sudden infant death syndrome
SWISS: South-West England Infant Sleep Study

PEDIATRICS (ISSN Numbers: Print, 0031-4005; Online, 1098-4275).

FINANCIAL DISCLOSURE: The authors have indicated they have no financial relationships relevant to this article to disclose.

FUNDING: Funding for the New Zealand Cot Death Study was provided by the Health Research Council of New Zealand and the Hawkes Bay Medical Research Foundation. Funding for the Chicago Infant Mortality Study was provided by the *Eunice Kennedy Shriver* National Institute of Child Health and Human Development, the National Institute on Deafness and Other Communication Disorders, the Centers for Disease Control and Prevention, and the Association of Teachers of Preventive Medicine. Funding for the German Sudden Infant Death Syndrome Study was provided by Germany's Federal Ministry for Science and Education. Funding for The Scottish Cot Death Trust Study was provided by The Scottish Cot Death Trust. Funding for the European Concerted Action on Sudden Infant Death Syndrome was provided by the European Union and the Foundation for the Study of Infant Deaths (now called the Lullaby Trust). Funding for the Irish Study of Infant Death was provided by Ireland's Department of Health and Children. Funding for the Confidential Enquiry into Stillbirth and Deaths in Infancy was provided by the National Advisory Body for the Confidential Enquiry into Stillbirths and Deaths in Infancy, the Foundation for the Study of Infant Deaths (now called the Lullaby Trust), and Babes in Arms. Funding for the South-West England Infant Sleep Study was provided by the Foundation for the Study of Infant Deaths (now called the Lullaby Trust), Babes in Arms, and The Charitable Trusts of University Hospitals Bristol.

POTENTIAL CONFLICT OF INTEREST: The authors have indicated they have no potential conflicts of interest to disclose.

REFERENCES

1. Ip S, Chung M, Raman G, Trikalinos TA, Lau J. A summary of the Agency for Healthcare Research and Quality's evidence report on breastfeeding in developed countries. *Breastfeed Med*. 2009;4(suppl 1):S17–S30

2. Vennemann MM, Bajanowski T, Brinkmann B, et al; GeSID Study Group. Does breastfeeding reduce the risk of sudden infant death syndrome? *Pediatrics*. 2009;123(3). Available at: www.pediatrics.org/cgi/content/full/123/3/e406

3. Hauck FR, Thompson JM, Tanabe KO, Moon RY, Vennemann MM. Breastfeeding and reduced risk of sudden infant death syndrome: a meta-analysis. *Pediatrics*. 2011;128(1):103–110

4. Mitchell EA, Taylor BJ, Ford RP, et al. Four modifiable and other major risk factors for cot death: the New Zealand study. *J Paediatr Child Health*. 1992;28(suppl 1):S3–S8

5. Hauck FR, Herman SM, Donovan M, et al. Sleep environment and the risk of sudden infant death syndrome in an urban population: the Chicago Infant Mortality Study. *Pediatrics*. 2003;111(5, pt 2):1207–1214

6. Vennemann MM, Findeisen M, Butterfass-Bahloul T, et al; GeSID Group. Modifiable risk factors for SIDS in Germany: results of GeSID. *Acta Paediatr*. 2005;94(6):655–660

7. Tappin D, Brooke H, Ecob R, Gibson A. Used infant mattresses and sudden infant death syndrome in Scotland: case-control study. *BMJ*. 2002;325(7371):1007–1012

8. Carpenter RG, Irgens LM, Blair PS, et al. Sudden unexplained infant death in 20 regions in Europe: case control study. *Lancet*. 2004;363(9404):185–191

9. McGarvey C, McDonnell M, Chong A, O'Regan M, Matthews T. Factors relating to the infant's last sleep environment in sudden infant death syndrome in the Republic of Ireland. *Arch Dis Child*. 2003;88(12):1058–1064

10. Matthews T, McDonnell M, McGarvey C, Loftus G, O'Regan M. A multivariate "time based" analysis of SIDS risk factors. *Arch Dis Child*. 2004;89(3):267–271

11. Fleming PJ, Blair PS, Pollard K, et al; CESDI SUDI Research Team. Pacifier use and sudden infant death syndrome: results from the CESDI/SUDI case control study. *Arch Dis Child*. 1999;81(2):112–116

12. Blair PS, Sidebotham P, Evason-Coombe C, Edmonds M, Heckstall-Smith EM, Fleming P. Hazardous cosleeping environments and risk factors amenable to change: case-control study of SIDS in south west England. *BMJ*. 2009;339:b3666

13. World Health Organization/UNICEF. *Global Nutrition Targets 2025: Breastfeeding Policy Brief (WHO/NMH/NHD/14.7)*. Geneva, Switzerland: World Health Organization; 2014

14. Paine SM, Jacques TS, Sebire NJ. Review: neuropathological features of unexplained sudden unexpected death in infancy: current evidence and controversies. *Neuropathol Appl Neurobiol*. 2014;40(4):364–384

15. Franco P, Scaillet S, Wermenbol V, Valente F, Groswasser J, Kahn A. The influence of a pacifier on infants' arousals from sleep. *J Pediatr*. 2000;136(6):775–779

16. Horne RS, Parslow PM, Ferens D, Watts AM, Adamson TM. Comparison of evoked arousability in breast and formula fed infants. *Arch Dis Child*. 2004;89(1):22–25

17. Ball HL. Breastfeeding, bed-sharing, and infant sleep. *Birth*. 2003;30(3):181–188

18. Blair PS, Ball HL. The prevalence and characteristics associated with parent-infant bed-sharing in England. *Arch Dis Child*. 2004;89(12):1106–1110

19. Duijts L, Jaddoe VW, Hofman A, Moll HA. Prolonged and exclusive breastfeeding reduces the risk of infectious diseases in infancy. *Pediatrics*. 2010;126(1). Available at: www.pediatrics.org/cgi/content/full/126/1/e18

20. Heinig MJ. Host defense benefits of breastfeeding for the infant. Effect of breastfeeding duration and exclusivity. *Pediatr Clin North Am*. 2001;48(1):105–123, ix

21. Kramer MS, Guo T, Platt RW, et al. Infant growth and health outcomes associated with 3 compared with 6 mo of exclusive breastfeeding. *Am J Clin Nutr*. 2003;78(2):291–295

22. Kinney HC, Brody BA, Finkelstein DM, Vawter GF, Mandell F, Gilles FH. Delayed central nervous system myelination in the sudden infant death

syndrome. *J Neuropathol Exp Neurol.* 1991;50(1):29–48

23. Byard RW, Makrides M, Need M, Neumann MA, Gibson RA. Sudden infant death syndrome: effect of breast and formula feeding on frontal cortex and brainstem lipid composition. *J Paediatr Child Health.* 1995;31(1):14–16

24. Ip S, Chung M, Raman G, et al. Breastfeeding and maternal and infant health outcomes in developed countries. *Evid Rep Technol Assess (Full Rep).* 2007;(153):1–186

25. Moon RY; Task Force on Sudden Infant Death Syndrome. SIDS and other sleep-related infant deaths: expansion of recommendations for a safe infant sleeping environment. *Pediatrics.* 2011;128(5):1030–1039

26. Public Health Agency of Canada. Joint statement on safe sleep: preventing sudden infant deaths in Canada. 2012. Available at: http://www.phac-aspc. gc.ca/hp-ps/dca-dea/stages-etapes/ childhood-enfance_0-2/sids/pdf/jsss-ecss2011-eng.pdf. Accessed June 1, 2017

27. Blair P, Inch S. *The Health Professional's Guide to: "Caring for Your Baby at Night".* London, England: UNICEF UK Baby Friendly Initiative; 2012

28. OECD Social Policy Division. Directorate of employment, labour and social affairs, OECD family database. Available at: https://www.oecd.org/els/family. Accessed June 1, 2017

29. Chen A, Rogan WJ. Breastfeeding and the risk of postneonatal death in the United States. *Pediatrics.* 2004;113(5). Available at: www.pediatrics.org/cgi/ content/full/113/5/e435

Supplemental Information

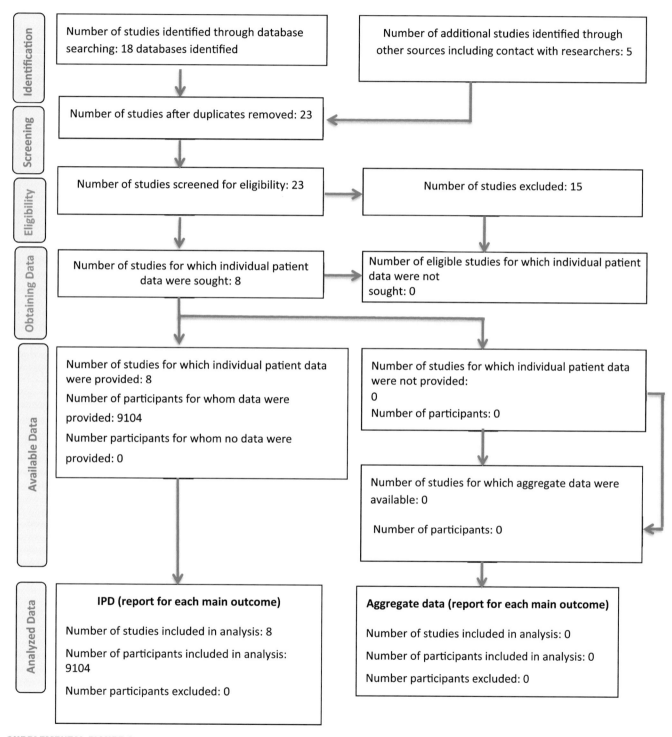

SUPPLEMENTAL FIGURE 2

Preferred Reporting Items for Systematic Reviews and Meta-Analyses flow diagram for pooled analyses using individual-level data. The Preferred Reporting Items for Systematic Reviews and Meta-Analyses individual patient data flow diagram. Reproduced with permission of the Preferred Reporting Items for Systematic Reviews and Meta-Analyses Individual Patient Data Group, which encourages sharing and reuse for noncommercial purposes.

Another Great Reason to Breastfeed: Decreased Risk of Kawasaki Disease

Dr Lewis First, MD, MS, Editor-in-Chief, *Pediatrics*

It is almost impossible to open an issue of *Pediatrics* and not find a study or policy in support of breastfeeding, many providing a look at a short- or long-term benefit of this nutritional practice for infants at least for the first year of life. This month we add to the support for breastfeeding with a somewhat unusual but important finding—the role of breastfeeding in reducing the risk of Kawasaki Disease (KD).

Yorifuji et al. (peds.2015-3919) used a longitudinal population-based cohort in Japan that began in 2010 and that had data on 37, 630 children and their feeding method at 6-7 months of age as well as data on hospital admission from 6 to 30 months of age. There were 232 hospitalizations for Kawasaki Disease and those infants who were breastfed exclusively or partially were found to be less likely to be hospitalized for KD.

Just why and how breastfeeding might be decreasing the risk of developing KD makes for an interesting discussion section of this article relative to the maturation of the immune system that may be occurring through this feeding method. The next time you have a patient with KD, you might want to ask about whether or not they were breastfed. If you're looking for yet another reason why breastfeeding is best, read this paper and add it to the overwhelming evidence that exists in our quest to promote breastfeeding to the mothers of all our newborns.

Breastfeeding and Risk of Kawasaki Disease: A Nationwide Longitudinal Survey in Japan

Takashi Yorifuji, MD, PhD,[a] Hirokazu Tsukahara, MD, PhD,[b] Hiroyuki Doi, MD, PhD[c]

BACKGROUND AND OBJECTIVES: Kawasaki disease (KD) is the most common cause of childhood-acquired heart disease in developed countries. However, the etiology of KD is not known. Aberrant immune responses are considered to play key roles in disease initiation and breastfeeding can mature immune system in infants. We thus examined the association between breastfeeding and the development of KD.

METHODS: We used a nationwide population-based longitudinal survey ongoing since 2010 and restricted participants to a total of 37 630 children who had data on their feeding during infancy. Infant feeding practice was queried at 6 to 7 months of age, and responses to questions about hospital admission for KD during the period from 6 to 30 months of age were used as outcome. We conducted logistic regression analyses controlling for child and maternal factors with formula feeding without colostrum as our reference group.

RESULTS: A total of 232 hospital admissions were observed. Children who were breastfed exclusively or partially were less likely to be hospitalized for KD compared with those who were formula fed without colostrum; odds ratios for hospitalization were 0.26 (95% confidence interval: 0.12–0.55) for exclusive breastfeeding and 0.27 (95% confidence interval: 0.13–0.55) for partial breastfeeding. Although the risk reduction was not statistically significant, feeding colostrum only also provided a protective effect.

CONCLUSIONS: We observed protective effects of breastfeeding on the development of KD during the period from 6 to 30 months of age in a nationwide, population-based, longitudinal survey in Japan, the country in which KD is most common.

[a]Department of Human Ecology, Okayama University Graduate School of Environmental and Life Science, Okayama, Japan; and Departments of [b]Pediatrics, and [c]Epidemiology, Okayama University Graduate School of Medicine, Dentistry, and Pharmaceutical Sciences, Okayama, Japan

Dr Yorifuji contributed to obtaining the data, the study design, data analysis and interpretation, and writing and revision of the manuscript; Dr Tsukahara contributed to the study design, data interpretation, and revision of the manuscript; Dr Doi contributed to the negotiation with the Ministry of Health to obtain the data, interpreting the data, revision of the manuscript, and study supervision; and all authors approved the final manuscript as submitted.

DOI: 10.1542/peds.2015-3919

Accepted for publication Mar 8, 2016

Address for correspondence to Takashi Yorifuji, MD, PhD, Department of Human Ecology, Okayama University Graduate School of Environmental and Life Science, 3-1-1 Tsushima-naka, Kita-ku, Okayama 700-8530, Japan. E-mail: yorichan@md.okayama-u.ac.jp

PEDIATRICS (ISSN Numbers: Print, 0031-4005; Online, 1098-4275).

WHAT'S KNOWN ON THIS SUBJECT: Kawasaki disease (KD), an acute self-limiting systemic vasculitis, is the most common cause of childhood-acquired heart disease in developed countries, but the etiology of the disease is unknown. Aberrant immune responses are considered to play key roles in disease initiation.

WHAT THIS STUDY ADDS: We observed protective effects of breastfeeding on the development of KD during the period from 6 to 30 months of age in Japan, the country in which KD is most common.

To cite: Yorifuji T, Tsukahara H, Doi H. Breastfeeding and Risk of Kawasaki Disease: A Nationwide Longitudinal Survey in Japan. *Pediatrics.* 2016;137(6):e20153919

Kawasaki disease (KD), an acute self-limiting systemic vasculitis of childhood, is the most common cause of childhood-acquired heart disease in most developed countries.[1-5] KD mainly occurs in young children[5]; ~88% of cases occurred under 5 years of age during the 2-year period of 2011 through 2012 in Japan.[6,7] The highest incidence of KD is reported in Japan.[8] Although the etiology of the disease is unknown,[1] KD may occur in genetically susceptible individuals with an aberrant immune response to some environmental trigger.[3,4,9]

Breastfeeding, a normative standard for infant feeding and nutrition, is considered to provide protection against infections and contain numerous factors that modulate and promote development of the immune system during infancy.[10] Immune maturation may relate to lifelong immunologic disorders[11]; thus, breastfeeding may be important to the development of the diseases in which the immune system plays a role in disease initiation, including KD. However, as far as we know, no studies have examined the association between breastfeeding and the development of KD.

In the current study, we therefore examined the association in children between breastfeeding and the development of KD from 6 to 30 months of age, using data from a nationwide, population-based, longitudinal survey in Japan, the country in which KD is most common.[8]

METHODS

Study Participants

Since 2010, the Japanese Ministry of Health, Labor, and Welfare has conducted an annual survey among newborn infants and their parents, known as the Longitudinal Survey of Babies in the 21st Century. Questionnaires were sent to all families in Japan who had

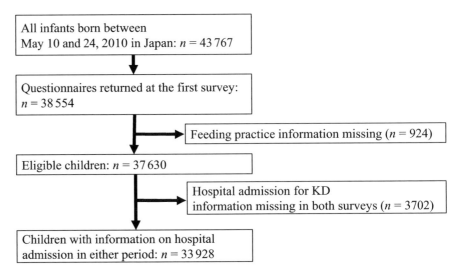

had an infant (or infants) born between May 10 and 24, 2010, to collect information of infants at 6 months of age. Among the 43 767 questionnaires mailed, 38 554 were completed and returned (response rate of 88.1%). Follow-up questionnaires were sent to participating families each year (at age 18 months, 30 months). Data from 2010–2012 (ie, the third survey at age 30 months) are currently available from the Ministry of Health, Labor, and Welfare. Birth records from the Japanese vital statistics system are also linked to each child surveyed. Birth record data include birth length; birth weight; gestational age; singleton, twin, or other multiple birth; gender; parity; and parental age at delivery.

In the current study, we used data from the first (age 6 months), second (age 18 months), and third surveys (age 30 months) because information on feeding practices during infancy was queried only in the first survey, and hospital admission for KD during the previous year was queried in the second and third surveys (ie, hospitalizations between the ages of 6 and 18 months and between

18 and 30 months). Children with information missing about feeding practices during infancy (n = 924) were excluded, leaving a total of 37 630 participants for the analysis (Fig 1). We then excluded 3702 participants who lacked information from the second and third surveys on hospital admission owing to KD. Among the remaining 33 928 participants, 27 735 had information on hospital admission for KD from both surveys: 31 355 participants only at the second survey, and 30 308 only at the third survey.

Infant Feeding Practices

The first survey at 6 months of age included questions on breastfeeding practices (infant was breastfed, only fed colostrum, or never breastfed) and formula feeding practices (infant was fed formula or never fed formula). Using information on both breastfeeding and formula feeding practices, we established the categories of "formula feeding without colostrum (and never breastfed)," "formula feeding (only) with colostrum," "partial breastfeeding," and "exclusive breastfeeding." We used category as a main exposure of interest.

Additionally, the duration (months) of breastfeeding and formula feeding was queried. We divided the category of "partial breastfeeding" based on breastfeeding duration (breastfeeding for 1–2 months, 3–5 months, or 6–7 months) in an additional analysis. Although the first survey was conducted at 6 months of age, children breastfed up to age 7 months were included owing to the timing of the survey.

Hospital Admission for KD

Hospital admission for KD during the previous 1 year was queried at the second and third surveys (ie, hospitalizations between the ages of 6 and 18 months and between 18 and 30 months). We used hospital admission at least once from age 6 to 30 months as the outcome of interest. We targeted KD incidence between age 6 and 30 months, owing to a high incidence of the disease during this period[7] and the availability of data. The diagnostic criteria for KD has not changed in Japan since 2002.[12,13]

Statistical Analyses

To evaluate the impact of loss to follow-up (Fig 1), we first compared baseline characteristics between children with information on breastfeeding (eligible children), children who were included in the analysis, and children who lacked information on hospital admission owing to KD at both surveys. We then compared baseline characteristics between the participants who were admitted for KD and those who were not.

We conducted logistic regression analyses to evaluate the relationships among the 4 infant feeding practice categories (formula feeding without colostrum, formula feeding with colostrum, partial breastfeeding, and exclusive breastfeeding) and hospital admission from age 6 to 30 months. We first estimated a crude odds ratio (OR) and a 95% confidence interval (CI) for the main outcome (model

1). We then examined the OR and 95% CI after controlling for child factors (model 2) and both child and maternal factors, in addition to residential information (model 3). Throughout the analyses, we used the formula feeding without colostrum category as our reference group.

Child factors included gender (dichotomous), singleton birth or not (dichotomous), term or preterm birth (<37 weeks' gestation; dichotomous), parity (0 and >1 birth; dichotomous). Maternal factors included maternal age at delivery (<30, 30–34, ≥35 years; categorical), maternal smoking habits (dichotomous), and maternal educational level (categorical). Residential information included the residential area where the participant was born (ward, city, and town or village; categorical). The child's gender, singleton birth or not, gestational age, parity, and maternal age at delivery were listed in the birth record. Maternal smoking status was ascertained at the first survey. Maternal educational level was used an indicator of socioeconomic status and obtained from the second survey (age 18 months). We reclassified the original 8 education categories into 3, as follows: university (4 years) or higher, junior college (2 years) or vocational school, and high school or less. Residential information was obtained from the national census conducted in 2010. We selected these potential confounders based on previous studies or previous knowledge of the association between breastfeeding and some allergic diseases.[14–16] We excluded cases with missing data and conducted our analyses with complete cases.

In further analyses, we divided the category "partial breastfeeding" based on breastfeeding duration (breastfeeding for 1–2 months, 3–5 months, or 6–7 months) and used the following categories: formula feeding without colostrum, formula feeding with colostrum,

partial breastfeeding for 1 to 2 months, partial breastfeeding for 3 to 5 months, partial breastfeeding for 6 to 7 months, and exclusive breastfeeding to 6 to 7 months of age. We then examined the association between infant feeding practices and hospital admission for KD.

Because of small numbers in the categories "formula feeding without colostrum" and "formula feeding with colostrum," we also combined these categories into 1 category designated "formula feeding" and repeated the analyses.

Furthermore, we stratified by gender and examined the association between infant feeding practices and hospital admission from age 6 to 30 months.

In the sensitivity analyses, we further adjusted for the following variables in addition to the same set of covariates as in model 3 because of possible potential confounding[17]: paternal annual income during the year the child was born as another indicator of socioeconomic status, obtained at the second survey (as a continuous variable), and day-care attendance. Persons who took care of the children during the daytime were queried at the first survey; children cared for by preschool teachers were classified as attending day care. Furthermore, most participants were considered to be of Japanese origin. We restricted participants to those whose father and mother are both Japanese and repeated the analyses because of high occurrence of KD among children of Japanese origin.[18]

In the additional analysis, to explore the possible mechanism between breastfeeding and the development of KD, we conducted logistic regression analyses to evaluate the relationships between breastfeeding and hospital admission for any cause excluding injuries, burn injuries, and fractures from 6 to 30 months of age. We adjusted for the same set of potential confounders.

All CIs were calculated at the 95% level. Stata statistical software Release 13 (StataCorp LP, College Station, TX) was used for all analyses. This study was approved by the Institutional Review Board at Okayama University Graduate School of Medicine, Dentistry, and Pharmaceutical Sciences (No. 1506-073).

RESULTS

Among eligible children, >34% were in the category of exclusive breastfeeding (Table 1). Children who lacked information on hospital admission for KD at the second and third surveys were more likely to be multiple births, preterm births, formula fed, and to have young mothers, mothers who smoked, mothers with lower educational level, and mothers who lived in rural areas (towns or villages) compared with children included in the analyses.

We show the baseline characteristics between the participants who were admitted for KD during the period of 6 to 30 months of age and those who were not in Table 2. Among 27 735 participants, a total of 232 admissions for KD were observed, that is, the incidence proportion of 0.84% for 2 years. The participants who were admitted tended to have more siblings, been formula fed, and older mothers compared with those who were not admitted. The same information among participants with information on hospital admission either at the second or third survey is shown in Supplemental Tables 5 and 6.

Children who were breastfed were less likely to be hospitalized for KD from 6 to 30 months of age (Table 3). Even after adjusting for all covariates (model 3), protective associations remained for exclusive and partial breastfeeding; ORs for hospitalization were 0.26 (95% CI: 0.12–0.55) for exclusive breastfeeding and 0.27 (95% CI: 0.13–0.55) for

TABLE 1 Demographic Characteristics of Eligible Children With or Without KD Hospital Admission Data (n = 37 630)

	Eligible Children	Included in the Analyses	Without Information in Both Periods	P^a
	(n = 37 630)	(N = 33 928)	(n = 3702)	
Characteristics of children				
Gender, n (%)[b]				
Male	19 346 (51.4)	17 442 (51.4)	1904 (51.4)	.98
Female	18 284 (48.6)	16 486 (48.6)	1798 (48.6)	
Singleton or multiple birth, n (%)[b]				
Singleton birth	36 918 (98.1)	33 307 (98.2)	3611 (97.5)	.008
Multiple birth	712 (1.9)	621 (1.8)	91 (2.5)	
Term or preterm birth, n (%)[b]				
Term birth	35 593 (94.6)	32 136 (94.7)	3457 (93.4)	.001
Preterm birth	2037 (5.4)	1792 (5.3)	245 (6.6)	
Parity, n (%)[b]				
0	17 682 (47.0)	15 895 (46.9)	1787 (48.3)	.10
≥1	19 948 (53.0)	18 033 (53.2)	1915 (51.7)	
Breastfeeding status[c]				
Formula feeding without colostrum	406 (1.1)	341 (1.0)	65 (1.8)	<.001
Formula feeding with colostrum	939 (2.5)	789 (2.3)	150 (4.1)	
Partial breastfeeding	23 399 (62.2)	21 003 (61.9)	2396 (64.7)	
Exclusive breastfeeding to 6–7 mo of age	12 886 (34.2)	11 795 (34.8)	1091 (29.5)	
Maternal characteristics				
Maternal age at delivery, y[b]				
<30	14 275 (37.9)	12 302 (36.3)	1973 (53.3)	<.001
30–35	13 892 (36.9)	12 848 (37.9)	1044 (28.2)	
≥35	9463 (25.2)	8778 (25.9)	685 (18.5)	
Maternal smoking status, n (%)[c]				
Nonsmoker	34 896 (93.0)	31 801 (94.0)	3095 (84.0)	<.001
Smoker	2634 (7.0)	2045 (6.0)	589 (16.0)	
Maternal educational attainment, n (%)[d]				
University or higher	8635 (26.5)	8581 (26.7)	54 (15.6)	<.001
Junior college	13 386 (41.1)	13 271 (41.2)	115 (33.2)	
Less than or equal to high school	10 524 (32.3)	10 347 (32.1)	177 (51.2)	
Residential area, n (%)				
Wards	10 739 (28.5)	9774 (28.8)	965 (26.1)	<.001
Cities	23 829 (63.3)	21 445 (63.2)	2384 (64.4)	
Towns or villages	3062 (8.1)	2709 (8.0)	353 (9.5)	

[a] The differences in the proportions of the group included in the analyses and the group without information in both periods were tested by using the χ^2 test.
[b] Obtained from the birth record.
[c] Obtained from the first survey (at age 6 mo).
[d] Obtained from the second survey (at age 18 mo).

partial breastfeeding. Although not statistically significant, a protective association was observed even for the category of formula feeding with colostrum: OR 0.39 (95% CI: 0.14–1.09). When we divided the category of "partial breastfeeding" based on breastfeeding duration, the ORs reached a plateau at a point estimate of around 0.26 for the category of breastfeeding for 3 to 5 months.

Even after we combined the categories of "formula feeding

without colostrum" and "formula feeding with colostrum" into 1 category of "formula feeding," we obtained similar findings. Protective associations remained for exclusive and partial breastfeeding (Table 4).

When stratified by sex, protective associations between breastfeeding and the development of KD did not change substantially between male and female participants; however, exclusive breastfeeding was more protective among male children (Supplemental Table 7).

In the sensitivity analyses, even after further adjusting for paternal income or day-care attendance, the main findings did not change substantially (data not shown). Among the 33 928 eligible children, the parents of 32 783 children (96.7%) were both Japanese. The results did not change even after restricting the analysis to these children, and ORs for hospitalization for KD were 0.27 (95% CI: 0.12–0.59) for exclusive breastfeeding and 0.27 (95% CI: 0.13–0.60) for partial breastfeeding, compared with the category of formula feeding without colostrum.

When we examined the relationships between breastfeeding and hospital admission for any cause in the additional analysis, exclusive breastfeeding and partial breastfeeding for longer months were protective for the risk of hospital admission (Supplemental Table 8).

DISCUSSION

In the current study, we examined the association in children between breastfeeding and the development of KD from 6 to 30 months of age, using data from a nationwide, population-based, longitudinal survey in Japan. We then observed that children who were breastfed exclusively or partially were less likely to be hospitalized for KD compared with those who were formula fed. Although the risk reduction was not statistically significant, feeding colostrum only also provided a protective effect. The protective associations did not change even after adjusting for an extensive list of potential confounders or in the sensitivity analyses. This is the first study examining the association between breastfeeding and development of KD.

TABLE 2 Demographic Characteristics of Eligible Children With Data of KD Hospital Admission From 6 to 30 Months of Age (n = 27 735)

	Total (n = 27 735)	No Admission (n = 27 503)	Admission (n = 232)	P[a]
Characteristics of children				
Gender, n (%)[b]				
Male	14 335 (51.7)	14 204 (51.7)	131 (56.5)	.14
Female	13 400 (48.3)	13 299 (48.4)	101 (43.5)	
Singleton or multiple birth, n (%)[b]				
Singleton birth	27 234 (98.2)	27 009 (98.2)	225 (97.0)	.16
Multiple birth	501 (1.8)	494 (1.8)	7 (3.0)	
Term or preterm birth, n (%)[b]				
Term	26 311 (94.9)	26 093 (94.9)	218 (94.0)	.53
Preterm	1424 (5.1)	1410 (5.1)	14 (6.0)	
Parity, n (%)[b]				
0	12 996 (46.9)	12 905 (46.9)	91 (39.2)	.02
≥1	14 739 (53.1)	14 598 (53.1)	141 (60.8)	
Breastfeeding status[c]				
Formula feeding without colostrum	262 (0.9)	254 (0.9)	8 (3.5)	.001
Formula feeding with colostrum	583 (2.1)	576 (2.1)	7 (3.0)	
Partial breastfeeding	17 097 (61.6)	16 958 (61.7)	139 (59.9)	
Exclusive breastfeeding to 6–7 mo of age	9793 (35.3)	9715 (35.3)	78 (33.6)	
Maternal characteristics				
Maternal age at delivery, y[b]				
<30	9438 (34.0)	9376 (34.1)	62 (26.7)	.008
30–35	10 799 (38.9)	10 711 (38.9)	88 (37.9)	
≥35	7498 (27.0)	7416 (27.0)	82 (35.3)	
Maternal smoking status, n (%)[c]				
Nonsmoker	26 292 (95.0)	26 080 (95.0)	212 (92.6)	.09
Smoker	1388 (5.0)	1371 (5.0)	17 (7.4)	
Maternal educational attainment, n (%)[d]				
University or higher	7735 (27.9)	7662 (27.9)	73 (31.5)	.45
Junior college	11 584 (41.8)	11 494 (41.9)	90 (38.8)	
Less than or equal to high school	8365 (30.2)	8296 (30.2)	69 (29.7)	
Residential area, n (%)				
Wards	7988 (28.8)	7909 (28.8)	79 (34.1)	.10
Cities	17 548 (63.3)	17 407 (63.3)	141 (60.8)	
Towns or villages	2199 (7.9)	2187 (8.0)	12 (5.2)	

[a] The differences in the proportions of the "no admission" group and the "admission" group were tested by using the χ^2 test.
[b] Obtained from the birth record.
[c] Obtained from the first survey (at age 6 mo).
[d] Obtained from the second survey (at age 18 mo).

We consider there to be at least 2 reasons for the protective effects of breastfeeding on development of KD. First, the mother may provide her own immunologic memory (ie, antimicrobial factors such as secretory immunoglobulin A, oligosaccharides, lactoferrin, nucleotides) to her infant via breast milk,[19,20] which may prevent the infant from contracting infections that trigger abnormal immune responses. Second, breastfeeding may support the maturation of immune system (ie, programming of the system),[17] which may limit potential damage from an uncontrolled inflammatory response.[19] Breast milk contains numerous factors, including allergens, which modulate and promote immune system development.[10,11,21] Moreover, breast milk is considered to mature the immune system through the establishment of intestinal microbiota.[10,11] We observed protective effects of breastfeeding on the risk of hospital admission excluding injuries, burn injuries, and fractures, which may indicate that breastfeeding has a generic effect rather than a specific effect

TABLE 3 Breastfeeding and KD Hospital Admission From 6 to 30 Month of Age

	KD Hospital Admission/Total Number	% of Hospital Admission	OR (95% CI)		
			Model 1: Crude	Model 2[a]	Model 3[b]
Breastfeeding status					
Formula feeding without colostrum	8/262	3.1	1 (reference)	1 (reference)	1 (reference)
Formula feeding with colostrum	7/583	1.2	0.39 (0.14–1.08)	0.39 (0.14–1.09)	0.39 (0.14–1.09)
Partial breastfeeding	139/17 097	0.8	0.26 (0.13–0.54)	0.27 (0.13–0.56)	0.27 (0.13–0.55)
Exclusive breastfeeding to 6–7 mo of age	78/9793	0.8	0.25 (0.12–0.53)	0.26 (0.12–0.54)	0.26 (0.12–0.55)
Breastfeeding duration					
Formula feeding without colostrum	8/262	3.1	1 (reference)	1 (reference)	1 (reference)
Formula feeding with colostrum	7/583	1.2	0.39 (0.14–1.08)	0.39 (0.14–1.09)	0.39 (0.14–1.09)
Partial breastfeeding, breastfeeding duration, mo					
1–2	20/2209	0.9	0.29 (0.13–0.67)	0.29 (0.13–0.67)	0.30 (0.13–0.68)
3–5	21/2689	0.8	0.25 (0.11–0.57)	0.25 (0.11–0.58)	0.26 (0.11–0.59)
6–7	98/12 199	0.8	0.26 (0.12–0.53)	0.27 (0.13–0.56)	0.26 (0.12–0.55)
Exclusive breastfeeding to 6–7 mo of age	78/9793	0.8	0.25 (0.12–0.53)	0.26 (0.12–0.54)	0.26 (0.12–0.55)

[a] Adjusted for children's factors (gender, preterm birth, parity, singleton or multiple birth).
[b] Adjusted for children's factors (gender, preterm birth, parity, singleton or multiple birth), maternal factors (maternal smoking status, maternal education, and maternal age category), and residential area.

TABLE 4 Associations Between Breastfeeding Duration and KD Hospital Admission From 7 to 30 Months of Age, Using the Category of Formula Feeding (Both With and Without Colostrum) as a Reference

	KD Hospital Admission/Total Number	% of Hospital Admission	OR (95% CI)		
			Model 1: Crude	Model 2[a]	Model 3[b]
Breastfeeding status					
Formula feeding[c]	15/845	1.8	1 (reference)	1 (reference)	1 (reference)
Partial breastfeeding	139/17097	0.8	0.45 (0.27–0.78)	0.47 (0.27–0.80)	0.46 (0.27–0.79)
Exclusive breastfeeding at 6–7 mo of age	78/9793	0.8	0.44 (0.25–0.78)	0.45 (0.25–0.78)	0.45 (0.25–0.80)
Breastfeeding duration					
Formula feeding[c]	15/845	1.8	1 (reference)	1 (reference)	1 (reference)
Partial breastfeeding, breastfeeding duration, mo					
1–2	20/2209	0.9	0.51 (0.26–0.99)	0.51 (0.26–0.99)	0.51 (0.26 – 1.00)
3–5	21/2689	0.8	0.44 (0.22–0.85)	0.44 (0.22–0.85)	0.44 (0.23–0.87)
6–7	98/12 199	0.8	0.45 (0.26–0.78)	0.47 (0.27–0.81)	0.45 (0.26–0.79)
Exclusive breastfeeding at 6–7 mo of age	78/9793	0.8	0.44 (0.25–0.78)	0.45 (0.25–0.78)	0.45 (0.25–0.80)

[a] Adjusted for children's factors (gender, preterm birth, parity, singleton or not).
[b] Adjusted for children's factors (gender, preterm birth, parity, singleton or not), maternal factors (maternal smoking status, maternal education, and maternal age category), and residential area.
[c] We combined the categories of "formula feeding without colostrum" and "formula feeding with colostrum" into a single category, "formula feeding."

on KD. The protective effects of breastfeeding on KD may be related to broad antiinfective functions of breast milk. In addition, a previous US cohort study suggested an increased risk of hospitalization for any cause among children who subsequently developed KD.[9] Although it is impossible to draw a definite conclusion as to the underlying mechanism, these observations may support the preceding theories.

Interestingly, both exclusive and partial breastfeeding had beneficial effects on the development of KD. In the category of partial breastfeeding

for 3 to 5 months, the magnitude of these effects reached a plateau, which means that breastfeeding for at least 3 to 5 months, even together with formula feeding, may provide some benefits. Moreover, although not statistically significant, feeding colostrum only also provided a protective effect. Colostrum, the mammary secretion during the first few days postpartum, also contains immunoglobulins and facilitates establishment of the intestinal microbiota,[22] which may provide some benefits in children.

The strength of the current study is that we had a nationally

representative sample, and roughly one-twentieth of the children born in 2010 were included in this survey. We thus had a relatively large number of KD cases, which allowed us to examine the dose-response relationship between breastfeeding and development of KD. In addition, the very high response rate at baseline (88.1%) strengthens the validity of our findings. The type and duration of feeding practices should be accurate because information on feeding was collected at the first survey, when children were 6 to 7 months old. However, we could not evaluate the effect of breastfeeding that continued beyond 6 to 7 months of age.

We have relatively smaller participants in the categories of "formula feeding without colostrum" and "formula feeding with colostrum" to the breastfed group, which may explain relatively wide 95% CIs. However, even after we combined the categories of "formula feeding without colostrum" and "formula feeding with colostrum" into 1 category ("formula feeding"), we obtained the similar findings (Table 4).

We cannot exclude the possibility of misclassification of hospital admission for KD because of the subjective nature of the questions used to assess this outcome. We could not directly confirm the admission by direct communication with the hospitals because the data set obtained from the Ministry was anonymized data that cannot be linked to any individual. However, the diagnostic criteria for KD in Japan has not changed since 2002[12,13]; therefore, the diagnostic method used by physicians would be similar throughout the country during the study period. Japan has a universal health insurance system that covers all of its citizens, so most patients with KD would have seen their physicians and then been hospitalized. Indeed, the incidence proportions of hospitalization for KD from 6 to 18 months (0.51%)

and from 18 to 30 months (0.37%) (Supplemental Tables 5 and 6) are close to or slightly higher than the age-specific incidences reported by the Nationwide Survey for KD in Japan: 0.33% to 0.41% from 6 to 17 months and 0.24% to 0.30% from 18 to 29 months of age.[6,7] The lower proportions in the Nationwide Survey may be due to its incomplete coverage. Even if there remain some misclassifications (eg, incomplete cases), they would be nondifferential, moving effect estimates toward the null.[23]

Loss to follow-up might be a concern. Because loss was more common among higher risk groups such as children who were formula fed and mothers who were smokers (Table 1), we may be underestimating the protective effects of breastfeeding on the development of KD.

There is the possibility of a biased association owing to residual confounding factors. However, we extensively adjusted for potential confounders in the main analyses. Furthermore, we examined other potential confounders (ie, paternal income and day-care attendance) in the sensitivity analyses, and the findings did not change substantially. Although familial susceptibility to KD has been reported,[24] we had no information on parental KD history. However, the possible number of parents with a past history of KD is considered insufficient to affect

the present findings. Therefore, it is unlikely that our findings can be fully explained by residual confounding.

Finally, we only included the admissions for KD from age 6 to 30 months of age because of data availability, which may limit the generalizability of the finding. However, ~50% of the KD cases occurred during this age-group during the 2-year period of 2011 to 2012 in Japan.[6,7]

CONCLUSIONS

We observed protective effects of breastfeeding on the development of KD from age 6 to 30 months in children using data of a nationwide longitudinal survey in Japan, where KD is most prevalent. Given the accumulated evidence on its short- and long-term protective advantages for other diseases,[25] breastfeeding should be recommended until such time as further confirmation on the association between breastfeeding and KD is obtained.

ACKNOWLEDGMENT

The authors thank Saori Irie for her help in data collection.

ABBREVIATIONS

CI: confidence interval
KD: Kawasaki disease
OR: odds ratio

FINANCIAL DISCLOSURE: The authors have indicated they have no financial relationships relevant to this article to disclose.

FUNDING: Supported in part by a grant for Strategies for Efficient Operation of the University (2007030201).

POTENTIAL CONFLICT OF INTEREST: The authors have indicated they have no potential conflicts of interest to disclose.

REFERENCES

1. Son MBF, Newburger JW. Kawasaki disease. In: Kliegman R, Behrman RE, Nelson WE, editors. *Nelson Textbook of Pediatrics*. 20th ed. Philadelphia, PA: Elsevier; 2016; 1209–1214

2. Kawasaki T, Kosaki F, Okawa S, Shigematsu I, Yanagawa H. A new infantile acute febrile mucocutaneous lymph node syndrome (MLNS) prevailing in Japan. *Pediatrics*. 1974;54(3): 271–276

3. Greco A, De Virgilio A, Rizzo MI, et al. Kawasaki disease: an evolving paradigm. *Autoimmun Rev.* 2015;14(8):703–709

4. Dimitriades VR, Brown AG, Gedalia A. Kawasaki disease: pathophysiology, clinical manifestations, and management. *Curr Rheumatol Rep.* 2014;16(6):423

5. Burns JC, Glodé MP. Kawasaki syndrome. *Lancet*. 2004;364(9433):533–544

6. Japan Kawasaki Disease Research Center. *The results of the 22nd Kawasaki disease nationwide survey* [in Japanese]. Tokyo, Japan; 2013

7. Makino N, Nakamura Y, Yashiro M, et al. Descriptive epidemiology of Kawasaki disease in Japan, 2011–2012: from the results of the 22nd nationwide survey. *J Epidemiol.* 2015;25(3):239–245

8. Uehara R, Belay ED. Epidemiology of Kawasaki disease in Asia, Europe, and the United States. *J Epidemiol.* 2012;22(2):79–85

9. Hayward K, Wallace CA, Koepsell T. Perinatal exposures and Kawasaki disease in Washington State: a population-based, case-control study. *Pediatr Infect Dis J.* 2012;31(10):1027–1031

10. Iyengar SR, Walker WA. Immune factors in breast milk and the development of atopic disease. *J Pediatr Gastroenterol Nutr.* 2012;55(6):641–647

11. M'Rabet L, Vos AP, Boehm G, Garssen J. Breast-feeding and its role in early development of the immune system in infants: consequences for health later in life. *J Nutr.* 2008;138(9):1782S–1790S

12. JCS Joint Working Group. Guidelines for diagnosis and management of cardiovascular sequelae in Kawasaki disease (JCS 2008)—digest version. *Circ J.* 2010;74(9):1989–2020

13. Kawasaki Disease Research Group. *Diagnostic criteria for Kawasaki disease, 5th version* [in Japanese]. 2002. Available at: http://www.jskd.jp/info/pdf/tebiki.pdf. Published Accessed Sep 24, 2015

14. Yamakawa M, Yorifuji T, Kato T, Yamauchi Y, Doi H. Breast-feeding and hospitalization for asthma in early childhood: a nationwide longitudinal survey in Japan. *Public Health Nutr.* 2015;18(10):1756–1761

15. Kramer MS. Does breast feeding help protect against atopic disease? Biology, methodology, and a golden jubilee of controversy. *J Pediatr.* 1988;112(2):181–190

16. Dogaru CM, Nyffenegger D, Pescatore AM, Spycher BD, Kuehni CE. Breastfeeding and childhood asthma: systematic review and meta-analysis. *Am J Epidemiol.* 2014;179(10):1153–1167

17. Kramer MS. Invited commentary: Does breastfeeding protect against "asthma"? *Am J Epidemiol.* 2014;179(10):1168–1170

18. Punnoose AR, Kasturia S, Golub RM. JAMA patient page. Kawasaki disease. *JAMA.* 2012;307(18):1990

19. Lawrence RM. Host-resistance factors and immunologic significance of human milk. In: Lawrence R, Lawrence R, eds. *Breastfeeding: A Guide for the Medical Profession.* 7th ed. Maryland Heights, MO: Mosby/Elsevier; 2011:153–195

20. Minniti F, Comberiati P, Munblit D, et al. Breast-milk characteristics protecting against allergy. *Endocr Metab Immune Disord Drug Targets.* 2014;14(1):9–15

21. Julia V, Macia L, Dombrowicz D. The impact of diet on asthma and allergic diseases. *Nat Rev Immunol.* 2015;15(5):308–322

22. Lawrence R, Lawrence R. Biochemistry of Human Milk. In: Lawrence R, Lawrence R, eds. *Breastfeeding: A Guide for the Medical Profession.* 7th ed. Maryland Heights, MO: Mosby/Elsevier; 2011:98–151

23. Rothman KJ. *Epidemiology: An Introduction.* 2nd ed. New York, NY: Oxford University Press; 2012

24. Uehara R, Yashiro M, Nakamura Y, Yanagawa H. Clinical features of patients with Kawasaki disease whose parents had the same disease. *Arch Pediatr Adolesc Med.* 2004;158(12):1166–1169

25. Section on Breastfeeding. Breastfeeding and the use of human milk. *Pediatrics.* 2012;129(3): e827–e841

Supplemental Information

SUPPLEMENTAL TABLE 5 Demographic Characteristics of Eligible Children With Data of KD Hospital Admission From 6 to 18 Months of Age (*n* = 31 355)

	Total	No Admission	Admission	P^a
	(*n* = 31 355)	(*n* = 31 194)	(*n* = 161)	
Characteristics of children				
Gender, *n* (%)[b]				
Male	16 168 (51.6)	16 076 (51.5)	92 (57.1)	.16
Female	15 187 (48.4)	15 118 (48.5)	69 (42.9)	
Singleton or multiple birth, *n* (%)[b]				
Singleton birth	30 780 (98.2)	30 625 (98.2)	155 (96.3)	.07
Multiple birth	575 (1.8)	569 (1.8)	6 (3.7)	
Term or preterm birth, *n* (%)[b]				
Term	29 712 (94.8)	29 564 (94.8)	148 (91.9)	.11
Preterm	1643 (5.2)	1630 (5.2)	13 (8.1)	
Parity, *n* (%)[b]				
0	14 706 (46.9)	14 652 (47.0)	54 (33.5)	.001
≥1	16 649 (53.1)	16 542 (53.0)	107 (66.5)	
Breastfeeding status[c]				
Formula feeding without colostrum	313 (1.0)	310 (1.0)	3 (1.9)	.40
Formula feeding with colostrum	699 (2.2)	694 (2.2)	5 (3.1)	
Partial breastfeeding	19 381 (61.8)	19 277 (61.8)	104 (64.6)	
Exclusive breastfeeding to 6–7 mo of age	10 962 (35.0)	10 913 (35.0)	49 (30.4)	
Maternal characteristics				
Maternal age at delivery, y[a]				
<30	11 118 (35.5)	11 067 (35.5)	51 (31.7)	.21
30–35	12 008 (38.3)	11 950 (38.3)	58 (36)	
≥35	8229 (26.2)	8177 (26.2)	52 (32.3)	
Maternal smoking status, *n* (%)[c]				
Nonsmoker	29 526 (94.4)	29 385 (94.4)	141 (88.1)	.001
Smoker	1758 (5.6)	1739 (5.6)	19 (11.9)	
Maternal educational attainment, *n* (%)[d]				
University or higher	8409 (26.9)	8357 (26.9)	52 (32.3)	.17
Junior college	12 946 (41.4)	12 890 (41.4)	56 (34.8)	
Less than or equal to high school	9936 (31.8)	9883 (31.8)	53 (32.9)	
Residential area, *n* (%)				
Wards	9036 (28.8)	8978 (28.8)	58 (36.0)	.08
Cities	19 830 (63.2)	19 735 (63.3)	95 (59.0)	
Towns or villages	2489 (7.9)	2481 (8.0)	8 (5.0)	

[a] The differences in the proportions of the "no admission" group and the "admission" group were tested by using the χ^2 test.
[b] Obtained from the birth record.
[c] Obtained from the first survey (at age 6 mo).
[d] Obtained from the second survey (at age 18 mo).

SUPPLEMENTAL TABLE 6 Demographic Characteristics of Eligible Children With Data of KD Hospital Admission From 18 to 30 Months of Age ($n = 30\,308$)

	Total	No Admission	Admission	P^a
	($n = 30\,308$)	($n = 30\,196$)	($n = 112$)	
Characteristics of children				
Gender, n (%)[b]				
Male	15 609 (51.5)	15 543 (51.5)	66 (58.9)	.12
Female	14 699 (48.5)	14 653 (48.5)	46 (41.1)	
Singleton or multiple birth, n (%)[b]				
Singleton birth	29 761 (98.2)	29 652 (98.2)	109 (97.3)	.49
Multiple birth	547 (1.8)	544 (1.8)	3 (2.7)	
Term or preterm birth, n (%)[b]				
Term birth	28 35 (94.8)	28 626 (94.8)	109 (97.3)	.23
Preterm birth	1573 (5.2)	1570 (5.2)	3 (2.7)	
Parity, n (%)[b]				
0	14 185 (46.8)	14 130 (46.8)	55 (49.1)	.62
≥1	16 123 (53.2)	16 066 (53.2)	57 (50.9)	
Breastfeeding status[c]				
Formula feeding without colostrum	290 (1.0)	285 (0.9)	5 (4.5)	.002
Formula feeding with colostrum	673 (2.2)	670 (2.2)	3 (2.7)	
Partial breastfeeding	18 719 (61.8)	18 653 (61.8)	66 (58.9)	
Exclusive breastfeeding to 6–7 mo of age	10 626 (35.1)	10 588 (35.1)	38 (33.9)	
Maternal characteristics				
Maternal age at delivery, y[b]				
<30	10 622 (35.1)	10 590 (35.1)	32 (28.6)	.16
30–35	11 639 (38.4)	11 597 (38.4)	42 (37.5)	
≥35	8047 (26.6)	8009 (26.5)	38 (33.9)	
Maternal smoking status, n (%)[c]				
Nonsmoker	28 567 (94.5)	28 461 (94.5)	106 (96.4)	.38
Smoker	1675 (5.5)	1671 (5.6)	4 (3.6)	
Maternal educational attainment, n (%)[d]				
University or higher	7907 (27.7)	7876 (27.7)	31 (30.1)	.85
Junior college	11 909 (41.7)	11 868 (41.7)	41 (39.8)	
Less than or equal to high school	8776 (30.7)	8745 (30.7)	31 (30.1)	
Residential area, n (%)				
Wards	8726 (28.8)	8689 (28.8)	37 (33.0)	.29
Cities	19 163 (63.2)	19 093 (63.2)	70 (62.5)	
Towns or villages	2419 (8.0)	2414 (8.0)	5 (4.5)	

[a] The differences in the proportions of the "no admission" group and the "admission" group were tested by using the χ^2 test.
[b] Obtained from the birth record.
[c] Obtained from the first survey (at age 6 mo).
[d] Obtained from the second survey (at age 18 mo).

SUPPLEMENTAL TABLE 7 Breastfeeding and KD Hospital Admission From 6 to 30 Months of Age, Stratified by Gender

	KD Hospital Admission/Total Number	% of Hospital Admission	OR (95% CI)		
			Model 1: Crude	Model 2[a]	Model 3[b]
Male					
Formula feeding without colostrum	4/140	2.9	1 (reference)	1 (reference)	1 (reference)
Formula feeding with colostrum	4/314	1.3	0.44 (0.11–1.78)	0.44 (0.11–1.79)	0.43 (0.11–1.76)
Partial breastfeeding	91/8857	1.0	0.35 (0.13–0.97)	0.36 (0.13–1.00)	0.35 (0.13–0.97)
Exclusive breastfeeding at 6–7 mo of age	32/5024	0.6	0.22 (0.08–0.62)	0.22 (0.08–0.63)	0.21 (0.07–0.62)
Female					
Formula feeding without colostrum	4/122	3.3	1 (reference)	1 (reference)	1 (reference)
Formula feeding with colostrum	3/269	1.1	0.33 (0.07–1.51)	0.34 (0.07–1.54)	0.33 (0.07–1.52)
Partial breastfeeding	48/8240	0.6	0.17 (0.06–0.49)	0.18 (0.06–0.51)	0.18 (0.06–0.51)
Exclusive breastfeeding at 6–7 mo of age	46/4769	1.0	0.29 (0.10–0.81)	0.29 (0.10–0.83)	0.30 (0.10–0.87)

[a] Adjusted for children's factors (preterm birth, parity, and singleton or not).
[b] Adjusted for children's factors (preterm birth, parity, and singleton or not), maternal factors (maternal smoking status, maternal education, and maternal age category), and residential area.

SUPPLEMENTAL TABLE 8 Breastfeeding and Hospital Admission for Any Cause Excluding Injuries, Burn Injuries, and Fractures From 6 to 30 Months of Age

	Hospital Admission for Any Cause/Total Number	% of Hospital Admission	OR (95% CI)		
			Model 1: Crude	Model 2[a]	Model 3[b]
Breastfeeding status					
Formula feeding without colostrum	54/262	20.6	1 (reference)	1 (reference)	1 (reference)
Formula feeding with colostrum	120/583	20.6	1.00 (0.70–1.43)	1.01 (0.70–1.45)	1.01 (0.70–1.46)
Partial breastfeeding	2823/17 097	16.5	0.76 (0.56–1.03)	0.80 (0.59–1.08)	0.80 (0.59–1.09)
Exclusive breastfeeding to 6–7 mo of age	1508/9793	15.4	0.70 (0.52–0.95)	0.72 (0.53–0.98)	0.72 (0.53–0.99)
Breastfeeding duration					
Formula feeding without colostrum	54/262	20.6	1 (reference)	1 (reference)	1 (reference)
Formula feeding with colostrum	120/583	20.6	1.00 (0.70–1.43)	1.01 (0.70–1.45)	1.02 (0.71–1.47)
Partial breastfeeding, breast feeding duration, mo					
1–2	431/2209	19.5	0.93 (0.68–1.28)	0.96 (0.70–1.32)	0.94 (0.68–1.30)
3–5	508/2689	18.9	0.90 (0.66–1.23)	0.92 (0.67–1.26)	0.91 (0.66–1.25)
6–7	1884/12 199	15.4	0.70 (0.52–0.95)	0.74 (0.55–1.01)	0.74 (0.55–1.01)
Exclusive breastfeeding to 6–7 mo of age	1508/9793	15.4	0.70 (0.52–0.95)	0.72 (0.53–0.98)	0.71 (0.52–0.97)

[a] Adjusted for children's factors (gender, preterm birth, parity, singleton or multiple birth).

[b] Adjusted for children's factors (gender, preterm birth, parity, singleton or multiple birth), maternal factors (maternal smoking status, maternal education, and maternal age category), and residential area.